Cesarean Delivery: A Practical Approach

Cesarean Delivery: A Practical Approach

Edited by Tianna Davis

AMERICAN
MEDICAL PUBLISHERS
www.americanmedicalpublishers.com

American Medical Publishers,
41 Flatbush Avenue,
1st Floor, New York,
NY 11217, USA

Visit us on the World Wide Web at:
www.americanmedicalpublishers.com

ISBN: 978-1-63927-150-4

Cataloging-in-Publication Data

Cesarean delivery : a practical approach / edited by Tianna Davis.
p. cm.
Includes bibliographical references and index.
ISBN 978-1-63927-150-4
1. Cesarean section. 2. Delivery (Obstetrics). 3. Obstetrics--Surgery. I. Davis, Tianna.
RG761 .C47 2022
618.86--dc23

Table of Contents

Preface

This book has been an outcome of determined endeavour from a group of educationists in the field. The primary objective was to involve a broad spectrum of professionals from diverse cultural background involved in the field for developing new researches. The book not only targets students but also scholars pursuing higher research for further enhancement of the theoretical and practical applications of the subject.

The use of surgery to deliver babies is known as cesarean delivery. It is performed when vaginal delivery can put the life of the mother or the baby at risk. Complicated cases such as twin pregnancy, obstructed labor, breech birth, high blood pressure in the mother often lead to cesarean delivery. Problems with umbilical cord can be another reason for choosing this technique. It can be done with a spinal block, where the mother is awake, or with general anesthesia. In the process of cesarean delivery, the bladder is drained using a urinary catheter and an antiseptic is used to clean the abdomen skin. An incision is made through the mother's lower abdomen, the uterus is opened with another incision and the baby is delivered. Both the incisions are stitched and closed in the end. This book outlines the processes and applications of the cesarean method of delivery in detail. From theories to research to practical applications, case studies related to all contemporary topics of relevance to this field have been included herein. Those in search of information to further their knowledge will be greatly assisted by this book.

It was an honour to edit such a profound book and also a challenging task to compile and examine all the relevant data for accuracy and originality. I wish to acknowledge the efforts of the contributors for submitting such brilliant and diverse chapters in the field and for endlessly working for the completion of the book. Last, but not the least; I thank my family for being a constant source of support in all my research endeavours.

Editor

1

Caesarean section by maternal age group among singleton deliveries and primiparous Japanese women: a secondary analysis of the WHO Global Survey on Maternal and Perinatal Health

Kyoko Yoshioka-Maeda[1], Erika Ota[2*], Togoobaatar Ganchimeg[2,3], Mariko Kuroda[1] and Rintaro Mori[2]

Abstract

Background: The rising caesarean section rate is an important public health concern that in turn increases maternal and perinatal risks of adverse effects, unnecessary medical consumption, and inequities in worldwide access. The aim of this study was to investigate caesarean section indications by maternal age group and examine the association between age and caesarean section in primiparous Japanese women with singleton births.

Methods: We analyzed the Japanese data of primiparous women with singleton births from the WHO Global Survey on Maternal and Perinatal Health to compare maternal and neonatal characteristics and outcomes between groups with and without caesarean section. Women were divided into 3 maternal age groups (≤29, 30 to 34 and ≥35 years). We performed multivariable logistic-regression analysis to identify characteristics associated with caesarean section.

Results: Of the 3245 women with singleton births were included in the Japanese data, 610 women (18.8 %) delivered by caesarean section, half of whom ($n = 305$) were nulliparous. We included singleton nulliparous women (1747 deliveries) in our analysis. The maternal age 35 years old was associated with higher risks for all caesarean section (adjusted odds ratio [AOR] 1.89, 95 % CI 1.28–2.78) and emergency antepartum caesarean section (AOR 2.26, 95 % CI 1.49–3.40). Intrapartum caesarean section, which is mainly performed for obstetric indications, was not higher among the older maternal age group.

Conclusion: In Japan, advanced maternal age significantly increased the risk for caesarean section; however, intrapartum caesarean section was not higher risk among the older age group. Management of maternal complications would help to reduce the rate of caesarean sections and associated unnecessary medical consumption.

Keywords: Advanced maternal age, Caesarean section, Pregnancy, Risk factors

Background

Despite a decline in the overall birth rate in many developed countries, delayed childbearing has increased in the last few decades as a result of social, educational and economic factors [1]. Childbearing at 35 years or older is commonly defined as advanced maternal age [2, 3]. Previous studies have shown higher risk of adverse pregnancy outcomes including preterm birth, low birth weight, stillbirth, pre-eclampsia, gestational hypertension, gestational diabetes, and delivery of small- or large-for-gestational-age neonates, and obstetric interventions like caesarean section (CS) and assisted vaginal delivery in women of advanced maternal age [4–9].

The World Health Organization (WHO) recommends that the appropriate rate of CS is not above 15 % [10]. However, data from the Organization for Economic Co-

* Correspondence: otaerika@gmail.com
[2]Department of Health Policy, National Center for Child Health and Development, Tokyo, Japan
Full list of author information is available at the end of the article

operation and Development (OECD) shows that the average rate of CS was 26 % in 2011, which has doubled over two decades [11]. In Japan, although the number of deliveries has decreased, the rate of CS increased 8 % in 1984, and doubled in 2008 to 23.3 % [12]. Previous studies on pregnancy outcomes in advanced maternal age have shown conflicting findings, although most have suggested an increased risk of CS in older women. These studies, however, featured different settings or small sample sizes, and failed to distinguish between elective and emergency CS, and adjustment for potential confounders [13–15]. To address this gap, we conducted a secondary analysis using Japanese data from the WHO Global Survey on Maternal and Perinatal Health (WHOGS), which included 10 health institutions from Japan. The aim of this study was to investigate CS indications by maternal age group, and examine the association between age and CS in primiparous Japanese women with singleton birth.

Methods

Study design and settings

The WHOGS was a multi-country facility-based cross-sectional study conducted between 2004 and 2008 including 24 countries and 373 facilities in Asia, Africa and Latin America [16]. The study methodology of the survey is explained elsewhere in detail [17–19]. In brief, a multi-stage stratified sampling design was used to select the sample of countries and health facilities across the world. Twenty-four countries were selected from 12 WHO regions, and in each country the capital city and two provinces were sampled randomly. Further, seven health facilities with at least 1000 deliveries per year that were capable of performing CS were randomly selected from each these areas. If there were less than 7 facilities, all facilities in that selected areas.

Data collection

We compiled data from the WHOGS of 3356 women and their infants collected from 10 facilities in Tokyo, Okayama and Nagano prefectures in 2008. All women giving birth in participating health institutions over a three-month period in 2008 were recruited in this study. Individual and health institution data were collected using standard forms. Individual data was obtained from medical records by trained health staff before hospital discharge or the 8th day postpartum for mothers and the 7th day after birth for neonates, with no identification of individuals involved. Collected data included maternal demographics, history of previous pregnancies, medical conditions and complications during the last pregnancy, mode of delivery and birth outcomes. Health institutional data were obtained by interview with the director or head of obstetrics. The data included were: infrastructure, basic emergency medical and obstetric care, availability of laboratory tests, anesthesiology resources, intensive care units, human resources and training. The study follow-up period was conducted at 8 days postpartum for mothers, and at 7 days after birth for newborns.

Study sample and variables

In our analysis, we included all primiparous women with singleton deliveries from the 10 participating health institutions in Japan. Women who gave birth for the first time were defined as primiparous. Multiple births, and women who had given birth one or more times, were excluded from the study sample.

The main exposure variable of maternal age was categorised into three groups: ages 20–29, 30–34 and 35 years or older. Outcomes were pregnancy and labour complications, and mode of delivery. The following pregnancy and labour complications were included: maternal hypertension (presence of having pregnancy-induced hypertension, preeclampsia and/or eclampsia), prelabour rupture of membranes, vaginal bleeding in 2nd half of pregnancy, fetal growth impairment, preterm birth (<37 weeks) and low birth weight (<2500 g). Mode of delivery was categorised as spontaneous vaginal delivery, instrumental vaginal delivery and CS. Further CS was categorised as elective CS (defined as CS performed before the onset of labour for medical and obstetric indications or at the request of the mother), emergency antepartum CS (defined as CS performed before onset of labour for medical and obstetric indications) and intrapartum CS (defined as CS performed after the onset of labour for failure to progress, failure of induction of labour, fetal distress or intrapartum hemorraghe). Available indications for CS in the dataset were as follows: pre-/eclampsia, suspected fetal growth impairment, fetal distress, failure to induction, cephalo-pelvic disproportion, breech or malpresentation, and other fetal, maternal and obstetric indications. We created the variable named "having two and more medical indications for CS" for women who presented with two and more indications for CS.

Available individual variables in the dataset were: marital status (married/cohabiting and single), maternal education, number of antenatal care visits, maternal pre-pregnancy body mass index (BMI) (25.0 and >25 kg/m^2), height (<1.5 m and >1.5 m), pre-existing medical conditions, gestational age at delivery (<37, 37 to 41 and ≥41 weeks) and birth weight (<2500, 2500 to 4000 and ≥4000 g). As maternal education was missing for approximately 25 % of women in the dataset, we excluded this variable from the analysis. A medical condition was defined as the presence of any of the following: chronic hypertension, cardiac/renal diseases, chronic respiratory conditions, diabetes mellitus, sickle cell anaemia, severe anaemia and pyelonephritis or urinary infection.

Type of health institution was categorised by ownership as public or private institutions. WHOGS data from Japan is not publicly available.

Ethical approval

Preceding this analysis, ethical approval was obtained from ethical review board of the WHO and each hospital.

Statistical analysis

We used frequencies to examine the study population characteristics, pregnancy and labour complications, and indications for CS among maternal age groups.

The risks of maternal age for all CS, elective CS, emergency antepartum CS and intrapartum CS were explored separately via multivariable logistic regression analysis. For each regression analyses, marital status, maternal height, pre-existing medical conditions, birth weight and type of health institution were considered as confounders. Because of strong correlation between maternal pre-pregnancy and maternal height (correlation coefficient = 0.9), only maternal height included in the regression analyses. The youngest age group (20 to 29 years of age) served as a reference group in the multivariable analyses. All estimates of association we accounted for the WHOGS study design as clustering of women within facilities and facilities with selected areas. The point and variance estimation were obtained by using the first-order Taylor linearization. Health institutions were considered as primary sampling units and areas as strata. Pearson x^2 statistics and multivariable logistic regression analysis were conducted accounting for multistage cluster sampling, using "svy" procedure in STATA 13.1 (Statacorp, College Station, TX, USA). Statistical significance was defined as $p < 0.05$.

Results

The WHOGS data included 3356 deliveries from 10 facilities in three prefectures in Japan during the study period. After excluding for multiple births (110 deliveries) and missing data on mode of delivery (1 delivery), 3245 singleton births remained. Of these singleton births, 610 (18.8 %) women delivered by CS, and half of them (n = 305) were nulliparous. A total of 1747 nulliparous women with singleton neonates were included in this analysis. The study population consisted of 702 (40.2 %) women aged 29 years or younger, 677 (38.8 %) aged 30–34 years, and 368 (21.0 %) aged 35 years or older (Fig 1).

Table 1 shows the characteristics of the study population. Women aged 35 years or older were more likely to have 12 or more antenatal care visits (47.7 % vs 36.3 % in women aged ≤29 years and 45.4 % in women aged 30–34 years), and a pre-existing medical condition (26.5 % vs 14.0 % in women aged ≤29 years and 15.1 % in women aged 30–34 years). Women aged ≤29 years

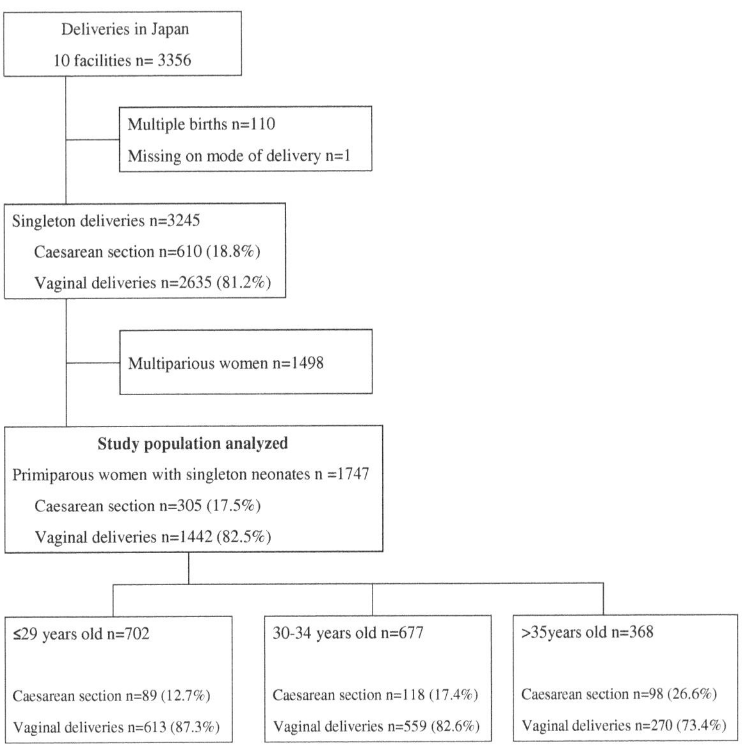

Fig. 1 Study flow chat

Table 1 Characteristics of nulliparous women with singleton birth $N = 1747$

Characteristics	Maternal age group, years						Adjusted x^2, P
	≤29		30–34		≥35		
	($n = 702$)		($n = 677$)		($n = 368$)		
	n	%	n	%	n	%	
Marital status							
Maried/cohabited	661	94.4	665	98.5	358	97.3	<0.001
Single	39	5.6	10	1.5	10	2.7	
Number of antenatal care visits							
< =12	440	63.7	361	54.6	186	52.3	<0.05
> 12	251	36.3	300	45.4	170	47.7	
BMI (kg/m^2)							
18.5 to 25.0	446	63.5	429	63.4	213	57.9	0.19
> 25	256	36.5	248	36.6	155	44.1	
Height							
< 1.5 m	30	4.3	23	3.4	13	3.5	0.44
> 1.5 m	672	95.7	654	96.6	355	96.5	
Pre-exiting medical conditions[a]	98	14.0	102	15.1	94	26.5	<0.001
Health institutional type							
Public	312	44.4	239	35.3	130	35.3	0.23
Private	390	55.6	438	64.7	238	64.7	

[a]Pre-exiting medical conditions was defined as presence of any of followings: chronic hypertension, cardiac/renal diseases, chronic respiratory conditions, diabetes mellitus, sickle cell anaemia, severe anaemia and pyelonephritis or urinary infection

Study-design based Pearson's chi-2 test was calculated

were less likely to deliver at private institutions (55.6 % vs 64.7 % in women aged 30–34 and >35 years).

Table 2 shows pregnancy and labour complications by age group in primiparous women with singleton births. The advanced maternal age group was more likely to have maternal hypertension (12.0 % vs 4.3 % in women aged ≤29 years and 6.1 % in women aged 30–34 years), preterm birth (8.7 % vs 4.5 % in women aged ≤29 years and 5.2 % in women aged 30–34 years), elective CS (10.3 % vs 4.1 % in women aged ≤29 years and 6.8 % in women aged 30–34 years) and emergency antepartum CS (6.5 % vs 2.3 % in women aged ≤29 years and 3.7 % in women aged 30–34 years) than other age groups.

Table 3 illustrated CS indications by age group in primiparous women with singleton births. The proportion of women who underwent CS for indication of pre-eclampsia/eclampsia, suspected fetal growth impairment and other obstetric and maternal complications were highest among women aged >35 years. However, these differences were not statistically significant. CS for indication of dystocia and other fetal complications were significantly higher in women aged 30–34 years, whereas a significantly higher proportion of women aged >35 years had two and more indications for CS (42.9 % vs 33.7 % in women aged ≤29 years and 26.3 % in women aged 30–34 years).

Table 4 showed risk factors for CS in primiparous women with singleton births. Compared to women aged ≤29 years after adjustment for marital status, maternal height, pre-existing maternal medical conditions, maternal hypertension, birth weight and type of health institution, risk of CS were 1.40 (95 % CI 1.02–1.92) and 1.89 (95 % CI 1.28–2.78) times higher in women aged 30–34 years and >35 years, respectively. Women aged >35 years had a significantly

Table 2 Pregnancy and labour complication by age groups in primiparous women with singleton births $N = 1747$

	Maternal age group, years						Adjusted x^2, P
	≤29		30–34		≥35		
	($n = 702$)		($n = 677$)		($n = 368$)		
	n	%	n	%	n	%	
Maternal hypertension[a]	30	4.3	41	6.1	44	12.0	<0.001
PROM	171	24.4	157	23.2	90	24.5	0.85
Fetal growth impairment	17	2.4	13	1.9	10	2.7	0.68
Preterm birth (<37 weeks)	32	4.5	35	5.2	32	8.7	<0.05
Low birth weight (<2500 g)	77	10.1	70	10.3	50	13.7	0.11
Instrumental vaginal delivery	53	7.6	59	8.7	43	11.7	0.08
Elective CS	29	4.1	46	6.8	38	10.3	<0.01
Emergency antepartum CS	16	2.3	25	3.7	24	6.5	<0.05
Intrapartum CS	44	6.3	47	6.9	36	9.8	0.20

CS caesarean section, *PROM* prelabour rupture of membrane

[a]Maternal hypertension was defined as presence of pregnancy-induced hypertension, preeclampsia and eclampsia

Study-design based Pearson's chi-2 test was calculated

Table 3 CS indication by age group in primiparious women with singleton births $N = 305^a$

CS Indications	Maternal age group, years						Adjusted x^2, P
	≤29 (*n* = 89)		30–34 (*n* = 118)		≥35 (*n* = 98)		
	n	%	*n*	%	*n*	%	
Pre-/eclampsia	3	3.4	10	8.5	13	13.3	0.05
Suspected fetal growth impairment	3	3.4	5	4.2	7	7.1	0.45
Fetal distress	30	33.7	28	23.4	32	32.6	0.22
Dystocia	20	22.5	40	33.9	17	17.4	<0.05
Failed induction	11	12.4	10	8.5	13	13.3	0.49
Breech/malpresentation	31	34.8	29	24.6	29	29.6	0.27
Other maternal medical indications	11	12.4	11	9.3	17	17.4	0.21
Other fetal indications	4	4.5	10	8.5	1	1.0	<0.05
Other obstetric indications	14	15.7	17	14.4	26	26.5	0.05
Having 2 and more indications	30	33.7	31	26.3	42	42.9	<0.05

CS caesarean section
[a]Total number of deliveries restricted to women who delivered by caesarean section
Other maternal medical indications included caesarean sections indicated for 3rd trimester vaginal bleeding, suspected/imminent uterine rupture, genital herpes/extensive condyloma and any other maternal medical complications. Other fetal indications included postmortem caesarean section and any other fetal indications. Other obstetric indications defined as conditions such as *placenta previa* without bleeding
Study-design based Pearson's chi-2 test was calculated

higher risk of emergency antepartum CS (AOR 2.26, 95 % CI 1.49–3.40) compared to women aged ≤29 years.

Discussion

To our knowledge, this is the first multiple facility-based study with a reasonable sample size focusing on the association between maternal age and CS in Japan. The strength of this secondary analysis was the pretested, standardised data collection form used to obtain individual and health facility risk factors for CS across randomly selected health facilities, therefore the study results could be generalisable to facilities in Japan.

We found that women having their first childbirth and aged >35 years more likely to have maternal hypertension and higher risk of all CS, elective CS and emergency antepartum CS.

After adjustment for potential confounding factors, risk of all CS and emergency antepartum CS were significantly higher in women aged >35 years compared to primiparous women aged ≤29 years with singleton births. The proportion of women having CS indicated for preeclampsia/eclampsia, suspected fetal growth impairment, other obstetric and maternal complications, and having multiple indications were significantly higher in women aged >35 years [20]. Previous research also highlights the effect of advanced maternal age increasing the risk for CS and operative vaginal delivery in the Asian population [21]. However, previous studies have not explored whether elective or emergency CS differs by

Table 4 The association between maternal age and caesarean section in primiparious women with singleton births. Results of multivariable logistic regression analyses

	Maternal age, years								
	≤29	30–34				≥35			
		Crude OR (95 % CI)		Adjusted OR (95 % CI)		Crude OR (95 % CI)		Adjusted OR (95 % CI)	
All CS	ref	1.45	(1.10–1.91)*	1.40	(1.02–1.92)*	2.50	(1.74–3.56)***	1.89	(1.28–2.78)**
Elective CS	ref	1.69	(1.11–2.55)*	1.55	(0.94–2.55)	2.67	(1.54–4.61)**	1.70	(0.88–3.30)
Emergency antepartum CS	ref	1.64	(0.68–3.97)	1.76	(0.73–4.25)	2.99	(1.94–4.61)***	2.26	(1.49–3.40)**
Intrapartum CS	ref	1.11	(0.63–1.98)	1.05	(0.56–1.97)	1.62	(0.97–2.69)	1.44	(0.92–2.25)

Multivariable logistic regression analysis with adjustment study design effect and risk factors. Risk factors were included: marital status, height, pre-exiting medical conditions, maternal hypertension, birthweight and health institutions ownership. Pre-exiting medical conditions was defined as presence of any of followings: chronic hypertension, cardiac/renal diseases, chronic respiratory conditions, diabetes mellitus, sickle cell anaemia, severe anaemia and pyelonephritis or urinary infection. Maternal hypertension was defined as presence of pregnancy-induced hypertension, preeclampsia and eclampsia
CS caesarean section, *ref* reference group
* < 0.05 ** < 0.01 *** < 0.001

indication [16, 20–22]. As well as increasing risk for CS, delaying family planning increases the use of assisted reproduction technology, medical costs, and adverse outcomes [3]. To promote safe pregnancy and delivery, the development of supportive health policies and a community healthcare system is needed for younger as well as older mothers.

This study has several important limitations. First, the study findings are not generalisable to the whole country as it includes few facilities out of thousands. Second, this is cross-sectional study and we were not able to identify the cause-effect relationship of CS. However, to the best of our knowledge, it is the first study on maternal age and caesarean section that obtained data from multi-facilities with most available data and indications on caesarean section in Japan.

Conclusion

In Japan, advanced maternal age significantly increased the risk for CS. However, intrapartum CS—which is generally undertaken for obstetric indications—was not higher risk among the older age group. Management of maternal complications would help to reduce the rate of CS and the associated medical consumption.

Competing interests

The authors declare that they have no competing interests.
This research was partially supported by the Ministry of Education, Science, Sports and Culture, Grant-in-Aid for Young Scientific Research (B), 2014–2015 (26860428). This research was supported by clinical research program for child health & development.

Authors' contributions

KMY conducted analysis and drafted the manuscript. EO conducted project design, methodological issues. GT partly conducted analysis and drafting additional method. EO, GT, MK and RM assisted in manuscript revision. All authors read and approved the final manuscript.

Acknowledgments

We appreciate the editorial support of Ms. Emma Barber.

Author details

[1]Department of Community Health Nursing, School of Nursing, Faculty of Medicine, Tokyo Medical University, Tokyo, Japan. [2]Department of Health Policy, National Center for Child Health and Development, Tokyo, Japan. [3]Faculty of Medicine, University of Tsukuba, Ibaraki, Japan.

References

1. Retherford RD, Ogawa N, Matsukura R. Late marriage and less marriage in Japan. Popul Dev Rev. 2001;27(1):65–102.
2. Astolfi P, Zonta LA. Delayed maternity and risk at delivery. Paediatr Perinat Epidemiol. 2002;16(1):67–72.
3. Tromp M, Ravelli AC, Reitsma JB, Bonsel GJ, Mol BW. Increasing maternal age at first pregnancy planning: health outcomes and associated costs. J Epidemiol Community Health. 2011;65(12):1083–90.
4. Bayrampour H, Heaman M. Advanced maternal age and the risk of cesarean birth: a systematic review. Birth. 2010;37(3):219–26.
5. Kenny LC, Lavender T, McNamee R, O'Neill SM, Mills T, Khashan AS. Advanced maternal age and adverse pregnancy outcome: evidence from a large contemporary cohort. PLoS One. 2013;8(2):e56583.
6. Kozinszky Z, Orvos H, Zoboki T, Katona M, Wayda K, Pal A, et al. Risk factors for cesarean section of primiparous women aged over 35 years. Acta Obstet Gynecol Scand. 2002;81(4):313–6.
7. Gibbons L, Belizan JM, Lauer JA, Betran AP, Merialdi M, Althabe F. Inequities in the use of cesarean section deliveries in the world. Am J Obstet Gynecol. 2012;206(4):331 e331–319.
8. Souza JP, Gülmezoglu AM, Lumbiganon P, Laopaiboon M, Carroli G, Fawole B, et al. Caesarean section without medical indications is associated with an increased risk of adverse short-term maternal outcomes: the 2004–2008 WHO Global Survey on Maternal and Perinatal Health. BMC Med. 2010;8(1):71.
9. Belizan JM, Althabe F, Cafferata ML. Health consequences of the increasing caesarean section rates. Epidemiology. 2007;18(4):485–6.
10. Organization WH. Appropriate technology for birth. Lancet. 1985;2(8452):436–7.
11. OECD, Health at a Glance 2011: OECD Indicators, OECD Publishing. Paris, France.http://dx.doi.org/10.1787/health_glance-2011-en.
12. Ministry of Health and Welfare , Japan. Trends in the number of deliveries and percentage of caesarean operations in healthcare facilities, 1984–2008. Health statistics of Japan in 2010. 2010: URL: http://www.mhlw.go.jp/toukei/saikin/hw/hoken/national/dl/22-00.pdf.
13. Chihara I, Uehara R, Kotani K, Sadakane A, Aoyama Y, Tsuboi S, et al. The effect of prepregnancy body mass index on singleton cesarean delivery among term nulliparous women in Japanese population. Arch Gynecol Obstet. 2011;284(5):1117–22.
14. Isono W, Nagamatsu T, Uemura Y, Fujii T, Hyodo H, Yamashita T, et al. Prediction model for the incidence of emergent cesarean section during induction of labor specialized in nulliparous low-risk women. J Obstet Gynaecol Res. 2011;37(12):1784–91.
15. Takahashi H, Watanabe N, Sugibayashi R, Aoki H, Egawa M, Sasaki A, et al. Increased rate of cesarean section in primiparous women aged 40 years or more: a single-center study in Japan. Arch Gynecol Obstet. 2012;285(4):937–41.
16. Bilano VL, Ota E, Ganchimeg T, Mori R, Souza JP. Risk factors of pre-eclampsia/eclampsia and its adverse outcomes in low- and middle-income countries: a WHO secondary analysis. PLoS One. 2014;9(3):e91198.
17. Bukola F, Idi N, M'Mimunya M, Jean-Jose WM, Kidza M, Isilda N, et al. Unmet need for induction of labor in Africa: secondary analysis from the 2004–2005 WHO Global Maternal and Perinatal Health Survey (A cross-sectional survey). BMC Public Health. 2012;12:722.
18. Karlsen S, Say L, Souza JP, Hogue CJ, Calles DL, Gulmezoglu AM, et al. The relationship between maternal education and mortality among women giving birth in health care institutions: analysis of the cross sectional WHO Global Survey on Maternal and Perinatal Health. BMC Public Health. 2011;11:606.
19. Lumbiganon P, Laopaiboon M, Gulmezoglu AM, Souza JP, Taneepanichskul S, Ruyan P, et al. Method of delivery and pregnancy outcomes in Asia: the WHO global survey on maternal and perinatal health 2007-08. Lancet. 2010; 375(9713):490–9.
20. Winkel S, Einsle F, Pieper L, Hofler M, Wittchen HU, Martini J. Associations of anxiety disorders, depressive disorders and body weight with hypertension during pregnancy. Archives of Women's Mental Health. 2015;18(3):473-483.
21. Hsieh TT, Liou JD, Hsu JJ, Lo LM, Chen SF, Hung TH. Advanced maternal age and adverse perinatal outcomes in an Asian population. Eur J Obstet Gynecol Reprod Biol. 2010;148(1):21–6.
22. Samuels-Kalow ME, Funai EF, Buhimschi C, Norwitz E, Perrin M, Calderon-Margalit R, et al. Prepregnancy body mass index, hypertensive disorders of pregnancy, and long-term maternal mortality. Am J Obstet Gynecol. 2007; 197(5):490 e491-496.

2

Caesarean delivery-related blood transfusion: correlates in a tertiary hospital in Southwest Nigeria

Fatimat M. Akinlusi*, Kabiru A. Rabiu, Idayat A. Durojaiye, Adeniyi A. Adewunmi, Tawaqualit A. Ottun and Yusuf A. Oshodi

Abstract

Background: Caesarean delivery carries a risk of major intra-operative blood loss and its performance is often delayed by non-availability of blood and blood products. Unnecessary cross-matching and reservation of blood lead to apparent scarcity in centres with limited supply. This study set out to identify the risk factors for blood transfusion in women who underwent caesarean delivery at a tertiary obstetric unit with a view to ensuring efficient blood utilization.

Methods: A prospective cohort analysis of 906 women who had caesarean deliveries at the Lagos State University Teaching Hospital, Nigeria between January and December, 2011. A comparison was made between 188 women who underwent blood transfusion and 718 who did not. Data were obtained on a daily basis by investigators from patients, clinical notes and referral letters using structured pre-tested data collecting form. Socio-demographic characteristics; antenatal, perioperative and intraoperative details; blood loss; transfusion; and puerperal observations were recorded. EPI-Info statistical software version 3.5.3 was used for multivariable analysis to determine independent risk factors for blood transfusion.

Results: Of the 2134 deliveries during the study period, 906 (42.5%) had caesarean deliveries and of which 188 (20.8%) were transfused. The modal unit of blood transfused was 3 pints (41.3%). The most common indication for caesarean section was cephalo-pelvic disproportion (25.7%).The independent risk factors for blood transfusion at caesarean section were second stage Caesarean Section (aOR = 76.14, 95% CI = 1.25–4622.06, $p = 0.04$), placenta previa (aOR = 32.57, 95% CI = 2.22–476.26, $p = 0.01$), placental abruption (aOR = 25.35, 95% CI = 3.06–211.02, $p < 0.001$), pre-operative anaemia (aOR = 12.15, 95% = CI 4.02–36.71, p < 0.001), prolonged operation time (aOR = 10.72 95% CI = 1.37–36.02, p < 0.001), co-morbidities like previous uterine scar (aOR = 7.02, 95% CI = 1.37–36.02, $p = 0.02$) and hypertensive disorders in pregnancy (aOR = 5.19, 95% CI = 1.84–14.68, p < 0.001). Obesity reduced the risk for blood transfusion (aOR = 0.24, 95% CI = 0.09–0.61, $p = 0.0024$).

Conclusion: The overall risk of blood transfusion in cesarean delivery is high. Paturients with the second stage Caesarean section, placenta previa, abruptio placentae and preoperative maternal anaemia have an increased risk of blood transfusion. Hence, adequate peri-operative preparations for blood transfusion are essential in these situations. Optimizing maternal hemoglobin concentration during antenatal period may reduce the incidence of caesarean-associated blood transfusion.

Keywords: Blood transfusion, Caesarean delivery, Risk factors, Case-control study, Blood loss

* Correspondence: fatimatakinlusi@yahoo.co.uk
Department of Obstetrics and Gynaecology, Lagos State University College of Medicine/Lagos State University Teaching Hospital, Ikeja, Lagos, Nigeria

Background

Research has consistently identified haemorrhage as a major cause of direct maternal death, maternal near miss and maternal morbidity. The majority of these deaths occur from postpartum hemorrhage often in association with caesarean section [1, 2], a procedure that carries a risk of major intra-operative blood loss [3]. This has made caesarean section a common indication for blood transfusion in obstetric practice. Its performance, however, is often delayed by non-availability of blood [1, 4].

Blood transfusion remains a life-saving intervention despite its attendant risks. Limited blood supplies due to poor donor response; anaemia; donor blood wastage from viral contamination [5]; and rising costs continue to hinder availability, timely provision and utilization of blood and blood products. With limited units of donor blood and blood-banking services, judicious utilization is required to achieve the overall goal of blood transfusion.

In our centre, it is common practice to cross-match two or more units of blood for patients undergoing caesarean section. This blood is reserved and unavailable to other users, a practice which is commonplace in many centres in this sub-region [6].

Unnecessary cross-matching and reservation of blood not only incur additional cost but also result in apparent blood scarcity in centres with limited blood supplies. Consequently, patients are deprived of blood even in life threatening situations [6]. In view of the foregoing and the dwindling health resources, it is important to identify risk factors for blood transfusion in patients undergoing caesarean delivery. This will prevent unnecessary routine cross-matching; ensure judicious and rational use; preserve limited blood supply; thus improve availability without compromising the quality of care.

This study aimed to identify and evaluate risk factors for blood transfusion in women who underwent caesarean delivery at the Obstetric Unit of Lagos State University Teaching Hospital, Ikeja, Nigeria.

Methods

This is a prospective observational study that was carried out at the obstetric unit of the Lagos State University Teaching Hospital (LASUTH), Nigeria. This hospital is a referral centre for private and public health institutions in Lagos and the neighboring states. Approximately 2000 deliveries take place per annum.

Pregnant women who attended the maternity unit for caesarean deliveries between January 1st and December 31st, 2011 were the participants.

Definition of terms

A patient was defined as "Transfused" or "Not transfused" when her caesarean delivery was associated or not associated with blood transfusion respectively; at any time prior to discharge. An 'unbooked patient' is one who is not registered for antenatal care at LASUTH. Pre-operative anaemia and pre-operative fever were defined as a packed cell volume of less than 30% and temperature of 37.5 °C or more respectively, occurring within 24 h of commencement of surgery. The duration of surgery (skin incision to last stitch) was regarded as 'prolonged' when it lasted more than one hour. An estimated blood loss of 1000mls or more at the conclusion of surgery was regarded as excessive. Obesity was defined as body mass index (BMI) equal to or greater than 30 kg/m^2. The period between 8.a.m. and 4.p.m. on weekdays are referred to as regular hours while call hours refers to all periods outside these hours.

Data collection

All women who had either elective or emergency caesarean deliveries during the study period consented to participation and were enrolled. Information was obtained directly from patients, their clinical notes and referral letters using structured pre-tested data collection form. Data were recorded on a daily basis by investigators and trained research assistants from admission through delivery till discharge. Women who had vaginal deliveries were excluded.

Socio-demographic data obtained included; age, parity, booking status, maternal weight, height, and educational status. Details of labour; pre-operative morbid conditions such as anaemia, presence of uterine fibroids, previous uterine surgery, chronic hypertension; and gestational age at delivery were amongst the perioperative conditions investigated. Intra-operative and post-operative characteristics obtained included indication for caesarean section, type of anaesthesia (general or regional), type of abdominal incision, cadre of surgeon, surgical events, and duration of surgery. The cadre of surgeon that carried out the caesarean delivery varied according to indication and unit protocol; either consultants or resident doctors. Placenta was delivered by controlled cord traction except where this was difficult in which case manual removal was performed.

Blood loss was estimated by counting the number of soaked abdominal packs and gauzes; measurement of volume of blood expelled from the vagina after caesarean section; and visual estimation of blood staining of the theatre linen and drapes. The intraoperative decision for blood transfusion was made by the attending anaesthesiologist based on preoperative haematocrit, the estimated blood loss and the clinical status of the patient. The attending obstetrician subsequently decided on the postoperative transfusion needs of patients. However, those with massive haemorrhage or consumption coagulopathy are jointly managed with the Haematologists. Though transfusion haematocrit threshold varies, patients in stable clinical condition hardly require transfusion at haematocrit levels of 26% or more. The units of blood transfused were recorded. The aforementioned were all explored as risk factors contributing to blood transfusion in caesarean deliveries.

Statistical analysis

Information obtained was entered into the computer and analysed with the EPI-Info statistical software 3.5.3 version (2011) of the Centre for Disease Control and prevention (CDC), Atlanta, USA. A comparison between transfused and non-transfused parturients was made using Chi-square, Student's t test and Mann-Whitney-U test where appropriate. A p value of <0.05 was considered statistically significant.

Univariable and multivariable logistic regression models were constructed to identify independent risk factors associated with blood transfusion in women with caesarean delivery.

Results

A total of 2134 deliveries occurred during the study period of which 906 had caesarean section. Thus a caesarean section rate of 42.5% was recorded. Of the 906 that had caesarean section, 188 (20.8%) received blood transfusion. The most common indication for caesarean section was cephalo-pelvic disproportion (25.7%) but only 15.9% of this group had blood transfused, whereas of the 12.2% women who under-went caesarean section for ante-partum haemorrhage 81.51% of the group were transfused.

Other common indications were malpresentation, fetal compromise, hypertensive disorders of pregnancy, repeat caesarean section and the transfusion rate was between 7.1% and 19.4% for these conditions.

The mean duration of surgery was 51.1 min (SD = 22.6) with a range of 20–334 min while the pre-operative packed cell volume (PCV) ranged from 20 to 39% with an overall mean of 32.9% (SD = 2.8). The median gestational age of women who had blood transfusion was 39.0 weeks (interquartile range, IR = 38–40) which was same as those who didn't receive blood transfusion. The highest frequency of blood units transfused was 3, occurring in 41.3% of patients as shown in Fig. 1.

The significant socio-demographic risk factors for transfusion in these women were; age (≥35), social class, parity and obesity with as many as 52.1% of patients who received blood transfusion being of unbooked status (cOR = 3.23, 95% CI = 2.3–4.5) as shown in Table 1.

After univariable analysis of all the factors, those found to be significantly associated with risk of blood transfusion at caesarean section were: previous uterine scar irrespective of elective or emergency C/S; cadre of surgeons; prolonged operation time; pre-operative anaemia; general anaesthesia, time of surgery and prolonged labour as depicted in Table 2.

Pre-existing conditions such as hypertension, pre- operative fever and uterine fibroids are shown in Table 3, while indications for caesarean section and second stage caesarean section (C/S) data are presented in Table 4.

Preoperative anaemia was a significant risk factor for blood transfusion (OR = 17.69). The mean packed cell volumes of transfused and non- transfused patients were 29.6% and 33.7% respectively and the difference was statistically significant.

Regional anaesthesia was a protective factor for blood transfusion (OR = 0.17, 95% CI 0.12–0.25) while co-existing uterine fibroid increased the odds of transfusion. (OR = 9.72, 95% CI 3.38–27.96).

Multiple logistic regression analysis of the significant factors was performed and independent risk factors were determined.

Second stage C/S (aOR = 76.14, 95% CI = 1.25–4622.06, $p = 0.04$), placenta previa (aOR = 32.57, 95% CI = 2.22–476.26, $p = 0.01$), placental abruption (aOR =

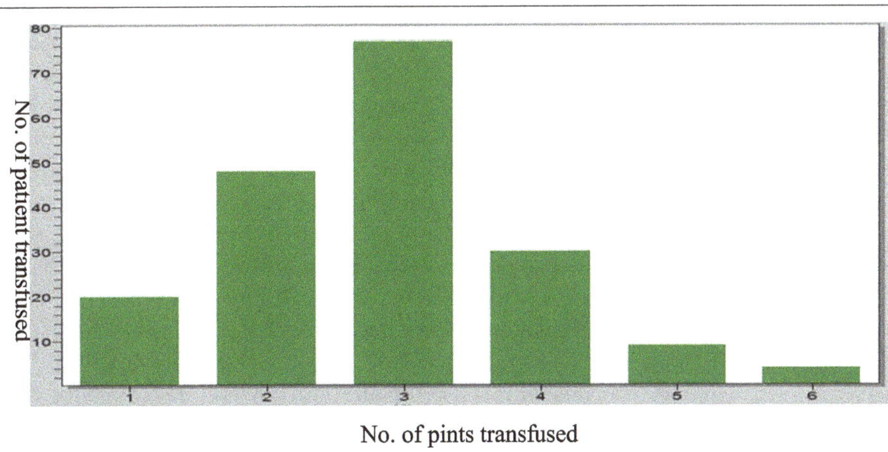

Fig. 1 Frequency of units of blood transfused

Table 1 Socio-demographic profile of blood transfused versus non-transfused patients

Variables	Transfused (*N* = 188)	Not transfused (*N* = 718)	Crude Odds Ratio(cOR)	95% CI	*P* value
Age group					
< 20	4(50%)	4(50%)	1.00	reference	reference
20–34	158(21.7%)	569(78.3%)	0.28	0.06–1.22	0.07
35 and above	26(15.2%)	145(84.8%)	0.18	0.04–0.76	0.02
Marital status					
Single	37(31.9%)	79(68.1%)	0.94	0.33–2.69	0.90
Married	134(18.8%)	577(81.2%)	0.46	0.17–1.26	0.13
Separated	6(16.2%)	31(83.8%)	0.39	0.10–1.44	0.16
Widowed	5(20.8%)	19(79.2%)	0.52	0.13–2.11	0.37
Divorced	6(33.3%)	12(66.7%)	1.00	reference	reference
Social class					
Upper	20(15.6%)	108(84.4%)	0.48	0.28–0.82	0.01
Middle	67(16.2%)	347(83.8%)	0.50	0.36–0.71	<0.001
Lower	101(27.7%)	263(72.3%)	1.00	Reference	Reference
Parity					
0	49(28%)	126(72%)	1.00	Reference	Reference
1–4	126(19.1%)	532(80.9%)	0.61	0.42–0.89	0.01
5 and above	3(17.8%)	60(82.2%)	0.56	0.28–1.11	0.09
Obesity					
Yes	77(17.5%)	362(82.5%)	0.68	0.49–0.95	0.02
No	111(23.8%)	356(76.2%)	1.00	Reference	Reference
Unbooked Status					
Yes	98(35.1%)	181(64.9%)	3.23	2.32–4.50	<0.001
No	90(14.4%)	537(85.6%)	1.00	Reference	Reference

*Significant p value < 0.05

25.35, 95% CI = 3.06–211.02, $p < 0.001$), pre-operative anaemia (aOR = 12.15, 95% CI = 4.02–36.71, p < 0.001), prolonged operation time (OR = 10.72 95% CI = 1.37–36.02, p < 0.001), previous uterine scar (aOR = 7.02, 95% CI = 1.37–36.02, $p = 0.02$) and hypertensive disorders in pregnancy (aOR = 5.19, 95% CI = 1.84–14.68, p < 0.001) were found to be significantly higher risk factors for blood transfusion at caesarean section while obesity was found to be a protective risk factor (aOR = 0.24, 95% CI = 0.09–0.61, $p = 0.002$) as depicted in Table 5.

Discussion

In this prospective study of 906 women undergoing caesarean delivery, we found an overall risk of caesarean-associated blood transfusion of 20.8%, which is high compared with 0.63% to 12.21% found in similar studies done in Australia, the United States of America, Denmark and India [3, 4, 7–9]. The high transfusion rate in this study may be explained by the high incidence of emergent cases such as prolonged labour, cephalo-pelvic disproportion and the relatively large number of cases of placenta previa, abruptio placentae and hypertensive disorders in pregnancy (pre-eclampsia/eclampsia).

In a study of blood transfusion in obstetric practice in Lagos University Teaching Hospital (LUTH), Lagos, a sister tertiary centre, the overall transfusion rate was 12.1% [6] lower than the 20.8% in this study. In an earlier study done in our centre by Akinola et al. [10], the blood transfusion rate was 12.5% which is significantly lower than the transfusion rate in this study. This lower figure may be explained by the shorter duration of that study (3 versus 12 month) and the potential underestimation and errors from incomplete data entries inherent in retrospective studies.

The caesarean section rate in this study was 42.5% which is high compared to the total U.S. caesarean delivery rate of 32.9% of all births in 2009 [11] and 5–21.8% reported in Sub-Saharan Africa [12]. The World Health Organization however recommends a caesarean section rate of 5–15% in any facility [13]. High caesarean delivery rates have been an issue of international concern, though most cases in this study were emergency surgeries with

Table 2 Obstetrics/Operative factors in blood transfused versus non-transfused patients

Variables	Transfused ($N = 188$)	Not transfused ($N = 718$)	Crude Odds Ratio (cOR)	95% CI	*P* value
Previous uterine scar					
Yes	42(14.1%)	256(85.9%)	0.52	0.36–0.76	<0.001
No	146(24.0%)	462(76.0%)	1.00	Reference	Reference
Elective c/s					
Yes	31(9.9%)	281(90.1%)	0.31	0.20–0.46	<0.001
No	157(26.4%)	437(73.6%)	1.00	Reference	Reference
No. of foetus					
Single	172(21.1%)	643(78.9%)	1.25	0.71–2.21	0.43
Multiple	16(17.6%)	75(82.4%)	1.00	reference	Reference
Cadre of surgeons					
Registrar	58(13.6%)	368(86.4%)	0.04	0.02–0.09	<0.001
Senior registrar	100(22.6%)	343(77.4%)	0.07	0.03–0.16	<0.001
Consultant	30(81.1%)	7(18.9%)	1.00	Reference	Reference
Time of surgery					
Regular hours	87(18.1%)	393(81.9%)	0.07	0.52–0.98	0.04
Call hours	101(23.7%)	87(18.1%)	1.00	Reference	Reference
Preoperative anaemia					
Yes	161(47.1%)	181(52.9%)	17.69	11.38–27.50	<0.001
No	27(4.8%)	537(95.2%)	1.00	Reference	Reference
Anaesthesia					
Regional	102(14.0%)	626(86.0%)	0.17	0.12–0.25	<0.001
General	86(48.3%)	92(51.7%)	1.00	Reference	Reference
Prolonged operation time					
Yes	111(55.5%)	89(44.5%)	10.19	7.07–14.69	<0.001
No	77(10.9%)	629(89.1%)	1.00	Reference	Reference
Prolonged labour					
Yes	38(46.9%)	43(53.1%)	3.46	2.09–5.75	<0.001
No	73(20.3%)	286(79.7%)	1.00	Reference	Reference

*significant $p = <0.05$

genuine indications. Our facility also serves as a major tertiary referral centre for Lagos metropolis with a population of about 18 million inhabitants which translates to a very large patient load.

The practice of routine cross matching of blood for women undergoing caesarean section in our centre, in anticipation of significant haemorrhage, irrespective of indication, may inadvertently result in unnecessary transfusions as the anaesthetist or obstetrician who might not have recommended a transfusion does so because the blood is available in the theatre.

In this study, second stage Caesarean delivery was an independent risk factor for blood transfusion (aOR = 76.14, 95% CI = 1.25–4622.06, $p = 0.04$). The risk of blood transfusion at second stage section was well stated in the study by Allen et al. that the maternal risks of second stage caesareans included major haemorrhage, greater risk of bladder trauma, and extension tears of the uterine angle leading to broad ligament haematoma [14]. Other studies have similarly reported increased frequency of uterine atony; the need for hysterectomy is also found to be more frequent in the Caesarean deliveries performed in the second stage of labour. This atony has been attributed to longer labour duration resulting in uterine hypotonia. The increased frequency may suggest that these operations are technically more difficult [14, 15]. In advanced cephalo-pelvic disproportion, when the head has entered deep into the pelvis, manipulating the trapped head may lead to lateral extension of the uterine incision with attendant massive haemorrhage [16]. Uterine atony and other causes of haemorrhage resulted in a significantly higher transfusion requirement

Table 3 Pre-pregnancy morbidities in transfused versus non- transfused patients

Variables	Transfused (N = 188)	Not transfused (N = 718)	(cOR)	95% CI	P value
Chronic Hypertension					
Yes	9(7.2%)	116(92.8%)	0.26	0.13–0.52	<0.001
No	178(23.0%)	596(77.0%)	1.00	Reference	Reference
Diabetes					
Yes	4(23.5%)	13(76.5%)	1.18	0.38–3.66	0.78
No	184(20.7%)	705(79.3%)	1.00	Reference	Reference
Pre-operative fever					
Yes	20(50%)	20(50%)	4.16	2.19–7.90	<0.001
No	168(19.4%)	698(80.6%)	1.00	Reference	Reference
HIV					
Yes	11(26.2%)	31(73.8%)	1.38	0.68–2.79	0.38
No	177(20.5%)	687(79.5%)	1.00	Reference	Reference
Uterine fibroids					
Yes	12(70.6%)	5(29.4%)	9.72	3.38–27.96	<0.001
No	176(19.8%)	713(80.2%)	1.00	Reference	Reference
Preoperative anaemia					
Yes	161(47.1%)	181(52.9%)	17.69	11.38–27.50	<0.001
No	27(4.8%)	537(95.2%)	1.00	Reference	Reference

Data presented as n (%), crude odds ratio (cOR) and 95% confidence intervals (CI)*Significant p = <0.05

in women undergoing Caesarean deliveries in the second stage of labour [17]. The Royal College of Obstetricians and Gynaecologists in the UK, suggests that a consultant be present at all second stage Caesarean deliveries to make an informed decision and to reduce complications arising from such operations [18].

Our antepartum haemorrhage indication for caesarean delivery of 12% is higher than 8–10% reported by a Medicins sans Frontiers multi-country analysis conducted in sub-Saharan Africa [19]. Incomplete evaluation for the aetiology of antepartum haemorrhage in unbooked patients coupled with obstetricians' reluctance to allow vaginal delivery even in cases of minor placental previa may be contributory. Placenta previa and Abruptio placentae are the major causes of ante-partum haemorrhage. This study shows that majority of the blood transfusions were indicated for antepartum haemorrhage (placenta previa and abruption) and much fewer transfusions for other indications. Of the 63 women with placenta previa, 51 were transfused (aOR = 32.57, 95% CI = 2.22–476.26, p = 0.01) and of the 56 women with abruptio placentae, 46 were transfused (aOR = 25.35, 95% CI = 3.06–211.02, p < 0.001). This shows a very significant risk for blood transfusion.

Pregnancies complicated by placenta previa are noted for increased blood loss and transfusion at surgery. Factors responsible include repeated ante-partum haemorrhage which may lower the haematocrit, thus putting the patient at a point close to transfusion threshold. Similarly, the low-lying placenta may provoke increased and uncontrollable intra-operative haemorrhage necessitating blood transfusion [5]. Abruptio placentae may be complicated by disseminated intravascular coagulopathy (DIC), couvelaire uterus, uterine atony and uterine rupture. These would further increase the risk of blood transfusion although these complications were not ascertained in the cases of ante-partum haemorrhage in this study.

In our centre, the most senior obstetrician conducts the delivery in cases of ante-partum haemorrhage as there might be recourse to hysterectomy. Research also suggests careful perioperative planning whenever placenta previa complicates a previous caesarean delivery. It can be inferred from this study that all patients with placenta previa or abruptio placentae should have blood cross matched for caesarean delivery.

Pre-operative anaemia was an independent risk factor for blood transfusion (aOR = 12.15, 95% CI = 4.02–36.71, p < 0.001). This was not surprising as a woman with anaemia will tolerate less any amount of blood loss and may develop cardiovascular compromise from haemodynamic instability. Antenatal care has been shown to positively influence haematocrit value in a population of Nigerian women [20]. Such care would identify complications of pregnancy and enable a goal-directed approach to labour and delivery. These risks also argue for optimizing maternal antenatal iron status to avoid severe

Table 4 Indications for caesarean section in transfused versus non-transfused patients

Variable	Transfused (*N* = 188)	Not transfused (*N* = 718)	Crude Odds Ratio(cOR)	95%CI	*P* value
Repeat C/S					
Yes	22(20.8%)	84(79.2%)	1.0	0.61–1.64	0.99
No	165(20.8%)	628(79.2%)	1.0	Reference	Reference
Cephalopelvic disproportion					
Yes	29(12.9%)	195(87.1%)	0.49	0.32–0.75	<0.001
No	158(23.4%)	517(76.6%)	1.0	Reference	Reference
Preeclampsia/Eclampsia					
Yes	64(30%)	149(70.0%)	0.26	1.38–2.80	<0.001
No	124(17.9%)	569(82.1%)	1.0	Reference	Reference
Placenta Previa					
Yes	51(81.0%)	12(19.0%)	21.88	11.36–42.11	<0.001
No	136(16.3%)	700(83.7%)	1.0	Reference	Reference
Abruptio Placenta					
Yes	46(82.1%)	10(17.9%)	22.94	11.31–46.52	<0.001
No	142(16.7%)	708(83.3%)	1.0	Reference	Reference
Non reassuring fetal status					
Yes	17(11.2%)	135(88.8%)	0.43	0.25–0.73	0.002
No	171(22.7%)	583(77.3%)	1.0	Reference	Reference
Malpresentation					
Yes	11(6.9%)	148(93.1%)	0.24	0.13–0.45	<0.001
No	177(23.7%)	570(76.3%)	1.0	Reference	Reference
Second stage C/S					
Yes	30(90.5%)	3(9.1%)	45.25	13.64–150.13	<0.001
No	158(18.1%)	715(71.9%)	1.0	Reference	Reference

anaemia and they suggest that informing severely anaemic iron deficient women about their high risk of transfusion should they undergo caesarean section might enhance compliance with iron supplementation. Thus, the panacea appears to be improved antenatal care. Meanwhile, patients who are presenting in labour without adequate prenatal care to mitigate anaemia should have donor blood cross-matched for caesarean delivery. Antenatal and preoperative anaemia should be corrected vigorously. Pregnant women should not approach term or go into spontaneous labour while still anaemic [20]. The role of oral iron supplements in correcting anaemia is well-documented [21].

In this study, multivariable analysis using the logistic regression model showed previous uterine scar as a risk factor for blood transfusion (aOR = 7.02, 95% CI = 1.37–36.02, $p = 0.02$) in contrast to the initial univariable analysis which suggested a reduced blood transfusion risk. (cOR = 0.52, 95% CI = 0.36–0.76, $P = 0.001$). The higher rate of transfusion in patients without uterine scar compared with those with scar (24.0% versus 14.1%) might be due to cases of abruptio placenta, preoperative anaemia and second stage sections occurring in those without uterine scars. The increased blood transfusion risk may be explained by the higher incidence of intra-operative complications such as adhesions, extension of uterine incision, atony and the need for hysterectomy. All these may be responsible for prolonged operation time (aOR = 10.72 95% CI = 1.37–36.02, $p < 0.001$) when compared to those without complications.

Obesity was found to reduce the risk for blood transfusion at caesarean section (aOR = 0.24, 95% CI = 0.09–0.61, $p = 0.002$). This finding appears surprising as one would expect more challenges at surgery and also the possibility of prolonged operation. However the reduced risk may be as a result of more experienced surgeon operating these patients because of the anticipated problem.

With an increasing incidence of abdominal delivery, the risk of requiring blood transfusion is still significant especially in high risk cases [22]. Improvements in obstetrics surgical techniques and practice, physicians' acceptance of lower peri-operative haemoglobin concentration and adoption of more restrictive indications for blood transfusion,

Table 5 Risk factors for caesarean-related blood transfusion: Multivariate analysis

Independent risk factors	aOR	95% CI	*P*-value
Age group (35 years or more versus <20 years)	0.02	0.00–1.79	0.09
Age group (20–34 versus <20 years)	0.02	0.00–1.67	0.09
Obesity (Yes/No)	0.24	0.10–0.61	<0.001
Pre-op anaemia (Yes/No)	12.15	4.02–36.71	<0.001
Anaesthesia (Regional/General)	0.37	0.13–1.07	0.07
Booked (Yes/No)	1.99	0.76–5.23	0.16
CPD (Yes/No)	0.57	0.08–3.93	0.57
Chronic Hypertension	0.60	0.07–5.30	0.64
Placenta previa (Yes/No)	32.57	2.23–476.26	0.01
Abruptio placentae (Yes/No)	25.35	3.05–211.02	<0.001
Fetal conditions (Yes/No)	1.13	0.13–9.47	0.91
Mal-presentation (Yes/No)	0.88	0.09–8.28	0.10
Prolonged labour (Yes/No)	1.90	0.62–5.87	0.26
2ndstageCs (Yes/No)	76.13	1.25–4622.06	0.04
Pre eclampsia/eclampsia (Yes/No)	5.19	1.84–14.68	<0.001
Pre-0pfever (Yes/No)	3.14	0.76–13.06	0.12
Fibroids (Yes/No)	1.31	0.11–15.75	0.84
Previous uterine scar (Yes/No)	7.02	1.37–36.02	0.02
Elective C/S (Yes/No)	0.03	0.00–46.39	0.34
Prolonged operation time (Yes/No)	10.72	4.20–27.33	<0.001
Cadre of surgeon (Registrar/Consultant)	5.32	0.10–285.63	0.41
Cadre of surgeon (Senior Registrar/Consultant)	1.21	0.02–70.36	0.93
Time of surgery (Regular hours/Call hours)	1.05	0.41–2.69	0.92
Parity grouped (1–4/0)	0.39	0.14–1.07	0.07
Parity grouped (5 and above/0)	0.30	0.03–2.66	0.28
Social class (middle/lower)	0.85	0.31–2.32	0.75
Social class (upper/lower)	0.52	0.13–2.09	0.36
CONSTANT	reference	reference	0.78

Adjusted odds ratio (aOR) and 95% confidence intervals (CI) *Significant p = <0.05

will no doubt contribute to a decrease in blood transfusion rate. Additionally, the challenge posed by patients' reluctance to receive homologous blood transfusion because of the risk of transmission of blood borne infectious agents and the fact that the obstetrics population is largely young and healthy [23] will by necessity compel obstetricians and anaesthetists [24] to consider a trend towards minimal transfusion.

Strengths and limitation

The strength of this study is the prospective nature of its design. Although this study was performed at a single institution, the data may be of a regional significance due to the institution's unique geographic location and patient volume. A larger sample size might have provided additional power to show statistically significant differences for some of the risk factors. Though a number of the factors appear to be statistically significant, caution has to be exercised in their interpretation because of the wide confidence intervals.

Conclusion

The overall risk of blood transfusion in cesarean delivery is high. Parturients with second stage Caesarean section, placenta previa, abruptio placentae and preoperative maternal anaemia have an increased risk of blood transfusion. Careful evaluation of patients for such risks factors prior to surgery coupled with adequate peri-operative preparations for blood transfusion would be expected to ensure optimal blood utilization and better maternal outcome. More so in settings with limited blood supplies and where haemorrhage plays a greater role in maternal mortality. Optimizing maternal hemoglobin concentration during antenatal period may reduce the incidence of caesarean-associated blood transfusion.

Abbreviations

CDC: Centre for Disease Control and prevention; LASUTH: Lagos State University Teaching Hospital; LUTH: Lagos University Teaching Hospital, Lagos

Acknowledgements

We appreciate all the women who participated in this study as well as the midwives and research assistants who helped with recruitment of participants.

Funding

No funding was received for this study.

Authors' contributions

KAR conceived the idea of the study. KAR, FMA, IAD, AAA, TAO, and YAO all participated in its design, data collection, coordination and analysis. FMA wrote the first draft of the paper and all six authors reviewed critically for content and approved the final manuscript.

Consent for publication

Not applicable.

Competing interests

The authors declare that they have no competing interests.

References

1. Onah HE, Ibeziako N, Umezulike AC, Effetie ER, Ogbuokiri CM. Decision-delivery interval and perinatal outcome in emergency caesarean sections. J Obstet Gynaecol. 2005;25(4):342–6.
2. Waterston M, Wolfe C, Hooper R, Bewley S. Postnatal morbidity after childbirth and severe obstetric morbidity. Br J ObstetGynaecol. 2003;110: 728–33.
3. Matot I, Einav S, Goodman S, Zeldin A, Weissman C, Elchalal U. A survey of physician's attitude towards blood transfusion in patients undergoing caesarean section. Am J ObstetGynecol. 2004;190:462–7.
4. Orji EO, Ojofeintimi EO, Esimai AO, Adejuyigbe E, Adeyemi AB, Owolabi OO. Assessment of delays in receiving delivery care at a tertiary healthcare delivery centre in Nigeria. J Obstet Gynaecol. 2006;26(7):643–4.
5. Imarengiaye CO, Ande ABA. Risk factors for blood transfusion during caesarean section in a tertiary hospital in Nigeria. Med SciMonit. 2006;12: CR269–72.
6. Anorlu RI, Orakwe CO, Abudu OO, Akanmu AS. Uses and misuse of blood transfusion in obstetrics in Lagos, Nigeria. West Afr J Med. 2003;22:124–7.
7. Chua SC, Joung SJ, Aziz R. Incidence and risk factors predicting blood transfusion in caesarean section. Aust N Z J Obstet Gynaecol. 2009;49:490–3.
8. Rouse DJ, MacPherson C, Landon M, Varner MW, Leveno KJ, Moawad AH, et al. Blood transfusion and caesarean delivery. ACOG. 2006;108(4):891–7.
9. Goundan A, et al. Descriptive study of blood transfusion practices in women undergoing cesarean delivery. J Obstet Gynecol Res. 2011;37(10): 1277–82.
10. Akinola OI, Fabamwo AO, Tayo AO, Rabiu KA, Oshodi YA, Onyekwere CA. Evaluation of blood reservation and use for caesarean sections in a tertiary maternity unit in south western Nigeria; BMC Pregnancy and Child birth. Vol. 2010:10.
11. Martin JA, Hamilton BE, Ventura SJ, et al. Births: Final data for 2009. National vital statistics reports; vol 60 no 1. Hyattsville, MD: National Center for Health Statistics. 2011.
12. Shah A, Fawole B, M'Imunya MJ, Amokrane F, Nafiu I, Wolomby JJ, Mugerwa K, Neves I, Nguti R, Kublickas M, Mathai M. Caesarean delivery outcomes from the World Health Organisation global survey on maternal and perinatal health in Africa. Int'l J ObstetGynaecol. 2009;107:191–7.
13. Chalmers B, Mangiaterra V, Porter R. World Health Organisation principles of perinatal care: the essential antenatal, perinatal and postpartum care course. Birth. 2001;28:202–7.
14. Allen VM, Connell CM O', Baskett TF. Maternal and perinatal morbidity of caesarean delivery at full cervical dilatation compared with caesarean delivery in the first stage of labour. Br J ObstetGynaecol. 2005;112:986–90.
15. Govender V, Panday M, Moodley J. Second stage caesarean section at a tertiary hospital in South Africa. J Matern Fetal Neonatal Med. 2010.
16. Fasuba OB, Ezechi OC, Orji EO, Ogunniyi SO, Akindele ST, Loto MN et al. Delivery of the impacted head of the foetus at caesarean section after prolonged obstructed labour: a randomized comparative study of two methods. Journal of Obstetrics and Gynaecology. 2002;22:375–78.
17. Sucak A, Celen S, Akbaba E, Soysal S, Moraloglu O, Danisman N. Comparison of Nulliparas Undergoing Cesarean Section in First and Second Stages of Labour: A Prospective Study in a Tertiary Teaching Hospital. Obstetrics and Gynaecology International. Vol, ID. 2011;986506
18. Royal College of Obstetricians and Gynaecologists. RCOG Clinical Effectiveness Support Unit. The National Sentinel Caesarean Section Audit Report. London; 2001.
19. Chu K, Cortier H, Maldonado F, Mashant T, Ford N, Trelles M. Cesarean section rates and indications in sub- Saharan Africa: a multi-country study from Medecins sans Frontiers. PLoS One. 2012;7(9)
20. Ogunbode O. Anaemia in pregnancy. Tropical Journal Obstetrics Gynaecology. 1995;12:19–25.
21. Young MW, Lupafya E, Kapenda E, Boboow EA. The effectiveness of weekly iron supplements in pregnant women of rural northern Malawi. Trop Dr. 2000;30:84–8.
22. Rebarber A, Lonser R, Jackson S, Copel JA, Sipes S. The safety of intra-operative autologous blood collection and auto transfusion during caesarean section. Am J ObstetGynecol. 1998;179:715–20.
23. Carmann WR, Datta S. Red cell use during caesarean delivery. Transfusion. 1991;31:12–5.
24. Rainaldi MP, Tazzari PL, Scagliarini G, Borghi B, Conte R. Blood salvage during caesarean section. Br J Anaesth. 1998;80:195–8.

3

Caesarean section rate and cost control effectiveness of case payment reform in the new cooperative medical scheme for delivery: evidence from Xi County, China

Shuang Liu[1†], Jing Wang[1,2†], Liang Zhang[1] and Xiang Zhang[1*]

Abstract

Background: In China, increases in both the caesarean section (CS) rates and delivery costs have raised questions regarding the reform of the medical insurance payment system. Case payment is useful for regulating the behaviour of health providers and for controlling the CS rates and excessive increases in medical expenses. New Cooperative Medical Scheme (NCMS) agencies in Xi County in Henan Province piloted a case payment reform (CPR) in delivery for inpatients. We aimed to observe the changes in the CS rates, compare the changes in delivery-related variables, and identify variables related to delivery costs before and after the CPR in Xi County.

Methods: Overall, 28,314 cases were selected from the Xi County NCMS agency from 2009 to 2010 and from 2014 to 2015. One-way ANOVA and chi-square tests were used to compare the distributions of CS and vaginal delivery (VD) before and after the CPR under different indicators. We applied multivariate linear regressions for the total medical cost of the VD and CS groups and total samples to identify the relationships between medical expenses and variables.

Results: The CS rates in Xi County increased from 26.1% to 32.5% after the CPR. The length of stay (LOS), total medical cost, and proportion of county hospitals increased in the CS and VD groups after the CPR, which had significant differences. The total medical cost in the CS and VD groups as well as the total samples was significantly influenced by inpatient age, LOS, and hospital type, and had a significant correlation with the CPR in the VD group and the total samples.

Conclusion: The CPR might fail to control the growth of unreasonable medical expenses and regulate the behaviour of providers, which possibly resulted from the unreasonable compensation standard of case payments, prolonged LOS, and the increasing proportion of county hospitals. The NCMS should modify the case payment standard of delivery to inhibit providers' motivation to render CS services. The LOS should be controlled by implementing clinical guidelines, and a reference system should be established to guide patients in choosing reasonable hospitals.

Keywords: Cost control, Integrated case payment, New cooperative medical scheme, Caesarean section rate, Delivery

* Correspondence: zhangchxiang@163.com
†Equal contributors
[1]Department of Health Management, School of Medicine and Health Management, Tongji Medical College, Huazhong University of Science and Technology, Wuhan, Hubei 430030, China
Full list of author information is available at the end of the article

Background

Caesarean delivery and its risk

The global rise in caesarean section (CS) rates has resulted in considerable concern. In 1985, the World Health Organization (WHO) first recorded the "highest" CS rate of 15% [1]. However, CS rates remain higher than what is considered reasonable in most areas [2]. In 2016, according to data collected from all continents, the highest CS rates were 40.5% for Latin America and the Caribbean region; these rates were above 15% for all other regions, except for Africa, which has a CS rate of 7.3% [3].

China has experienced remarkable increases in the number of CS procedures, and the CS rate has grown by more than 30% since 1992 [4]. Before the 1990s, the CS rate was below 10% because the development of modern medicine in China was in the early stages. However, this rate rose rapidly. Between 1988 and 2008, the CS rate increased from 3 to 39%, which initially occurred in urban areas and then later in the rural areas with the improvement of the health system [5]. The rapid increase in CS has evoked concern about the health system in China. Therefore, a series of measures have been taken to reduce the unreasonable CS rates, including the reformation of the payment system, the normalization of clinical guidelines, and the strengthening of health education. Accordingly, the growth of the CS rate has slowed and reached 34.9% in 2014 [6].

High CS rates have led to a series of problems. CS is a costly operation compared to vaginal delivery (VD); consequently, it could aggravate the financial burden for households and health care systems and lead to unnecessary risks for maternal and neonatal health [7, 8]. Because CS are subsidized to different degrees, the increased use of CS in many developing countries has resulted in an increase in government funding and a substantially higher proportion of government funding in the total health-care expenditures [9]. From a global perspective, excess use of CS has had considerable costs [10]. Additionally, CS has been linked to a risk of surgical site infections, as described by Eriksen et al. [11], and CS increases the risk of early childhood anaemia compared with VD, as confirmed by Li et al. [12].

Although many objective factors led to the CS rate increase, such as the obstetric care system, provider factors, and pregnant factors, it is likely that social factors, not medical factors, are the main cause for the rate increase in China [13]. These non-medical reasons for the high proportion of CS could be motivated by the preferences of pregnant women and providers. In the absence of medical indications, many pregnant women who insist on requiring CS generally mistakenly believe that CS is less painful and more convenient than VD [14]. Physicians often favour the rapid surgical turnover over a potentially long labour and have incentives to perform CS because they fear charges of malpractice [15]. High medical insurance coverage could also be a key reason for the high CS rates among both providers and patients. Bogg et al. [16] found that the unhealthy increases in CS rates in rural China resulted from the design of the NCMS, the payment systems, and revenue-related bonus systems for doctors. Hu et al. [17] previously emphasised that providers and patients were less likely to avoid excessive tests and medication when a large proportion of the costs were shifted to third-party payers, which leads to increased medical expenses.

To reduce the CS rates and control delivery costs, many countries have adopted various measures and methods, which can be roughly classified into 3 strategies: (1) health education and teaching correct delivery concepts in society, (2) payment reform, and (3) medical malpractice reform [18]. China aims to modify and improve the medical insurance payment system in many places to reduce the CS rates and control delivery costs.

Medical insurance in China and payment reform in Xi County

Through the end of 2016, the health insurance system in China has had three main parts: (1) the Urban Employee Basic Medical Insurance Scheme, (2) the Urban Resident Basic Medical Insurance Scheme, and (3) the NCMS. The NCMS, which was established in 2003, aims to cover the medical expenses of rural residents through financial assistance from the central government, local government, and rural residents themselves, with a separate pool of funds for each county. The annual premium per capita of the NCMS was raised from 30 Chinese Yuan (¥) (USD 4.35, according to the exchange rate of USD 1 = ¥6.89 in April 1, 2017) in 2003, of which ¥20 (USD 2.90) came s from the government and ¥10 (USD 1.45) came from the rural residents, to an average of ¥410(USD 59.50) in 2014 and ¥570 (USD 82.72) in 2016, of which ¥420 (USD 60.95) came from the government and ¥150 (USD 21.77) came from the rural residents. Until 2015, the NCMS covered 99% of all rural residents. However, in 2017, the NCMS began gradually being integrated into the Urban Resident Basic Medical Insurance scheme.

To control the increase in medical expenses, the NCMS agencies in some counties have attempted to implement payment reform for providers by transforming the fee-for-service (FFS) payment into case payment. Because of the FFS payment, which is the most popular method of paying providers in the NCMS, incentivizes health providers to generate unnecessary procedures for high profits and resulted in the inefficient utilization of health services, it has played an important role in the increasing medical expenses in China [19–21]. Therefore, case payment, which is a prospective payment system (PPS), is considered a useful measure for regulating the behaviour of health providers and ultimately controlling the unreasonable increases in medical expenses. Both experts and governors consider the use of case payment more suitable than the use of diagnosis-related groups in rural China because of the limitation of the medical information system and providers' ability to code procedures. McCue et al. [22] testified that the case payment approach reduces costs by approximately 6%–10% compared with FFS arrangements.

Accordingly, the NCMS agencies in some counties, such as Xi County, Henan Province, China, have explored the use of case payment through some support policies to control the increase in medical expenses. In Xi County, which is predominantly occupied by rural residents who are covered by the NCMS, a pilot CPR for inpatients in the NCMS began in 2009 and was implemented for the entire county in 2011. Delivery was the first case covered by the CPR in Xi County. The effectiveness of the CPR to control costs in Xi County requires further examination.

To provide insight into the reform and determine its value as a model for other districts that intend to implement such policies, we take delivery as a research object and investigated the effectiveness of the CPR on CS rate reduction and delivery cost control. In the present study, we aim to (1) observe the changes in the CS rates and delivery costs before and after the CPR, (2) compare the changes in delivery-related variables between CS and VD before and after the CPR, and (3) identify variables related to delivery costs in Xi County.

Methods

Data collection

Data were obtained from the inpatient information database of the Xi County NCMS agency. This database contains the claim information of individuals residing in Xi County, which was covered by the NCMS from January 1, 2009, to December 31, 2010, and from January 1, 2014, to December 31, 2015. In total, 34,210 admissions for delivery were found among a total 295,796 inpatient admission cases over the past four years. In China, township hospitals are grass-root institutions, only providing basic medical services and treating. County hospitals are higher level institutions than township hospital in the county. County hospital could provide comprehensive medical services and treat both ordinary delivery without complication and severe case with complication, because their medical service capacity is stronger than township hospitals.

To focus on studying the effectiveness of the CPR, we excluded patients who were not covered by the case payment for unknown reasons in the hospital, patients for whom the delivery method (VD vs. CS) could not be determined, and patients who visited from outside Xi County. A total of 28,314 deliveries were analysed.

We considered hospital deliveries from January 1, 2009, to December 31, 2010, as the pre-CPR patients and deliveries from January 1, 2014, to December 31, 2015, as the post-CPR patients. There were 12,705 deliveries in the pre-CPR group and 15,609 in the post-CPR group.

Statistical analysis

To ensure the comparability of the medical costs of delivery, we adjusted the medical costs using the consumer price index (2010, 2014, and 2015 = 102.8, 101.8, and 101.1, respectively) in Henan Province.

The variables in this study included inpatient age, LOS, total medical cost, CPR, hospital type, and delivery type. The inpatient age, LOS, and total medical cost were the continuous variables, whereas CPR, hospital type and delivery type were the categorical variables. Total medical cost refers to the full costs of hospitalization. CPR includes the pre-CPR and the post-CPR, and there were two types of hospitals: township and county hospitals. Two types of delivery: VD and CS.

We compared the variables of the VD and CS groups between the pre-CPR and post-CPR, respectively. The variables include the inpatient age, LOS, total medical cost and hospital type. The continuous variables were analysed using a one-way ANOVA to compare the differences in the means, and the categorical variables were analysed using a chi-squared test to compare the differences in proportions.

We applied multivariate linear regressions for the total medical cost of the VD and CS groups and total samples to identify the relationship between medical expenses and variables. The variables include age, CPR, LOS, hospital type and delivery type. Delivery type was only taken into Model 3 (total samples). CPR, hospital type and delivery type are dichotomy variables. Dummy variables can quantify the dichotomy variables and be incorporated in regression models [23]. In order to set reference variables for these three dichotomy variables in multivariate linear regressions, we set (1. the pre-CPR = 0 versus the post-CPR = 1, (2. township hospital = 0 versus county hospitals = 1, and (3. VD = 0 versus and CS = 1, respectively [24]. All data were analysed using SPSS 19.0. All *P* values used in these tests were two-tailed, with 0.05 indicating statistical significance.

Results

Table 1 shows the CS rate of Xi County before and after the CPR. The number of cases in the VD and CS groups increased after the CPR, but there was a statistically significant increase in the CS rates of rural women in Xi

Table 1 Cesarean rate of Xi County before and after CPR

Mode of delivery	pre-CPR	post-CPR	total	% change in CS rate	*p*-value
Total	12,705	15,609	28,314		
CS (N (%))	3319 (26.124)	5069 (32.475)	8388	+ 6.351%	<0.001
VD (N (%))	9386 (73.876)	10,540 (67.525)	19,926		

County from 26.1% before the CPR to 32.5% after the CPR.

Table 2 presents the variable differences between the pre-CPR and post-CPR of the CS and VD groups, respectively. All the variables, except age, showed significant differences in the CS and VD groups between the pre-CPR and post-CPR, respectively. The LOS of the post-CPR is longer than that of the pre-CPR in each group, especially for the VD group, which increased from 2.79 days to 4.59 days. Similarly, the total medical cost post-CPR was higher than pre-CPR for each group. Another phenomenon that should be noticed is that the proportion of county hospitals increased markedly from 70.50% to 95.86% in the CS group and 71.26% to 80.89% in the VD group after the CPR.

Table 3 presents the results of the multivariate linear regression analysis to explain the relationships among the variables and the total medical costs of the CS and VD groups and the total sample. In the CS group (Model 1), almost all variables, including inpatient age, LOS, and hospital type but not the CPR, were significantly correlated with the total medical cost. Additionally, these three factors are risk factors that affect the total medical cost. Furthermore, in the VD group (Model 2), all variables were significantly related to the total medical cost. The LOS and hospital type are also risk factors for the total medical cost. The CPR is also a risk factor. However, age becomes is a protective factor for the total medical costs. In the total samples (Model 3), all variables have a relationship with the total medical cost; CPR, LOS, hospital type, and delivery type are risk factors, but age is a protection factor. Accordingly, the total medical cost among the three regression models were significantly influenced by inpatient age, LOS, and hospital type, but the LOS and hospital type were the risk factors in each model, whereas age was a protection factor for the VD group and total samples. In addition, the total medical cost in the CS group had no relation to the CPR, despite showing a significant correlation with costs in the VD group and the total samples. The higher the level of the delivery was in hospitals, the longer the LOS was and the higher the total medical cost was.

Discussion

The CS rates in Xi County remained high, and the total medical costs of delivery increased, even after the implementation of the CPR in 2011. Furthermore, the medical costs of delivery increased in the CS and VD groups after adjusting the price inflation by using the consumer price index. The proportion of county hospitals in the CS and VD groups increased markedly after the CPR. Therefore, CPR failed to achieve its objective of controlling the growth of excessive medical expenses and regulating the behaviour of providers.

The consistently high CS rates in Xi County could be related to the unreasonable case compensation standards for CS and VD. The case compensation standard for CS is substantially higher than that of VD. For example, the standard total medical cost of VD and CS were set at ¥1360 (USD 197.39) and ¥3400(USD 493.47), respectively, for a delivery without complications. Therefore, the providers prefer CS for economic incentives [5]. McCue et al. [22] testified that the case payment reduces costs by approximately 6%–10% compared with the FFS arrangements, although this scenario may require many years of research to elicit determine whether there is an apparent effect on costs, depending on how high the payment levels were initially set [25, 26]. However, the gap between the reimbursement standards of CS and VD may not be sufficiently narrow to eliminate the economic

Table 2 Descriptive variables comparison between pre-CPR and post-CPR of Xi County

	pre-CPR		post-CPR		*p*-value ((1) VS (3))	*p*-value ((2) VS (4)
	CS (1) (*N* = 3319)	VD (2) (*N* = 9386)	CS (3) (*N* = 5069)	VD (4) (*N* = 10,540)		
Age (years) (mean(SD))	25.92 (5.577)	25.50 (5.194)	25.99 (4.738)	25.598 (4.324)	0.551	0.142
LOS (days) (mean/SD)	6.55 (6.737)	2.786 (6.784)	6.94 (5.099)	4.590 (7.675)	0.004	<0.001
Total medical cost (USD) (mean/SD)	502.12 (950.967)	170.32 (643.585)	558.90 (507.763)	242.31 (514.039)	<0.001	<0.001
Type of hospital					<0.001	<0.001
Township Hospital (*N* (%))	979 (29.500)	2716 (28.936)	210 (4.142)	2014 (19.108)		
County Hospital (*N* (%))	2340 (70.500)	6670 (71.063)	4859 (95.856)	8526 (80.892)		

*α = 0.05

Table 3 Multivariate linear regressions on total medical cost in Xi County

	Factor		B	S.E.[a]	Beta[b]	t	p-value[b]
Model 1 (CS)	Constant		578.684	41.200		14.046	< 0.001
	Age		3.496	1.049	0.024	3.332	< 0.001
	CPR	pre-CPR[c]					
		post-CPR	−21.090	11.715	−0.014	−1.800	0.072
	LOS		4.924	0.929	0.039	5.298	< 0.001
	Hospital type	Township hospital[c]					
		County hospital	1617.581	16.538	0.761	97.811	< 0.001
	R^2		0.566				
Model 2 (VD)	Constant		− 215.343	22.027		−9.776	< 0.001
	Age		−5.800	0.652	−0.044	−8.895	< 0.001
	CPR	pre-CPR[c]					
		post-CPR	405.942	6.309	0.322	64.343	< 0.001
	LOS		1.446	0.432	0.017	3.349	< 0.001
	Hospital type	Township hospital[c]					
		County hospital	895.982	7.431	0.606	120.567	< 0.001
	R^2		0.518				
Model 3 (total)	Constant		−493.046	20.014		−24.635	< 0.001
	Age		−2.474	0.577	−0.010	−4.289	< 0.001
	CPR	pre-CPR[c]					
		post-CPR	315.185	5.779	0.128	54.540	< 0.001
	LOS		2.610	0.413	0.015	6.325	< 0.001
	Hospital type	Township hospital[c]					
		County hospital	1030.098	7.131	0.341	144.457	< 0.001
	Delivery type	VD[c]					
		CS	2130.934	6.317	0.793	337.314	< 0.001
	R^2		0.853				

[a]S.E. = Standard Error
[b]$\alpha = 0.05$
[c]Reference group of categorical predictor variables in multivariate linear regressions

incentives for doctors, and doctors may still be prompted to choose CS instead of VD. The CPR cannot solve the problem of service regulation when the compensation standards are not designed reasonably, even if the payment reform could affect the service choice of the providers. Controlling the CS rate requires strict clinical indications and guidelines to serve as regulatory tools. Althabe et al. confirmed that clinical guidelines and the policy of a mandatory second opinion decreased the CS rate by 25%, showing that clinical guidelines have a clear effect on reducing the CS rate [27].

The increasing total medical cost of delivery could be a result of not only the increase of the CS rate in Xi County but also the unreasonable compensation standards for case payment, the prolonged LOS, and the increasing proportion of county hospitals. Besides the fact that the case compensation standard of CS was higher than that of VD, the case compensation of CS and VD in Xi County was set to be higher than the average level from the past years, promoting the involvement of a substantial number of hospital and health providers in the CPR. For example, the standard total medical cost of VD was set to ¥1360 (USD 197.39) for delivery without complication and ¥1632 (USD 236.87) for delivery with complications, which were both higher than the real average total medical cost of VD (¥1297.94, USD 188.38) before the CPR. The standard total medical cost of CS was set to ¥3400 (USD 493.47) for delivery without complication and ¥4080 (USD 592.16) for delivery with complication, but the average total medical cost of CS before the CPR was ¥3304.57 (USD 479.62). Consequently, the average medical cost of delivery was substantially higher after the CPR than it was before the CPR.

The prolonged LOS was another reason for the total medical cost increase because the LOS is proportional to the total medical cost [28]. Taheri et al. emphasised that the LOS is a mature indicator of hospital cost reduction and that reducing LOS by 1 day reduces the overall cost of care by an average of 3% or less, which demonstrates a direct link between the LOS and cost [29]. The LOS in CS and VD patients in Xi County increased after the CPR to 6.94 and 4.59 days, respectively. Additionally, the change of the LOS in VD is more significant compared to CS. However, in the United States, the LOS for CS and VD was only 3.01 and 1.74 days, respectively [30]. Generally, case payment can shorten the LOS, but the Xi County case payment extended the LOS, possibly because the LOS can be affected by the availability or lack of local medical level services, social culture, and postpartum family care [31]. However, in this study, no specific evidence was found to explain the prolonged LOS.

A phenomenon that should not be ignored is that the proportion of county hospitals increased tremendously, which may lead to excessive growth in the total medical cost because the cost standards of county hospitals are higher than those of township medical institutions. For example, the standard total medical cost of VD was set to ¥1050 (USD 152.40) for delivery without complication in township hospitals, but in county hospitals, the cost was set to ¥2400 (USD 348.33). Additionally, the standard total medical cost of CS without complications was set to ¥2800 (USD 406.39) in township hospitals and was set to ¥3400 (USD 493.47) in county hospitals. Therefore, the total medical cost of CS and VD increased with an increase in the delivery hospital level. In China, a study verified that the higher the hospital's level, the more it might cost, which could be explained by the fact that high-level hospitals are much more likely to use expensive drugs and diagnostic tests [32].

Our study has several limitations. First, we used claim data, which lacked vital information on the severity of the pregnancy and ex-experience of the delivery. Therefore, we could not determine the effects of previous medical history on our results. Furthermore, the limited information regarding the social-economic characteristics of the inpatients resulted in the lack of an extensive analysis of residents to explain the conclusion. Additionally, because there was no control group to compare with Xi County, the effectiveness of the CPR in Xi County was tested using only a before-and-after contrast analysis. It was not confirmed with a difference-in-difference estimation, which is an effective method for reducing bias when comparing groups and can produce considerably accurate and effective estimates [33].

Conclusion

The purpose of the CPR was to control the unreasonable growth of medical expenses and regulate the behaviour of providers. However, our results confirmed that it failed to achieve its goal because the CS rate remained at a high level and the total medical cost continued to increase. The consistently high level of CS rates in Xi County could be related to the unreasonable case compensation standards of CS. The continuing increase in the total medical cost of delivery could be a result not only of the growth in CS rates in Xi County but also the unreasonable compensation standards for case payment, the prolonged LOS, and the increasing number of county hospitals. Therefore, the NCMS should modify the case payment standard of delivery for CS and VD to inhibit the motivation of providers to offer CS services. The LOS should be strictly controlled by implementing clinical guidelines, and a reference system should be established to guide patients to choose reasonable hospitals.

Abbreviations

CPR: Case payment reform; CS: Caesarean section; FFS: Fee for service; LOS: Length of stay; NCMS: New Cooperative Medical Scheme; PPS: Prospective payment system; VD: Vaginal delivery

Funding

The research design and data collection were supported by the Research in Model of Interaction Mechanism of Rural Health Service Network and based on the continuity of service as well as research on the Vertical Integration Management Model of the Chinese Rural Medical Service based on the Complex Adaptive System Theory, and Research on multi-dimension risk identification of health poverty vulnerability of elderly individuals in rural areas and targeted poverty alleviation strategies funded by National Natural Science Foundation of China (grant number 71371091, 71273099,71673093).

Authors' contributions

SL and JW proposed the study, contributed to acquisition, analyses and interpretation of data and drafted the manuscript. ZL contributed to the conception and design of the study. XZ supervised the study design, statistical analysis and critical review of important intellectual content in this manuscript. All authors read and approved the final manuscript.

Consent for publication

Not applicable.

Competing interests

The authors declare that they have no competing interests.

Author details

[1]Department of Health Management, School of Medicine and Health Management, Tongji Medical College, Huazhong University of Science and Technology, Wuhan, Hubei 430030, China. [2]The Key Research Institute of Humanities and Social Science of Hubei Province, Huazhong University of Science and Technology, Wuhan, Hubei 430030, China.

References

1. WHO. Monitoring emergency obstetric care: a handbook. Journal of Obstetrics & Gynaecology. 2010;30(4):430.
2. Robson SJ, de Costa CM. Thirty years of the World Health Organization's target caesarean section rate: time to move on. Med J Aust. 2017;206(4):181.
3. Betrán AP, Ye J, Moller AB, Zhang J, Gülmezoglu AM, Torloni MR. The increasing trend in caesarean section rates: global, regional and National Estimates: 1990-2014. PLoS One. 2016;11(2):e0148343.

4. National Bureau of Statistics of China.Statistical report on the implementation of the "outline of Chinese women's development (2011–2020)" in 2014.2015. http://www.stats.gov.cn/tjsj/zxfb/201511/t20151127_1282257.html. Accessed 27 Nov 2015.
5. Hellerstein S, Feldman S, Duan T. China's 50% caesarean delivery rate: is it too high? BJOG Int J Obstet Gynaecol. 2015;122(2):160.
6. Li HT, Luo S, Trasande L, Hellerstein S, Kang C, Li JX, Zhang Y, Liu JM, Geographic Variations BJ. Temporal trends in cesarean delivery rates in China, 2008-2014. JAMA. 2017;317(1):69–76.
7. Lumbiganon P, Laopaiboon M, Gülmezoglu AM, Souza JP, Taneepanichskul S, Ruyan P, et al. Method of delivery and pregnancy outcomes in Asia: the WHO global survey on maternal and perinatal health 2007-08. Lancet. 2010;375(9713):490.
8. Long Q, Klemetti R, Wang Y, Tao F, Yan H, Hemminki E. High caesarean section rate in rural China: is it related to health insurance (new co-operative medical scheme)? Soc Sci Med. 2012;75(4):733–7.
9. Kruk ME, Galea S, Prescott M, Freedman LP. Health care financing and utilization of maternal health services in developing countries. Health Policy Plan. 2007;22(5):303–10.
10. Gibbons L, Belizán JM, Lauer JA, Betrán AP, Merialdi M, Althabe F. The global numbers and costs of additionally needed and unnecessary caesarean sections performed per year: overuse as a barrier to universal coverage. World health report. 2010;30:1–31.
11. Eriksen HM, Saether AR, Løwer HL, Vangen S, Hjetland R, Lundmark H, et al. Infections after caesarean sections. Journal of the Norwegian Medical Association. 2009;129(7):618–22.
12. Li HT, Trasande L, Zhu LP, Ye RW, Zhou YB, Liu JM. Association of cesarean delivery with anemia in infants and children in 2 large longitudinal Chinese birth cohorts. Am J Clin Nutr. 2015;101(3):523–9.
13. Tang S, Li X, Wu Z. Rising cesarean delivery rate in primiparous women in urban China: evidence from three nationwide household health surveys. American Journal of Obstetrics & Gynecology. 2006;195(6):1527–32.
14. He Z, Cheng Z, Wu T, Zhou Y, Chen J, Fu Q, Feng Z. The costs and their determinant of cesarean section and vaginal delivery: an exploratory study in Chongqing municipality, China. Biomed Res Int. 2016; https://doi.org/10.1155/2016/5685261.
15. Hellerstein S, Feldman S, Duan T. Survey of obstetric care and cesarean delivery rates in shanghai, China. Birth. 2016;43(3):193–9.
16. Bogg L, Huang K, Long Q, Shen Y, Hemminki E. Dramatic increase of cesarean deliveries in the midst of health reforms in rural China. Soc Sci Med. 2010;70(10):1544–9.
17. Hu S, Tang S, Liu Y, Zhao Y, Escobar ML, de Ferranti D. Reform of how health care is paid for in China: challenges and opportunities. Lancet. 2008;372(9652):1846–53.
18. Stafford RS. Alternative strategies for controlling rising cesarean section rates. JAMA. 1990;263(5):683–7.
19. Yip WC, Hsiao W, Meng Q, Chen W, Sun X. Realignment of incentives for health-care providers in China. Lancet. 2010;375(9720):1120–30.
20. Yip WC-M, Hsiao WC, Chen W, Hu S, Ma J, Maynard A. Early appraisal of China's huge and complex health-care reforms. Lancet. 2012;379(9818):833–42.
21. Eggleston K, Ling L, Qingyue M, Lindelow M, Wagstaff A. Health service delivery in China: a literature review. Health Econ. 2008;17(2):149–65.
22. McCue MJ, Thompson JM. Early effects of the prospective payment system on inpatient rehabilitation hospital performance. Arch Phys Med Rehabil. 2006;87(2):198–202.
23. Usman AU, Hassan SA, Tukur K. Application of dummy variables in multiple regression analysis. International Journal of Recent Scientific Research. 2015;7(11):7440–2.
24. Sapkota S, Kobayashi T, Kakehashi M, Baral G, Yoshida I. In the Nepalese context, can a husband's attendance during childbirth help his wife feel more in control of labour? Bmc Pregnancy & Childbirth. 2012;12(1):1–10.
25. Cavalieri M, Gitto L, Guccio C. Reimbursement systems and quality of hospital care: an empirical analysis for Italy. Health policy. 2013;111(3):273–89.
26. Rosko MD, Mutter RL. Inefficiency differences between critical access hospitals and prospectively paid rural hospitals. J Health Polit Policy Law. 2010;35(1):95–126.
27. Althabe F, Belizán JM, Villar J, Alexander S, Bergel E, Ramos S, et al. Mandatory second opinion to reduce rates of unnecessary caesarean sections in Latin America: a cluster randomised controlled trial. Lancet. 2004;363(9425):1934–40.
28. Wei JW, Heeley EL, Jan S, Huang YN, Huang QF, Wang JG, et al. Variations and determinants of hospital costs for acute stroke in China. PLoS One. 2010;5(9):4439–51.
29. Taheri PA, Butz DA, Greenfield LJ. Length of stay has minimal impact on the cost of hospital admission. J Am Coll Surg. 2000;191(2):123.
30. Eggleston K, Ling L, Quingyue M, Lindelow M, Wagstaff A. Health service delivery in China: a literature review. Health Econ. 2008;17(2):149.
31. Petrou S, Henderson J, Glazener C. Economic aspects of cesarean section and alternative modes of delivery. Best Practice & Research Clinical Obstetrics & Gynaecology. 2001;15(1):145.
32. Yip WCM, Hsiao W, Meng Q, Chen W, Sun X. Realignment of incentives for health-care providers in China. Lancet. 2010;375(9720):1120.
33. Grabich SC, Robinson WR, Engel SM, Konrad CE, Richardson DB, Horney JA. County-level hurricane exposure and birth rates: application of difference-in-differences analysis for confounding control. Emerging Themes in Epidemiology. 2015;12(1):19.

4

Paradox lost on the U.S.-Mexico border: U.S. Latinas and cesarean rates

Theresa Morris[1*], Amanda Gomez[2], Miriam Naiman-Sessions[3] and Christine H. Morton[4]

Abstract

Background: We apply Intersectional Theory to examine how compounded disadvantage affects the odds of women having a cesarean in U.S.-Mexico border hospitals and in non-border hospitals. We define U.S. Latinas with compounded disadvantage as those who have neither a college education nor private health insurance.

Results: Analyzing quantitative and qualitative data from Childbirth Connection's Listening to Mothers III Survey, we find that, consistent with the notion of the Latinx Health Paradox, compounded disadvantage serves as a protective buffer and decreases the odds of cesarean among women in non-border hospitals. However, the Latinx Health Paradox is absent on the border.

Conclusion: Our data show that women with compounded disadvantage who give birth on the border have significantly *higher* odds of a cesarean compared to women without such disadvantage. Further, women with compounded disadvantage who give birth in border hospitals report receiving insufficient prenatal, pregnancy, and postpartum information, providing a direction for future research to explain the border disparity in cesareans.

Keywords: Cesarean, Childbirth, Hispanic health paradox, U.S-Mexico border, Listening to Mothers III, Intersectional theory

Background

The U.S.-Mexico border region is a politically significant geographical region, as evidenced by its centrality in the 2016 United States presidential campaign. In fact, this strip of land, which spans 2000 miles, 48 counties, and four states, is often used to highlight hot-button political issues like immigration, crime, and poverty [1]. The region is ethnically, culturally, and economically distinct from the rest of the U.S. population. For instance, in 2000, Latinos and Latinas comprised 49% of the population in border counties—a far greater percentage than the 12.6% of Latinos in the general population in 2000 [2][1]. Further, compared to the overall U.S. population, individuals in the border region have a lower income per capita. This income disparity is greater for Latinos and Latinas in the border region, who make less than both whites in the border region and Latinos and Latinas in non-border regions. Border residents also have a lower level of educational attainment than the general population and are less likely to have private health insurance, suggesting the importance of looking at compounded disadvantage, especially in the border region [2].

However, despite Latinos' and Latinas' lower socioeconomic status, Latinx ethnicity in the United States is often correlated with positive health outcomes – a phenomenon referred to as the Hispanic or Latinx Health Paradox [3][2]. This phenomenon has been applied to maternal-fetal health, although findings typically focus on fetal rather than maternal outcomes. For example, studies have found that Latinas have lower pre-term birth, low-birth weight, and maternal mortality rates compared to non-Latinas in the U.S. [4–9].

Thinking about the border and the Latinx Health paradox led us to wonder how this geographic and socioeconomic context might affect maternal outcomes on the border, specifically women's odds of having a cesarean, an important maternal outcome because cesareans carry greater health risks than vaginal birth [10]. Thus, in this study we examine how compounded disadvantage—defined as being Latina without private health insurance or a college degree—affects the odds of cesarean in border and in non-border hospitals. Does the Latinx Paradox protect Latinas, especially Latinas with compounded disadvantage, from cesareans? If it

* Correspondence: theresa.morris@tamu.edu
[1]Department of Sociology, Texas A&M University, MS4351, College Station, TX 77843, USA
Full list of author information is available at the end of the article

does, is this paradox present in border and in non-border hospitals?

The World Health Organization concludes that "[a]t the population level, caesarean section rates higher than 10% are not associated with reductions in maternal and newborn mortality rates" [11]. U.S. Healthy People 2020 sets a target for a low-risk, first birth cesarean rate of 23. 9% [12]. Despite these goals and statements, the cesarean rate has increased in both developing and developed nations and for all groups of women [13]. As of 2016, the United States' cesarean rate was 31.9% [14]. This rate varies greatly among women, hospitals, and states. For example, certain individual health conditions, prior cesarean, hospital characteristics, and state have all been shown to affect a woman's chance of having a cesarean [15, 16]. The likelihood of cesarean is also affected by social factors like race, ethnicity, and socioeconomic status [15, 17]. African American women have a higher risk-adjusted rate of cesarean than white women; but the data are inconsistent for Hispanic and Pacific Islander women, with studies indicating equivalent, lower, and higher rates than white women [18–21][3]. The few studies that have analyzed educational attainment—a proxy measure of socioeconomic status—and its effect on cesarean rates have provided mixed results, but the majority of national and state studies find that the probability of having a cesarean increases with level of maternal educational attainment [22–24], although some studies show just the opposite effect [25][4]. Further, women with private insurance have higher rates of cesareans compared to those with Medicaid and those who are uninsured [15, 26–28].

A few studies have analyzed cesarean rates on the U.S-Mexico border. An analysis of birth certificate data compared cesarean rates in Mexico to the cesarean rate of Hispanics in the United States and residents in border regions (both south and north of the border). This study found that U.S. border residents have a higher cesarean rate than the U.S. Hispanic cesarean rate. Both of these groups have a lower cesarean rate than the Mexican rate of 44.5% (in 2009). Additionally, a Texas-based study found that border residents, particularly Hispanic women, have a higher rate of cesareans than non-border residents [29]. Although these studies shed light on border-region cesarean rates, they neither explore the reason for the difference in border rates nor integrate women's voices into their analysis.

Our study fills a gap in this literature in two ways. First, we focus on how compounded disadvantage affects the odds of Latinas having a cesarean in border and non-border hospitals, which allows us to add nuance to the application of the Latinx Health Paradox on maternal outcomes. Second, we include an analysis of qualitative data on women's birth experiences to better explore whether the Latinx paradox with regard to cesarean rates persists on the border.

Methods

We used data from Childbirth Connection's Listening to Mothers III survey: a nationally representative survey of 2400 women who gave birth in U.S. hospitals in 2011 and 2012 [30]. This was an online survey of women aged 18–45 who had given birth between July 1, 2011 and June 30, 2012 and who could complete the survey in English. Participants took the survey between October and December 2012. Women who completed the survey were re-contacted and invited to complete a follow-up survey between January 29, 2013 and April 15, 2013. Almost half of the women (1072 or 45%) completed this follow-up survey, which included open-ended questions about their pregnancy and birth experiences and questions asking in what hospital, city, and state they gave birth. We analyzed data from this follow-up survey because it includes the geographic location of the women's birth. Although the post-partum dataset is weighted to make the data representative of the national population of English-speaking women aged 18–45 who gave birth to a singleton baby in hospitals in 2011 and 2012, we do not use the weight due to deletion of 138 women from the dataset because they did not provide the hospital, city, and/or state of the birth. For the quantitative analysis, we drop cases list-wise to allow for the most data to be used in each analysis. In order to provide a greater number and variety of experiences to analyze for the qualitative data, we analyze responses from women who provided information for hospital location and ethnicity, even if they did not provide information for educational attainment and/or insurance status.

The dependent variable is mode of delivery, with attributes of cesarean or vaginal birth. The independent variable in this study is compounded disadvantage, measured as being Latina, without a college degree and without private insurance. We also ran analyses that examine the independent effect of ethnicity (Latina or non-Latina), educational attainment (four-year college degree and above or less than four-year college degree), and private health insurance status (absent or present). We further integrated border region into our analysis. We used the Centers for Disease Control and Prevention's definition of the border, which is based on the La Paz Agreement and defined as "the area situated 100 kilometers on either side of the inland and maritime boundaries between [the United States and Mexico]" [1]. Our study focuses on the United States border region (i. e. 100 km north of the U.S. Mexico border). In order to contextualize the study, we included descriptive measures of average parity and age, as well as the percent of births involving pre-term infants (less than 37 weeks' gestation), term infants (37–42 weeks' gestation), and post-term infants (42 weeks' or more gestation), and percent of cesareans for malpresentation, the closest measure in the dataset to indicate non-vertex presentation.

The qualitative measures of birth experiences are derived from two questions in the post-partum survey: 1) If you have a baby in the future, would you want to give birth again in the same hospital? Why or why not? 2) If you could go back in time and give yourself any advice or information as you were going into your birth, what would it be?

We analyzed the data in two ways: quantitatively and qualitatively. For the quantitative analysis, we used multiple logistic regression models to examine the association between individual characteristics in the full sample (Model 1), compared to how those same individual characteristics interact to create a compounded disadvantage in the non-border (Model 2) and border (Model 3) subsamples. Compounded disadvantage is measured using an interaction term (coded as being Latina with no private insurance and no college education). Results are presented as odds ratios (i.e. exponentiated coefficients). We used SPSS version 24.0 to analyze the quantitative data.

For the qualitative analysis, due to relatively short responses, we coded overall answers as positive or not positive. The responses coded as 'not positive' included those that were neutral-to-negative, as they were a stark contrast to the glowing responses provided by happy, satisfied women. After coding overall responses as positive or not positive, we examined the themes that emerged from the data related to birth experiences. Women did not provide their names in the survey. Thus, all names used in the analysis are fictitious. We used Dedoose Version 7.5.10 (SocioCultural Research Consultants, LLC, Manhattan Beach, California), a mixed-methods software program, to code and analyze the qualitative data.

Results

Quantitative results

Univariate and Bivariate analysis

Table 1 contains descriptive statistics from our sample, which we separate by whether women gave birth in hospitals located on the U.S.-Mexico border or not on the border. While Latinas are greatly outnumbered by non-Latinas in the non-border region (14.9% Latinas), they only slightly out number Latinas in the border region (45.1% Latinas). A little more than half (51.5%) of the women had a college degree in the non-border region while fewer than half (46.2%) of the women in the border region had a college degree. Sixty-nine percent of women in the non-border region had private health insurance compared to 56.9% of women in the border

Table 1 Descriptive statistics by region

	Border Region	Non-Border Region
Ethnicity		
Latina	45.1%	14.9%
Health Insurance Status		
Private	56.9%	69.3%
Education		
College Degree or more	46.2%	51.5%
Compounded Disadvantage	25.5%	6.4%
Cesarean Rate	32.7%	28.7%
Gestational Age		
Pre-term (< 37 weeks)	7.7%	8.0%
Term (37–41 weeks)	92.3%	91.0%
Post-term (42 or more weeks)	0.0%	1.0%
Mean Parity	1.9	1.9
Mean Maternal Age	28.4	30.6
Previous Cesarean	25%	19%
Cesarean for Malpresentation	0%	2.4%
	N = 52	*N* = 941

region. These results are expected based on previous demographic studies conducted on the border region. Historically, the border region has been an area with low educational attainment and income per capita (a measure of socioeconomic status) [2]. As evidence, 26% of the women in the border region fell into the compounded disadvantaged group, while only 6% of non-border women fell into this group. We also include indictors of parity (1. 9 for both groups); mean maternal age (28.4 for the border group and 30.6 for the non-border group); gestational age (Nearly all women delivered at term in both groups with 7.7% and 8% having pre-term births and 0% and 1% having post-term births in the border and non-border groups, respectively); previous cesarean (25% for the border group and 19% for the non-border group); and cesarean for malpresentation (0% for the border group and 2.4% for the non-border group).

Figure 1 examines whether region affects the cesarean rate. Cesarean rates for the non-border region and border region were 28.7% and 32.7% respectively, a non-significant difference. According to CDC 2012 birth data, the national cesarean section rate was 33% in 2012 [31].

Multivariate analysis

Table 2 contains the multivariate analysis. First, we examined the effect of women's individual characteristics on the cesarean rate for the entire sample (Model 1). We find that none of these characteristics individually are significantly related to the cesarean rate. This is not surprising as cesarean rates increased for women of all races and ethnicities until 2009; although recently rates

Table 2 Odds Ratios for logistic regression analysis of cesarean section delivery

	Model 1 Entire Sample	Model 2 Non-Border Sample	Model 3 Border Sample
Latina	.920		
Private Health Insurance	1.162		
College Degree	1.133		
Border	1.194		
Compounded Disadvantage		.532*	3.759*
Constant	.354**	.422**	.310**
	N = 960	*N* = 933	*N* = 51

(* $p \leq 0.05$; ** $p \leq 0.01$; one-tailed test)

of low-risk cesareans have declined slightly among non-Hispanic white, non-Hispanic black, and Hispanic women [8]. Then, we separated the data into border and non-border subsamples by hospital location where women gave birth and used an interaction term to analyze the effect of compounded disadvantage on the odds of cesarean section. Through these analyses, we find that compounded disadvantage is statistically significant and negative for the non-border sample (Model 2)—compounded disadvantage (i.e. being Latina with no private insurance and no college education) decreases the odds of a cesarean section by 47%—and statistically significant and positive for the border sample (Model 3)—compounded disadvantage increases the odds of cesarean by 276%. In regard to cesarean rates, the Latinx Paradox is lost along the border. That is to say, Latinas with public health insurance and low educational attainment—compounded disadvantage—are more likely to have cesareans in the border region, while women with these same characteristics are less likely to have a cesarean in the non-border region.

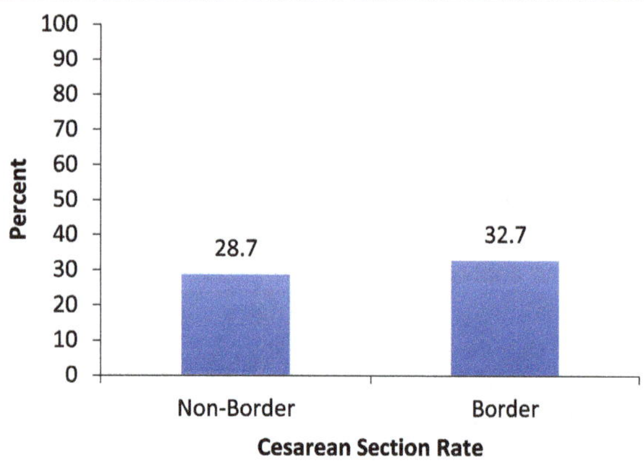

Fig. 1 Cesarean Section Rate by Region, LTMIII, 2011–2012. Cesarean Section Rate

Qualitative results

We analyzed the qualitative data to contextualize the quantitative findings by analyzing the experience of (1) Non-Latinas in the border region; (2) Latinas in the border region; (3) Non-Latinas in the non-border region; and (4) Latinas in the non-border region. Within each of these groups, we focus upon themes we see in the compounded advantaged or compounded disadvantaged groups. Recall that for the qualitative analysis, we focused on the experiences of the group with compounded advantaged (non-Latinas with private health insurance and a college degree) compared to the group with compounded disadvantage (Latinas without private health insurance or college degree).

Birth experiences for non-Latinas in the border region

Overall response The vast majority of non-Latina women on the border (twenty out of twenty-eight) were positive about their births while six provided either neutral or non-responses and two were negative. Michelle, a college-educated mother with private health insurance and in her late thirties, reflected a commonly shared sentiment among non-Latina women on the border: "Yes, I love the hospital and staff. They are so attentive and friendly. They give you the sensation that you are the only person in the hospital [with] needs and that my birth is special and important." The majority of those who responded positively about their births were non-Latinas in the advantaged group on the border who had given birth vaginally (eleven out of twenty). Out of the three non-Latinas in the disadvantaged group on the border, two had vaginal births and gave positive responses. The remaining woman, Kristin, had a cesarean and did not give a positive response. When asked whether she would return to the same hospital, she responded: "I have no choice which hospital I give birth at. Our military medical makes us go to the [hospital] if we can make it. And, with c-sections with both living children, my third will most likely be a repeat c-section." While Kristin's answer is not inherently negative, it does reflect constrained hospital choice and a resignation with her history of repeat cesarean.

Reactions to cesarean All five women who spoke about cesareans indicated that they either wished they had not had a cesarean in the past or that they did not want a cesarean in the future. For instance, Iliana, a college educated mother with private health insurance in her late twenties, simply stated that if she could go back in time and give herself advice, she "would have attempted a natural birth instead of a 2nd c-section." Another mother, also in the advantaged group, took her cesarean history and her hospital's vaginal birth after cesarean (VBAC) rate into consideration when deciding whether she would return to her hospital for future births: "I might. I want to do a vbac and a midwife center is the best place to do one. The hospital I went to is not known for its great vbac success rate. I am afraid I would end up with another c-section if I went back to the same hospital." Two women equated their cesareans with a loss of efficacy. Sharing a similar sentiment to Kristin's response above, Melanie, a privately insured mother with an associate's degree, did not have any advice for past self: "I don't think there is anything I would tell myself. I had a c-section and did not push or anything, so I doubt anything I would tell myself would have an effect."

Remarks about staff While most non-Latinas were happy with the staff attending their birth, one woman had a surprising comment about the staff at her hospital. When asked if she would return to this facility, Jessica, a college educated mother on government insurance, said, "No. The staff spoke very broken English and seemed to get upset with me when I didn't understand them."

Birth experiences for Latinas in the border region

Overall response Similar to non-Latina women on the border, most Latinas on the border (nineteen out of twenty-three) had positive birth experiences. Cassandra, a teenage mother insured through Medicaid, gave a typical response: "I would give birth to my next child at the same hospital. The staff were so great with me. I enjoyed their presence in the room. I know many say hospital food is the worst but I loved it. I miss hospital food the most." Like Cassandra, Latinas on the border in the disadvantaged group who had vaginal births had the highest number of positive responses (six out of nineteen). Latinas on the border in the disadvantaged group who had cesareans, however, had the highest number of non-positive responses (three out of four). Further, all four border Latinas who had responses that were non-positive had cesareans. Two women directly stated that they would not return to the hospital, one woman noted that she had a tubal ligation and thus would not be having children again (no comment about hospital experience), and one woman did not give a clear answer about returning to her hospital. All Latinas on the border who had vaginal births gave positive responses.

Tubal ligation While a few non-Latinas on the border mentioned that they were "not planning" on having any more children, none of them directly referred to tubal ligations. Two Latinas on the border who had cesareans, however, directly commented on having this procedure. Both of these mothers were in the disadvantaged group. Another border Latina, a mother in her early to mid-twenties without a college degree, wanted information about when she could get a tubal ligation.

Requesting information While no non-Latinas on the border indicated that they wanted more information from their healthcare providers or other resources, two Latinas on the border expressed a desire for more information during pregnancy, birth, and postpartum. Laura, a high school educated mother insured through Medicaid, mentioned communication with staff more generally: "i would ask nurses when im unsure." Ida, a mother in her early to mid-twenties without a college degree, had a list of specific topics she wanted information about: "How many C-sections can you have at a certain age, information on preeclampsia, exercise tips after having a c-section, when can I get my tubes tied, etc." Both Laura and Ida had cesareans. Briana, a mother without a college degree and insured through Medicaid, provided the most negative response: "The doctor's attentiveness could have been a little better, and they didn't have to wait so long. If a patient says that they don't feel well, it is because they don't feel well – not because they want to be stupid and wait for hours in the waiting room"[5]. Brianna had a cesarean.

Birth experiences for Latinas in the non-border region

Overall response The majority of Latinas in non-border regions (79.1%) provided positive comments about their births. Nina, a mother with a high school diploma and Medicaid, gave a characteristic response: "yes i would love too give birth in the same place because i love how the doctors and nurses were with me. they were so nice and respectful and helpful. cause being a first time mommy is kinda scare you dont know whats going to happen in the labor room but they sure cheered me up. god bless them." Out of all non-border Latinas, women in the disadvantaged group who had vaginal births had the highest percentage of positive responses (35.8%). Interestingly, this same group of women had the highest percentage of neutral to negative responses (25.0%). Although some women cited reasons that they would not return to their hospital for another birth (dissatisfaction with staff, rooms, facility), the majority of them did not give a specific reason. Examples of responses coded as non-positive (neutral to negative) are "I don't know," "no," and "maybe." However, one of these non-positive responses was from Kayla, a mother with her associate's degree and insured through Medicaid, who stated, "The hospital i went to was in the poor part of town. i would like to go where the rich go, downtown [city]."

Not having any more babies Similar to the border non-Latinas, nine non-border Latinas stated that they were not planning on having any more children. When asked if she would return to her hospital, Rosa, a mother in her forties with a high school diploma and private insurance, responded, "I can't have anymore children but if I could I would use the same hospital. They took excellent care of me and my baby." Like Rosa, many women said they "can't" or "won't" be giving birth again without providing further explanation. We cannot say whether or not these women had a tubal ligation performed, but it is interesting that, in contrast, every border Latina explained that they were not having more babies specifically because they had a tubal ligation.

Reactions to cesarean Only two non-border Latinas mentioned cesareans at all in their responses. And unlike border Latinas, non-border Latinas did not give their past selves advice about avoiding the procedure. Rather, both women brought up their cesareans to highlight interactions with hospital staff. For instance, Lidia, a mother with an associate's degree and Medicaid, said that she loved her hospital because "they informed me of the reasons why they recommended certain things, including the c-section." Karla, a mother with an associate's degree and private insurance, said she would not go back to her hospital partly because she had to "deal with a c-section all by [herself]" and because her "dr didn't discharge [her] or visit [her] after [her] c section." However, both of these women appear to have understood that cesareans are serious procedures. This explains why Lidia appreciated her hospital staff's thorough information about the need for surgery and why Karla was dissatisfied with her doctor's absence after the procedure.

Information Five non-border Latina women spoke directly about issues regarding information. Two of these responses were negative, two were positive, and one was neutral. Similar to Lidia's experience above, a woman in her early twenties with Medicaid said that she would return to her hospital because she was "given all the information." Conversely, Olivia, a mother who completed some college and has Medicaid, gave herself the following advice: "Fight like the Mama bear you are. Do not let anyone tell you how to parent your child, especially doctors that try to bully you by giving misleading information. You can do it, because you have maternal instincts that will overcome so much in the future." When asked whether she would return to her hospital, another woman who provided a negative response said she would not because she felt "rushed" and did not know who to ask for help. Both of these negative responses are not simply about information. Lack of information (and misleading information) resulted in these women feeling dissatisfied with their health care providers and hospital. The non-border Latina who provided a neutral response said that she wanted to take a natural birth class.

Discussion

Intersectional Theory posits that social identities, such as race, class, and gender, interact simultaneously to create multidimensional systems of oppression and lead to different experiences and outcomes [32]. That is, social disadvantage can have a multiplicative effect, as individuals with social identities belonging to multiple oppressed groups experience compounding social disadvantage. In terms of maternal health, our data show that women's individual characteristics of ethnicity and SES do not independently affect their chance of cesarean. However, we find that the likelihood of cesareans is influenced by intersecting identities in particular geographic contexts. In the non-border region, Latinas with low levels of education and public health insurance have a lower rate of cesareans than non-Latinas or Latinas with high education levels and private insurance. However, in border regions, Latinas with compounded disadvantage (low education/no private health insurance, have a higher cesarean rate than other women. This finding provides validity for applying Intersectional Theory to explain mode of delivery in certain contexts, since most studies tend to look at these factors individually. In this study, we find that the Latinx Health Paradox for cesarean outcome is lost on the border.

A strength of our study lies in our use of Intersectional Theory, which informed our creation of a "compounded disadvantage" variable. Using this variable, our analysis shows that intersecting statuses affect cesarean rates in particular geographic contexts for particular women. Research on variations in cesarean rates have found differences by hospital and geographic regions [15] that cannot be fully explained by medical or pregnancy characteristics of women. Our analysis goes further to demonstrate that Latinas who are multiply disadvantaged in terms of education and health-insurance status have greater risks of cesarean if they give birth in border hospitals. Future studies that examine drivers for disparities in mode of birth could apply similar methods and theories to better understand reasons for variation in or overuse of cesareans.

There are limitations to our study that should be considered in analyzing the results. First, we are limited to the LTMIII methodology, which required women to take the survey in English, a major consideration for a study focused on the border region where some women may be primarily Spanish speakers. New data from the 2017 Listening to Mothers California may solve this problem by oversampling Latinas and also by fielding the survey in both English and Spanish, though only in one state. While we cannot generalize our study to the U.S. population as a whole, the application of Intersectional

Theory to investigate disparities in mode of birth provides an innovative way to explore non-medical factors that contribute to an overuse of cesareans. Second, the survey from which we draw our data has the limitation of selection bias, which is very difficult to control. However, all surveys, particularly those in which participation is voluntary, share this problem. In short, some women are more inclined than others to respond. However, the data we use are the only data from a representative sample of U.S. women who gave birth that also include the geographic location in which they gave birth.

Conclusions

These findings deserve further exploration. First, it is important for clinicians working in the border region to understand the increased risk for disadvantaged Latinas to have cesareans. Hospital leaders already working to reduce cesarean rates may want to analyze their institutional rates by using these intersecting statuses to understand the processes and policies that produce these outcomes. Our qualitative analysis shows that Latinas who give birth in border hospitals desire more information throughout pregnancy and childbirth. Interestingly, this desire for information is less visible among non-Latinas who gave birth in a border hospital and among Latinas who gave birth in a non-border hospital, perhaps reflecting their lower rates of cesarean overall. Thus, clinicians and birth professionals should make an extra effort to get relevant information about childbirth and cesarean prevention to Latinas on the border. Second, Latinas on the border were the only group of women in our analysis to discuss tubal ligation. Because of the history of forced sterilization of Latinas in the United States, it is concerning to find a pattern of Latinas on the border discussing sterilization, whereas this topic is absent from the responses of other groups of women [33]. We do not know the circumstances of these sterilizations. It is beyond our data to determine whether sterilizations were coerced or chosen because women understand that they can be done easily during a cesarean or for some other reason. However, again, hospitals should be cautious of how sterilization is discussed with patients and make sure that the discussion is culturally sensitive.

Endnotes

[1]The 2000 Census includes the most recent survey of the U.S. southern border. The 2010 Census Brief on the Hispanic population does not report the ethnic composition of the border region.

[2]Although this phenomenon is commonly referred to as the "Hispanic Paradox," we choose to use the term "Latinx Paradox" because our study centers on women from Latina America.

[3]The Centers for Disease Control and Prevention does not provide separate analysis for women who are both Black and Hispanic.

[4]One should also note that this effect may be complicated by the effect of age; primiparous women (those who give birth for the first time) with higher levels of educational attainment are generally older than primiparous women with lower levels of education.

[5]This response was translated from Spanish to English. The original response was: "que la atencios de los medicos fuera un poco mejo y no tubieran que esperar mucho, siun paciente dice me siento mal es porque de verdad se siete mal, no pruqe se quiera hacer tonta y la dejen esperando horas sentadas en la sala de espera."

Abbreviations

LTMIII: Listening to Mothers III; VBAC: Vaginal Birth After Cesarean

Acknowledgements

We thank Childbirth Connection for giving us access to the restricted data in this survey, the W.K. Kellogg Foundation for funding the LTMIII survey, and Ophra Leyser-Whalen for comments on previous drafts.

Funding

Texas A&M College of Liberal Arts provided start-up funds to TM. Funds were used to purchase hospital data from the American Hospital Association and to pay AG as an undergraduate research assistant. The open access publishing fees for this article have been covered by the Texas A&M University Open Access to Knowledge Fund (OAKFund), supported by the University Libraries and the Office of the Vice President for Research.

Authors' contributions

TM, AG, and MNS analyzed and interpreted the data. MNS managed the data set. TM, AG, and CM were major contributors in writing the manuscript. All authors read and approved the final manuscript.

Competing interests

The authors declare that they have no competing interests.

Author details

[1]Department of Sociology, Texas A&M University, MS4351, College Station, TX 77843, USA. [2]Independent Scholar, Bryan, TX, USA. [3]Independent Scholar, Helena, MT, USA. [4]Independent Scholar, Redwood City, CA, USA.

References

1. About the Border Region [https://www.cdc.gov/usmexicohealth/about-border-region.html]. Accessed 20 Mar 2018.
2. United States-Mexico Border Health Commission: Healthy border 2010. 2003.
3. McCarthy M. CDC report confirms "Hispanic paradox". Br Med J. 2015;350 https://doi.org/10.1136/bmj.h2467.
4. Brown HL, Chireau MV, Jallah Y, Howard D. The "Hispanic paradox": an investigation of racial disparity in pregnancy outcomes at a tertiary care medical center. Am J Obstet Gynecol. 2007;197(2):197.e1–7. discussion 197.e197-199

5. Cervantes A, Keith L, Wyshak G. Adverse birth outcomes among native-born and immigrant women: replicating national evidence regarding Mexicans at the local level. Matern Child Health J. 1999;3(2):99–109.
6. Gonzalez-Quintero VH, Tolaymat L, Luke B, Gonzalez-Garcia A, Duthely L, O'Sullivan MJ, Martin D. Outcome of pregnancies among Hispanics: revisiting the epidemiologic paradox. J Reprod. Med. 2006;51(1):10–4.
7. McGlade MS, Saha S, Dahlstrom ME. The Latina paradox: an opportunity for restructuring prenatal care delivery. Am J Public Health. 2004;94(12):2062–5.
8. Osterman MJ, Martin JA. Trends in low-risk cesarean delivery in the United States, 1990-2013. Natl Vital Stat. Rep. 2014;63(6):1–16.
9. U.S. Department of Health and Human Services: Women's Health USA 2010. 2010.
10. American College of Obstetricians and Gynecologists, Society for Maternal-Fetal Medicine, Caughey AB, Cahill AG, Guise JM, Rouse DJ. Safe prevention of the primary cesarean delivery. Am J Obstet Gynecol. 2014;210(3):179–93.
11. World Health Organization and Human Reproduction Programme: WHO Statement on Caesarean Section Rates. April, 2015 WHO/RHR/15.02. http://www.who.int/reproductivehealth/publications/maternal_perinatal_health/cs-statement/en/. Accessed 20 Mar 2018.
12. Health People 2020 [https://www.healthypeople.gov/2020/topics-objectives/topic/maternal-infant-and-child-health/objectives]. Accessed 20 Mar 2018.
13. Betran AP, Ye J, Moller AB, Zhang J, Gulmezoglu AM, Torloni MR. The increasing trend in caesarean section rates: global, regional and National Estimates: 1990-2014. PLoS One. 2016;11(2):e0148343.
14. Hamilton BE, Martin JA, Osterman MJK, Driscoll AK, Rossen LM: Births: provisional data for 2016. National Vital Statistics Rapid Release June 2017, Report No. 002.
15. Kozhimannil KB, Law MR, Virnig BA. Cesarean delivery rates vary tenfold among US hospitals; reducing variation may address quality and cost issues. Health Aff. 2013;32(3):527–35.
16. Medical Reasons for a C-Section [http://www.marchofdimes.org/pregnancy/c-section-medical-reasons.aspx]. Accessed 20 Mar 2018.
17. Osterman MJK, Martin JA. Primary cesarean delivery rates, by state: results from the revised birth certificate, 2006-2012. Natl Vital Stat. Rep. 2014;63(1):1–10.
18. Aron DC, Gordon HS, DiGiuseppe DL, Harper DL, Rosenthal GE. Variations in risk-adjusted cesarean delivery rates according to race and health insurance. Med Care. 2000;38(1):35–44.
19. Edmonds JK, Hawkins SS, Cohen BB. The influence of detailed maternal ethnicity on cesarean delivery: findings from the U.S. birth certificate in the state of Massachusetts. Birth (Berkeley, Calif). 2014;41(3):290–8.
20. Getahun D, Strickland D, Lawrence JM, Fassett MJ, Koebnick C, Jacobsen SJ. Racial and ethnic disparities in the trends in primary cesarean delivery based on indications. Am J Obstet Gynecol. 2009;201(4):422.e1–7.
21. Martin JA, Hamilton BE, Osterman MJ, Driscoll AK, Matthews TJ. Births: final data for 2015. Natl. Vital Stat. Rep. 2017;66(1):1–69.
22. Henry DE, Rabinowitz SS, Berger GA, American Bar Association. Law practice division: finding bliss : innovative legal models for happy clients & happy lawyers. Chicago: American Bar Association, Law Practice Division; 2015.
23. Moscariello M, Bol K. Cesarean section deliveries and inductions of labor in Colorado: an analysis of current trends and demographics. In: CDoPHa E, editor. Health watch; 2011.
24. Wang T, Schoen LD, Melnik TA, Kacica MA, Shields E. Primary cesarean delivery in New York state, 2003-2012. In: New York State Department of Health, Office of Quality and Patient Safety, Bureau of Vital Statistics; 2013.
25. Roth LM, Henley MM. Unequal motherhood racial-ethnic and socioeconomic disparities in cesarean sections in the United States. Soc Probl. 2012;59(2):207–27.
26. Haas JS, Udvarhelyi S, Epstein AM. The effect of health coverage for uninsured pregnant women on maternal health and the use of cesarean section. JAMA. 1993;270(1):61–4.
27. Attanasio L, Kozhimannil KB, Jou J, McPherson ME, Camann W. Women's experiences with Neuraxial labor analgesia in the listening to mothers II survey: a content analysis of open-ended responses. Anesth Analg. 2014; https://doi.org/10.1213/ANE.0000000000000546.
28. Stafford RS. Cesarean section use and source of payment: an analysis of California hospital discharge abstracts. Am J Public Health. 1990;80(3):313–5.
29. Walker LO, Cheng HR, Brown A. Birth outcomes of Hispanic women and risks or strengths associated with ethnicity and Texas border residence. J Obstet Gynecol Neonatal Nurs. 2014;43(4):422–34.
30. Declercq ER, Sakala C, Corry MP, Applebaum S, Herrlich A. Listening to mothers III:new mothers speak out. New York: Childbirth Connection; 2013.
31. Martin JA, Hamilton BE, Osterman MJK, Curtin S, Matthews TJ. Births: final data for 2012. Natl Vital Stat Rep. 2013;62(9):1–67.
32. Crenshaw K. Mapping the margins: Intersectionality, identity politics, and violence against women of color. Stanford Law Rev. 1991;43(6):1241–99.
33. Stern AM. STERILIZED in the name of public health: race, immigration, and reproductive control in modern California. Am J Public Health. 2005;95(7):1128–38.

5

Vaginal birth after caesarean versus elective repeat caesarean delivery after one previous caesarean section: a cost-effectiveness analysis in four European countries

Maaike Fobelets[1,2*], Katrien Beeckman[2,3], Gilles Faron[4], Déirdre Daly[5], Cecily Begley[5,6] and Koen Putman[1,2]

Abstract

Background: The OptiBIRTH study incorporates a multicentre cluster randomised trial in 15 hospital sites across three European countries. The trial was designed to test a complex intervention aimed at improving vaginal birth after caesarean section (VBAC) rates through increasing women's involvement in their care. Prior to developing a robust standardised model to conduct the health economic analysis, an analysis of a hypothetical cohort was performed to estimate the costs and health effects of VBAC compared to elective repeat caesarean delivery (ERCD) for low-risk women in four European countries.

Methods: A decision-analytic model was developed to estimate the costs and the health effects, measured using Quality Adjusted Life Years (QALYs), of VBAC compared with ERCD. A cost-effectiveness analysis for the period from confirmation of pregnancy to 6 weeks postpartum was performed for short-term consequences and during lifetime for long-term consequences, based on a hypothetical cohort of 100,000 pregnant women in each of four different countries; Belgium, Germany, Ireland and Italy. A societal perspective was adopted. Where possible, transition probabilities, costs and health effects were adapted from national data obtained from the respective countries. Country-specific thresholds were used to determine the cost-effectiveness of VBAC compared to ERCD. Deterministic and probabilistic sensitivity analyses were conducted to examine the uncertainty of model assumptions.

Results: Within a 6-week time horizon, VBAC resulted in a reduction in costs, ranging from €3,334,052 (Germany) to €66,162,379 (Ireland), and gains in QALYs ranging from 6399 (Italy) to 7561 (Germany) per 100,000 women birthing in each country. Compared to ERCD, VBAC is the dominant strategy in all four countries. Applying a lifetime horizon, VBAC is dominant compared to ERCD in all countries except for Germany (probabilistic analysis, ICER: €8609/QALY). In conclusion, compared to ERCD, VBAC remains cost-effective when using a lifetime time.

Conclusions: In all four countries, VBAC was cost-effective compared to ERCD for low-risk women. This is important for health service managers, economists and policy makers concerned with maximising health benefits within limited and constrained resources.

Keywords: Cost-effectiveness analysis, Elective repeat caesarean delivery (ERCD), Vaginal birth after caesarean (VBAC)

* Correspondence: maaike.fobelets@vub.ac.be
[1]I-CHER (Interuniversity Centre for Health Economics Research), Faculty of Medicine and Pharmacy, Vrije Universiteit Brussels, Laarbeeklaan 103, 1090 Brussels, Belgium
[2]Department of Public Health, Faculty of Medicine and Pharmacy, Vrije Universiteit Brussel, Laarbeeklaan 103, 1090 Brussels, Belgium
Full list of author information is available at the end of the article

Background

Rates of caesarean section have increased steadily in Europe [1, 2], and in many countries worldwide [3] in the past three decades. This rise in rates, and the wide variation in rates between and within countries has led to research exploring the factors contributing to the increase, and into the comparative risks of giving birth by caesarean section and vaginally [4]. One factor contributing to the increasing rates of caesarean section is elective repeat caesarean delivery (ERCD), a term used to indicate that the caesarean birth is deemed necessary prior to the start of labour, and is not performed as an emergency procedure. Nowadays, more women who had one previous caesarean section are being offered the possibility of having a subsequent birth vaginally. Studies have shown that vaginal birth after caesarean (VBAC) for low-risk women is associated with benefits compared to an ERCD [4–7]. Coupled with this is a growing interest in costs, and results from health economic analyses have demonstrated the cost effectiveness of VBAC compared to ERCD [8–12]. VBAC was found to be a dominant strategy, i.e. less expensive and more effective than the ERCD strategy [9–11, 13]. The underlying reasons for this finding is that VBAC results in a reduced length of hospital stay postpartum and is associated with fewer long-term maternal morbidities such as hysterectomy, placenta praevia and mortality [9, 11, 14–18]. Conversely, VBAC was associated with higher rates of uterine ruptures, long term neonatal morbidities such as cerebral palsy, and neonatal death [14, 16, 17, 19–21].

Internationally, several health economic analyses have been performed by using different costing techniques i.e. different perspectives, variation in perinatal outcomes accounted for in the analyses and differences in time horizons [8–12, 22]. The health services perspective is the most frequently used [7]. However, this perspective has some limitations; it excludes important items such as direct costs borne by women and their families, indirect costs associated with welfare losses and productivity losses. Perinatal outcomes included in health economic analyses vary considerably, both for the mother and newborn. Some studies do not include the neonatal outcomes [23], though the need to include these outcomes has been demonstrated previously [5, 6, 11, 13]. Including some perinatal outcomes in health economic analysis on mode of birth requires a longer time horizon than the commonly used perinatal care episode. Some longer-term conditions affecting the newborn, e.g. cerebral palsy, are associated with significant costs and major losses of quality of life for both the newborn/child and the parents. Conditions affecting the woman in subsequent pregnancies, e.g. placenta accreta or praevia are a cause of maternal morbidity of women with multiple ERCDs. Including these outcomes would mean using a lifetime horizon. However, using a more standardised health economic analysis model for one prior low transverse caesarean delivery, with a core set of outcomes and a lifetime horizon, would already increase the comparability across models.

Clinicians and health policy makers, concerned about the rising rates of caesarean sections, are seeking ways of stopping these rates from rising further, and reducing the number of caesarean sections being performed [7]. An example of the growing interest in VBAC is the OptiBIRTH project [24, 25], a part of which is an international multicentre trial that aims to increase the proportion of women having VBAC by increasing women-centred care and facilitating women's empowerment in their choice of birth in three countries, Germany, Ireland and Italy. As a part of this project, a health economic evaluation was planned to evaluate the cost effectiveness across these three countries. Performing a health economic analysis on mode of birth is challenging, especially in the context of a multi-country study, because of the variability in the content of usual care, the organisation of the healthcare system and the availability of appropriate data on costs [9]. Using a more uniform health economic model applied in a multi-country context would be beneficial, increasing the comparability and external validation of the results. To our knowledge, no such uniform health economic model comparing VBAC with ERCD, from societal perspective, with a time horizon starting from pregnancy recognition up to 6 weeks postpartum, and including the costs and consequences for both the mother and newborn, has been published. The model was conducted for four European Union (EU)-countries, Germany, Ireland, Italy where the trial was being conducted, and Belgium, where the health economic analysis was being conducted.

Methods

Model

A decision analytic model was developed to compare the costs and consequences of VBAC and ERCD. The decision tree (Fig. 1) was built based on previously published models and expert opinion (GF) [7, 9]. A hypothetical cohort of 100,000 women was used for each country (Belgium, Germany, Ireland and Italy). Women included in the model were low-risk (i.e. without pre-existing medical conditions or risk factors), with a singleton pregnancy, at term gestation who had one previous caesarean section that was performed using low uterine transverse incision. The assumption is that in this cohort of women, there are no contraindications to VBAC [26] at time of admission for giving birth. The time horizon of the model was from pregnancy recognition up to 6 weeks postpartum for short-term consequences and a lifetime horizon was applied for long-term consequences. The

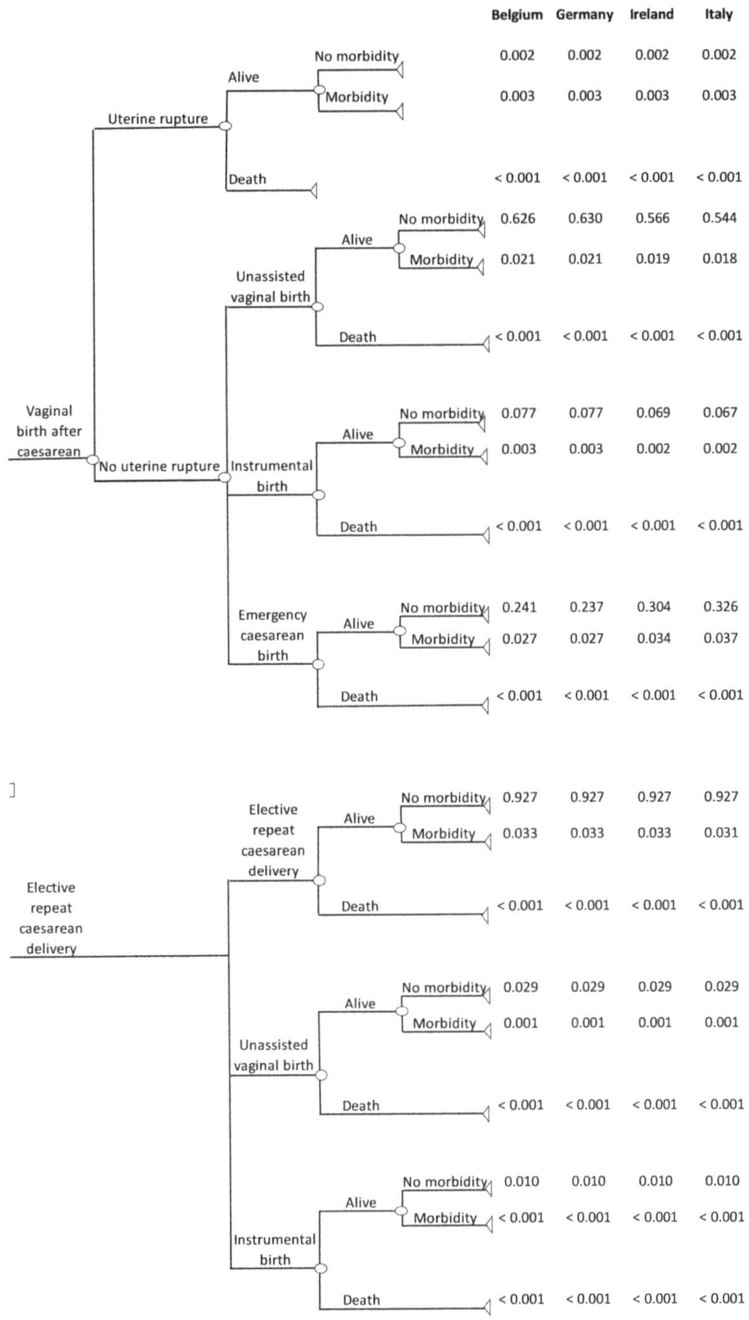

Fig. 1 Decision tree comparing vaginal birth after caesarean with elective repeat caesarean delivery

decision tree consisted of two main arms, VBAC and ERCD. Women in the VBAC arm may have a successful VBAC resulting in an unassisted vaginal birth or instrumental vaginal birth. Women in this arm may also experience an emergency caesarean section or uterine rupture. In the ERCD arm, women may have an ERCD, and a small proportion of women might go into labour spontaneously resulting in an unassisted vaginal birth or instrumental vaginal birth. Women planning an ERCD may also suffer uterine rupture but, as it occurs only rarely, we have not included it in the model. In all cases, women could have no morbidity, suffer a morbidity, or die. To account for maternal morbidity, the maternal outcomes included were: uterine rupture, endometritis, peripartum hysterectomy, blood transfusion, thrombotic events, operative injury and wound complications [11, 15–21, 27–30]. Neonatal health outcomes were not built directly into the decision tree but accounted for via the health state of the women (see below) [11]. A neonate could be born alive and have no morbidity, suffer a morbidity or die. In cases of neonatal morbidity, the following neonatal outcomes were evaluated: hypoxic ischemic encephalopathy (HIE), sepsis and respiratory conditions including transient tachypnoea of the newborn (TTN) and respiratory distress syndrome (RDS) [5, 6, 11, 17, 20, 31–38]. Cerebral palsy was included in the model as a long-term consequence of HIE, assuming that 12% of the infants would finally be diagnosed with cerebral palsy [11, 39]. Country-specific data on the VBAC success rates were available for Germany (74%), Ireland (66%) and Italy (64%), and the overall European success rate was used for Belgium (73%) [9, 40–42]. All other probabilities, including maternal and neonatal morbidities and mortality, were based on data obtained from the literature, and were identical for all countries (Additional file 1: Table S2) [5, 6, 9, 11, 15–21, 27–38, 43, 44]. Based on the probability data, the probability per arm was calculated by multiplying the probability of each branch to calculate the final probability of the endnodes e.g. for unassisted vaginal birth: probability of unassisted vaginal birth (VBAC success rate * proportion of unassisted vaginal birth * probability to be alive * probability to have no morbidities) (Fig. 1).

Costs and utilities

The analysis was performed from a societal perspective and included maternal and neonatal health outcomes and costs. The costs included direct medical costs for the ante-, peri- and postnatal periods and non-medical costs and indirect costs. An overview of all costs and their respective sources can be found in Table 1 and in Additional file 1: Tables S1 and S2. For each country, antenatal resource usage calculations were based on the national antenatal/neonatal guidelines and were validated by an expert in each country. One extra consultation with an anaesthesiologist was included when an ERCD was planned. Ambulatory costs, i.e. costs for outpatient care, were obtained from country specific ambulatory tariff lists and linked to resource use. Inpatient costs of the mother and newborn were calculated per health-state based on country-specific Diagnostic Related Groups (DRG) data. Two extra visits with an obstetrician and paediatrician were included in cases of short-term maternal and/or neonatal morbidities, and direct non-medical costs (i.e. travel costs) were also included. The average distance to ambulatory centres and hospitals was multiplied by the unit cost for transportation. The cost of HIE was estimated as half of the yearly cost of CP, for 2 years [11]. For long-term consequences such as cerebral palsy and maternal and neonatal mortality, lifetime costs were calculated including the lifetime societal cost for cerebral palsy for 50 years [13] and lifetime productivity loss for maternal and neonatal mortality. National discount rates for costs and utilities were used: Belgium (3%, 1.5%), Germany (5%, 5%), Ireland (5%, 5%) and Italy (3%, 3%) [45–48]. The Harmonized Indices of Consumer Prices (HICP) - health were used to convert all costs to 2016 euros [49].

Quality-adjusted life years (QALYs) were used to measure outcomes for the different health states (Table 2 and Additional file 1: Table S2). The country-specific utilities for normal health were considered as the base-case utility [50, 51]. Ireland did not have country-specific values available, and UK utility values were used. Utility values during the antenatal period were assumed to be equal for both groups, VBAC and ERCD. Thereafter, utilities were calculated for each maternal and neonatal outcome separately by reducing the country-specific utilities for normal health with the corresponding disutility of the maternal and neonatal outcome. No country-specific disutilities could be obtained, consequently, the disutility values were based on data obtained from the literature [9, 11, 12, 52].

The primary outcome was the incremental cost-effectiveness ratio (ICER) per QALY gained using the expected costs and QALYs gained by using the following formula:

$$\text{ICER} = \frac{(\text{Expected Cost VBAC} - \text{Expected Cost ERCD})}{(\text{Expected Utility VBAC} - \text{Expected Utility ERCD})}$$

The cost-effectiveness threshold was country dependent. For Belgium, Germany and Italy, the gross domestic product (GDP) per capita was used, with an ICER of €36,633/QALY, €37,719/QALY and €27,219/QALY respectively [53]. The cost-effectiveness threshold for Ireland was historically set at €45,000/QALY [9]. Additionally, the incremental net monetary benefit (INMB) between VBAC versus ERCD was calculated applying various thresholds in order to evaluate the cost-effectiveness (Additional file 1: Figure S2).

Sensitivity analysis

To identify the uncertainty of parameters and the robustness of the results of the base-case model, sensitivity analyses were performed. Both one-way and probabilistic sensitivity analyses were conducted on the input parameters for all costs, probabilities and utilities used in the model. In the one-way sensitivity analysis, input parameters were varied by 30% of their initial value, and parameters with the highest impact are presented in Tornado diagrams. Simulations were conducted by using beta and Dirichlet distributions for probabilities and utilities, and gamma distributions for costs. A probabilistic sensitivity analysis was performed using Monte Carlo simulations with 5000 iterations.

Results

Base-case scenario analysis

The base-case analysis comparing VBAC with ERCD for this hypothetical cohort resulted in an average of 32,312

Table 1 Cost estimates, €[a]

	Belgium	Germany	Ireland	Italy
Antenatal care				
Intention: vaginal birth after caesarean	535	791	1656	1017
Intention: elective repeat caesarean delivery	563	826	1844	1095
Mode of birth				
Unassisted vaginal birth				
Without complications	2948	1745	2337	1315
With complications	3363	2394	4065	1674
Instrumental vaginal birth				
Without complications	3363	2049	3063	2956
With complications	4790	2394	4065	2956
Elective repeat caesarean delivery				
Without complications	4083	2659	4805	2163
With complications	5105	3180	6242	2876
Emergency caesarean section				
Without complications	5105	3661	4805	2163
With complications	8261	3903	6242	2876
Uterine Rupture				
Without complications	5105	3903	4805	2876
With complications	8261	3903	6242	2876
Neonatal HIE/CP (six-week time horizon)	12,347	7587	10,275	4052
Neonatal HIE (first 2 years)	16,926	16,423	17,093	15,250
Neonatal CP (lifetime)	846,309	821,171	854,688	762,516
Neonatal Sepsis	7266	19,413	15,408	4052
Neonatal respiratory conditions				
Transient tachypnoea	3007	788	1485	579
Respiratory distress syndrome	11,392	19,413	15,408	13,478
Neonatal mortality	4712	7198	7036	5579
Postnatal care				
Without complications	182	622	135	308
With complications	329	782	885	643
Productivity loss (per year)	48,511	46,373	46,607	35,272

HIE hypoxic ischemic encephalopathy, *CP* cerebral palsy
[a]Currency in 2016 euros (€) [49]
Total costs, travel costs included. More detailed costs and their sources are described in Additional file 1: Table S1 and S2

fewer caesarean sections per 100,000 women in each of the four countries (Additional file 1: Table S3). The ICER results of the deterministic analysis for a 6-week time horizon demonstrated that VBAC was a dominant strategy in all four countries, which means less costly and more effective than ERCD. This results in a negative ICER of -€441/QALY for Germany, −€2035/QALY for Belgium, −€3042/QALY for Italy and -€9891/QALY for Ireland (Table 3). When considering a lifetime time-horizon, VBAC was a dominant strategy in Ireland (−€96,753/ QALY) and Italy (−€15,965/QALY). Compared to ERCD, VBAC remained a cost-effective strategy, which means slightly more costly and more effective, for Belgium (€3669/QALY) and Germany (€12,817/QALY). The overall maternal morbidity rate was higher in the VBAC arm compared to the ERCD arm (5.64% versus 3.25%) due to the morbidity related to performing emergency caesarean sections. The neonatal morbidity rate, 6.82% for VBAC and 5.14% for ERCD, and mortality rate, 0.02% for VBAC and 0.00% for ERCD, were higher in the VBAC arm due to the higher amount of complications in case of an emergency caesarean section or uterine rupture. The overall maternal mortality rate was comparable for both groups (0.01% and 0.00% in both groups).

Table 2 Utilities by country and disutilities by mode of birth or outcome[a]

Country	Utility (per day[b])	Duration (days)	References
Belgium	0.98	42	[51]
Germany	0.99	42	[50]
Ireland	0.99	42	[50]
Italy	0.99	42	[50]
Mode of birth/outcome	Disutility (per day)	Duration (days)	References
Successful vaginal birth after caesarean	0.41	7	[9]
Elective repeat caesarean delivery	0.58	21	[9]
Emergency caesarean birth	0.58	21	[9]
Hysterectomy	0.58	21	[9]
Uterine rupture	0.58	21	[9]
Endometritis	0.38	14	[9]
Blood transfusion	0.41	7	[9]
Thrombotic events	0.41	14	Assumption
Operative injury	0.53	21	[9]
Wound complication	0.53	21	Assumption
Well (no adverse outcome)	0	42	[12]
HIE	0.75	21	[11]
CP	0.53	All	[11]
Sepsis	0.01	42	[52]
Respiratory conditions	0.01	14	[52]
Maternal/neonatal death	1	All	[12]

HIE hypoxic ischemic encephalopathy, *CP* cerebral palsy
[a] parameter distributions can be found in Additional file 1: Table S2
[b] daily utilities were derived from annual utilities

The costs and QALYs saved differ between the four countries. Within a 6-week time horizon, the total costs saved (per 100,000 women) were €3,334,052 in Germany, €15,271,888 in Belgium, €19,465,446 in Italy and €66,162,379 in Ireland and the total number of QALYs were 6399 in Italy, 6689 in Ireland, 7503 in Belgium and 7561 in Germany more per 100,000 women. When considering lifetime costs and consequences, the total cost of the VBAC strategy was €1,386,210 in Belgium and €8,481,119 in Germany with 376 QALYs and 662 QALYs more in Belgium and Germany. The total costs saved were €53,955,166 in Ireland and €6,558,036 in Italy and the total number QALYs were 558 in Ireland and 411 in Italy.

Sensitivity analyses

The results of the one-way sensitivity analysis showed the robustness of the models when varying the input parameters. Overall, the model was robust, i.e. varying parameters by the sensitivity analysis did not result in large variations of the ICERs. Four of the most influential drivers on the ICERs were similar for all four countries: the costs of antenatal care in both ERCD and VBAC, cost of an ERCD and unassisted vaginal birth without complications. For Belgium, Ireland and Italy, the (dis) utility associated with emergency caesarean birth was found to be sensitive variables for the ICER result. The probability of an unassisted vaginal birth was sensitive for Belgium, Germany and Italy. For the two latter countries, the disutility of an ERCD was also a sensitive variable. For Germany, the model was also sensitive for the probability of an ERCD and for the disutility of unassisted vaginal birth in Ireland (Additional file 1: Figure S2). The probabilistic sensitivity analysis resulted in a mainly dominant ICER with a reduction of the costs and increased effects when comparing VBAC with ERCD. The results differed between countries, ranging from -€423/QALY in Germany to -€9886/QALY in Ireland for a 6 week time horizon (Table 3), and from €8609/QALY in Germany to -€60,905 in Ireland for a lifetime time horizon. The most favourable ICER was for Ireland which can be explained by the high incremental cost of an ERCD compared to a vaginal birth. The lowest ICER was for Germany, as a result of the high probability and cost of neonatal sepsis in case of an emergency caesarean section or uterine rupture. The Monte Carlo simulations (6-week time horizon) are graphically presented as cost-effectiveness planes (Fig. 2), and are mainly plotted in the south-east quadrant for all four countries. For Belgium and Germany 7.34% and 34. 50% of all simulations were plotted in the north-east quadrant, with the latter showing VBAC to be slightly more expensive compared to ERCD. All simulations remained far below the national cost-effectiveness thresholds [53] and the likelihood of cost-effectiveness at the national thresholds were 100% for all four countries. For the lifetime model, VBAC was the preferred strategy for 98.66% (Belgium) and 100.00% (Germany, Ireland and Italy) of all Monte-Carlo simulations.

Discussion

We developed a standardised theoretical decision analytic model for four EU-countries comparing two strategies, attempting a VBAC and a planned ERCD. This model was adjusted to take into account more realistic clinical scenarios compared with previous health economic models, including the possibility of having a vaginal birth even when an ERCD had been planned. The results from these analyses confirm the cost-effectiveness of VBAC compared to ERCD in low-risk women. The probability of VBAC being cost-effective was almost 100% for the 6 weeks and lifetime time horizon for all four countries, and resulted in fewer caesarean sections.

Table 3 Cost-effectiveness results of vaginal birth after caesarean versus elective repeat caesarean per woman, €[a]

Model	Vaginal birth after caesarean		Elective repeat caesarean delivery		ICER	Total costs (€)	Total utilities (QALY)
	Cost (€)	Utility (QALY)	Cost (€)	Utility (QALY)	(€/QALY)		
Six-week time horizon							
Belgium						−15,271,888	7503
Deterministic	4862	0.84	5167	0.69	− 2035		
Probabilistic	4852	0.84	5171	0.69	− 2127		
Germany						−3,334,052	7561
Deterministic	4921	0.85	4988	0.70	−441		
Probabilistic	4921	0.85	4985	0.70	−423		
Ireland						−66,162,379	6689
Deterministic	6056	0.84	7379	0.70	− 9890		
Probabilistic	6057	0.84	7380	0.70	−9886		
Italy						−19,465,446	6399
Deterministic	4167	0.83	4556	0.70	−3042		
Probabilistic	4163	0.83	4552	0.70	− 3026		
Litetime time horizon							
Belgium						1,386,210	376
Deterministic	5281	34.79	5254	34.79	3669		
Probabilistic	5239	34.79	5251	34.77	− 596		
Germany						8,481,119	662
Deterministic	5222	19.12	5052	19.11	12,817		
Probabilistic	5147	19.12	5051	19.10	8609		
Ireland						−53,955,166	558
Deterministic	6363	18.64	7442	18.63	−96,753		
Probabilistic	6363	18.64	7442	18.63	−60,905		
Italy						−6,558,036	411
Deterministic	4488	26.44	4619	26.43	−15,965		
Probabilistic	4414	26.44	4618	26.42	−10,633		

QALY quality adjusted life year, *ICER* incremental cost-effectiveness ratio
[a] Currency in 2016 euros (€) [49]

Comparing these results with previously published health economic evaluations is difficult because of the variation in the models used, and the probabilities, utilities and costs included in these models [11]. We found four studies comparing VBAC with ERCD following one previous caesarean section of which one was European [9] and three from the United States of America [8, 10, 12]. Additionally, two cost-effectiveness studies compared VBAC with ERCD after one previous caesarean section over a lifetime horizon, and considered outcomes from subsequent pregnancies [11, 13]. All studies found the VBAC strategy to be cost-effective. Fawsitt et al.'s study [9], based on a hypothetical cohort in Ireland, found VBAC to be a dominant strategy resulting in an ICER -€15,773/QALY, comparable to our result of -€9886/QALY. However, their study included a limited number of maternal outcomes, e.g. thrombotic events and wound complications were not taken into consideration, and no neonatal outcomes (and associated costs) were included. The remaining health economic analyses included neonatal outcomes [8, 10–12]. Gilbert et al. [10] found that VBAC was a dominant strategy compared to ERCD and showed savings of $139 million, and gains of 1703 QALYs per 100,000 women. Grobman et al. [12] and Chung et al. [8] did not report the total number of QALYs gained; their cost-effectiveness analysis estimated $179 million saved per 100,000 women and $112,023/QALY respectively. Gilbert's et al. [11] lifetime cost-effectiveness analysis resulted in $164 million saved and 500 QALYs gained per 100,000 women, with an ICER of $-328,200/QALY. The lifetime cost-effectiveness study of Wymer et al. [13] showed VBAC to be a dominant strategy compared to ERCD with an incremental cost and effectiveness of -$4700,00 and 0.073 QALYs per patient (mother and neonate) for the sixth delivery. Findings from our study of VBAC being cost-effective are comparable with previous studies [9–11]. When incorporating a lifetime

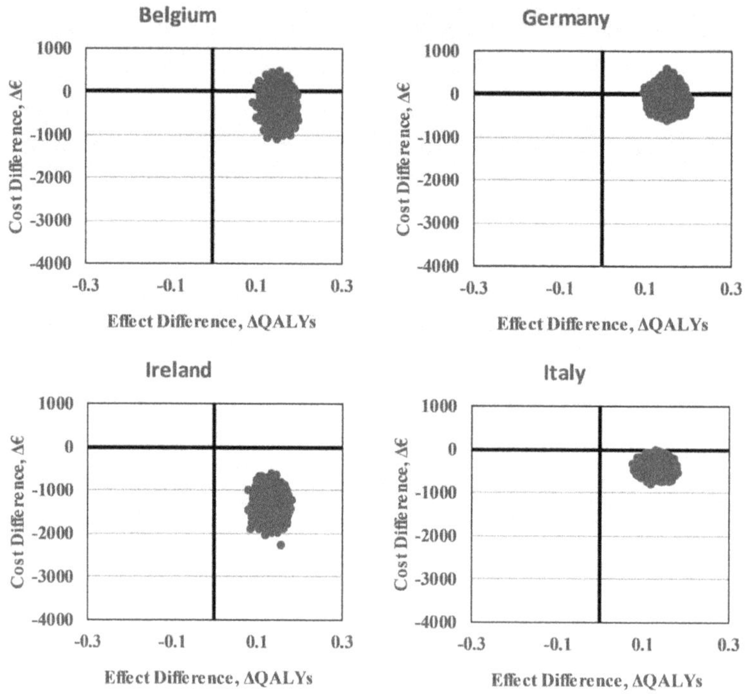

Fig. 2 Cost-effectiveness planes (6 weeks time horizon). Distribution of incremental costs and outcomes of vaginal birth after caesarean versus elective repeat caesarean delivery for Belgium, Germany, Ireland and Italy. 5000 Monte Carlo simulations were conducted for every country. QALY, quality adjusted life year

time horizon, the VBAC strategy was found to be more effective for all four countries but also slightly more costly for Germany. Previous studies showed the VBAC strategy to become less costly and more effective when including more subsequent deliveries [11, 13]. For all four countries and for both time horizons (6 weeks and lifetime), the VBAC strategy was cost-effective compared to ERCD, and the ICER results remained far below the national cost-effectiveness thresholds.

To the best of our knowledge, our model is the first to be used in multi-country context. We performed the health economic analysis from a societal perspective by including direct medical costs and non-medical costs, such as costs borne by the women, and indirect costs such as productivity loss. This societal approach includes costs related to the society's welfare, whereas the health services perspective considers only direct medical costs. We included costs and health effects for all three episodes of perinatal care, the ante-, peri- and postnatal periods for both the mother and newborn. Therefore, we believe this model is more comprehensive and better reflects the clinical situation in real life compared to previous models. All costs included in our model were country specific and, where possible, based on national data sources. Neonatal outcomes were included because mode of birth can impact some adverse neonatal outcomes such as cerebral palsy and sepsis. In addition, we developed a standardised model for application in all four countries. Our model builds on previously published models and offers a unique contribution to performing international health economic analyses. We have included all the model's input parameters, thus giving other researchers the opportunity to test and use our model for future health economic evaluations in other countries which, ultimately, will increase the comparability of study results.

This study has limitations, primarily because our findings are based on a hypothetical cohort. However, wherever possible, we used country-specific probabilities, particularly for variables described as important in previous studies [8]. Health-effects were measured as QALYs, and country specific QALYs of the general population were reduced with the corresponding disutility of the maternal and neonatal outcome. In our method of calculating disutilities, we consider the mode of birth and neonatal outcome to be independent. As a consequence, this may lead in some scenarios to an over/under estimation of the disutilities due to double counting health effects. In our opinion, there is no clear method available to overcome this methodological issue. Further studies are needed, which attempt to disentangle the health effects on the mother and child, and give guidance on how the health effects of neonates can be considered separately in health economic evaluations. While all costs included in our model were country specific, for some costs, such as the in-patient DRG costs, we were unable to find a specific DRG cost for every arm of the decision tree. Some countries such as Italy and Ireland had only two DRGs for a caesarean section, one with and one without complications. Therefore, the cost of an ERCD or emergency caesarean, could only be distinguished based on the appearance of complications. We considered these uncertainties in the deterministic and probabilistic sensitivity analyses and found they did not have a high impact on the estimated ICER. In addition, we limited our cohort to women with only one previous caesarean section and included only the major short and long-term consequences.

The main strength of this study is the development of a standardised health economic analysis model which can be used for cost-effectiveness studies of VBAC versus ERCD in an international context. Other researchers may consider developing and advancing this model, and including more subsequent deliveries and more long-term consequences.

Conclusions

This model is the first health economic analysis model that can be used to calculate the cost-effectiveness of VBAC and ERCD in an international context. The results of this study suggests that, compared to ERCD, VBAC is cost-effective in Belgium, Germany, Ireland and Italy. This model, and its underlying methods and assumptions can be applied to more EU-countries, or even beyond. This model can easily be used by researchers to calculate the cost-effectiveness of new strategies comparing VBAC with ERCD by inputting probability, costs and utility data collected during the study.

Additional file

Additional file 1: Additional tables and files including an overview of resource use, costs and model parameters used in the models; overview of the distribution over maternal and infant outcomes per 100,000 women by mode of birth, by country; results of the incremental net monetary benefit per country; country specific tornado diagrams as a result of the one-way sensitivity analysis. **Table S1**. Healthcare utilisation and unit costs antenatal and postnatal care. **Table S2**. Model parameters and distributions probabilistic sensitivity analysis. **Table S3**. Distribution mode of birth by country. **Figure S1**. Incremental Net Monetary Benefit (lifetime horizon). **Figure S2**. Country specific tornado diagrams as a result of the one-way sensitivity analysis (6-week time horizon)

Abbreviations

CP: Cerebral palsy; DRG: Diagnostic related groups; ERCD: Elective repeat caesarean delivery; EU: European Union; HICP: Harmonized indices of consumer prices; HIE: Hypoxic ischemic encephalopathy; ICER: Incremental cost-effectiveness ratio; QALY: Quality adjusted life years; VBAC: Vaginal birth after caesarean

Acknowledgments

We would like to thank the following experts for sharing their knowledge: Prof. Dr. Mechthild Groβ, Susanne Grylka-Baeschlin, Andrea Matterne and Ulrike Geppert-Orthofer for Germany; Prof. Dr. Declan Devane, Dr. Patricia Healy and Christopher Fawsitt for Ireland; Prof. Dr. Sandra Morano, Dr. Jane Nicoletti, Dr. Lucia Arrata, Prof. Dr. Marcello Montefiori, Dr. Mauro Occhi for Italy.

Funding

We are grateful to the European Commission for funding this study under the European Union's Seventh Framework Programme (FP7/2007–2013) through grant agreement no. 305208, and to the Wetenschappelijk Fonds Willy Gepts (UMC Brussels) for providing funding for the additional time required for the lead author to conduct additional analyses and finalise the manuscript.

The funding bodies had no role in study design, data collection, data analyses and interpretation, or writing the manuscript. The opinions expressed here are those of the study team.

Authors' contributions

MF drafted and revised the manuscript for content, performed the analysis, handled the study coordination, and is the guarantor for the overall content. KB revised the manuscript for content. GF validated the model, revised the manuscript for content. DD and CB contributed to initial planning of the study and revised the manuscript for clinical applicability. KP validated the model, revised the manuscript for content and supervised the study. All authors gave final approval for publication of this manuscript.

Consent for publication

Not applicable

Competing interests

The authors declare that they have no competing interest.

Author details

[1]I-CHER (Interuniversity Centre for Health Economics Research), Faculty of Medicine and Pharmacy, Vrije Universiteit Brussels, Laarbeeklaan 103, 1090 Brussels, Belgium. [2]Department of Public Health, Faculty of Medicine and Pharmacy, Vrije Universiteit Brussel, Laarbeeklaan 103, 1090 Brussels, Belgium. [3]Department of Nursing and Midwifery, Nursing and Midwifery research group, Universitair Ziekenhuis Brussel, Laarbeeklaan 103, 1090 Brussels, Belgium. [4]Department of Obstetrics, Universitair Ziekenhuis Brussel, Vrije Universiteit Brussel, Laarbeeklaan 101, 1090 Brussels, Belgium. [5]School of Nursing and Midwifery, Trinity College Dublin, 24 D'Olier Street, Dublin D02 T283, Ireland. [6]Institute of Health and Care Sciences, Sahlgrenska Academy, University of Gothenburg, Gothenburg, Sweden.

References

1. Declercq E, Young R, Cabral H, Ecker J. Is a rising cesarean delivery rate inevitable? Trends in industrialized countries, 1987 to 2007. Birth. 2011;38: 99–104.
2. EURO-PERISTAT Project with SCPE and EUROCAT. European perinatal health report. The health and care of pregnant women and babies in Europe in 2010. 2013. www.europeristat.com. Accessed 14 June 2016.
3. Betran AP, Ye J, Moller AB, Zhang J, Gulmezoglu AM, Torloni MR. The increasing trend in caesarean section rates: global, regional and National Estimates: 1990-2014. PLoS One. 2016;11:e0148343.
4. Guise JM, Eden K, Emeis C, Denman MA, Marshall N, Fu RR, et al. Vaginal birth after cesarean: new insights. Report Number; 2010. p. 1530–4396.

5. Fisler RE, Cohen A, Ringer SA, Lieberman E. Neonatal outcome after trial of labor compared with elective repeat cesarean section. Birth. 2003;30:83–8.
6. Hook B, Kiwi R, Amini SB, Fanaroff A, Hack M. Neonatal morbidity after elective repeat cesarean section and trial of labor. Pediatrics. 1997;100:348–53.
7. Liu S, Liston RM, Joseph KS, Heaman M, Sauve R, Kramer MS. Maternal mortality and severe morbidity associated with low-risk planned cesarean delivery versus planned vaginal delivery at term. CMAJ. 2007;176:455–60.
8. Chung A, Macario A, El-Sayed YY, Riley ET, Duncan B, Druzin ML. Cost-effectiveness of a trial of labor after previous cesarean. Obstet Gynecol. 2001;97:932–41.
9. Fawsitt CG, Bourke J, Greene RA, Everard CM, Murphy A, Lutomski JE. At what price? A cost-effectiveness analysis comparing trial of labour after previous caesarean versus elective repeat caesarean delivery. PLoS One. 2013;8:e58577.
10. Gilbert SA, Grobman WA, Landon MB, Spong CY, Rouse DJ, Leveno KJ, et al. Cost-effectiveness of trial of labor after previous cesarean in a minimally biased cohort. Am J Perinatol. 2013;30:11–20.
11. Gilbert SA, Grobman WA, Landon MB, Varner MW, Wapner RJ, Sorokin Y, et al. Lifetime cost-effectiveness of trial of labor after cesarean in the United States. Value Health. 2013;16:953–64.
12. Grobman WA, Peaceman AM, Socol ML. Cost-effectiveness of elective cesarean delivery after one prior low transverse cesarean. Obstet Gynecol. 2000;95:745–51.
13. Wymer KM, Shih YC, Plunkett BA. The cost-effectiveness of a trial of labor accrues with multiple subsequent vaginal deliveries. Am J Obstet Gynecol. 2014;211:56 e1–e12.
14. Curtin SC GK, Korst LM, Uddin SFG. Maternal morbidity for vaginal and cesarean deliveries, according to previous cesarean history: new data from the birth certificate, 2013. Report number. 2015.
15. Gregory KD, Korst LM, Fridman M, Shihady I, Broussard P, Fink A, et al. Vaginal birth after cesarean: clinical risk factors associated with adverse outcome. Am J Obstet Gynecol. 2008;198:452 e1–12.
16. Nair M, Soffer K, Noor N, Knight M, Griffiths M. Selected maternal morbidities in women with a prior caesarean delivery planning vaginal birth or elective repeat caesarean section: a retrospective cohort analysis using data from the UK obstetric surveillance system. BMJ Open. 2015;5:e007434.
17. Spong CY, Landon MB, Gilbert S, Rouse DJ, Leveno KJ, Varner MW, et al. Risk of uterine rupture and adverse perinatal outcome at term after cesarean delivery. Obstet Gynecol. 2007;110:801–7.
18. Wen SW, Rusen ID, Walker M, Liston R, Kramer MS, Baskett T, et al. Comparison of maternal mortality and morbidity between trial of labor and elective cesarean section among women with previous cesarean delivery. Am J Obstet Gynecol. 2004;191:1263–9.
19. Cahill AG, Stamilio DM, Odibo AO, Peipert JF, Ratcliffe SJ, Stevens EJ, et al. Is vaginal birth after cesarean (VBAC) or elective repeat cesarean safer in women with a prior vaginal delivery? Am J Obstet Gynecol. 2006;195:1143–7.
20. Loebel G, Zelop CM, Egan JF, Wax J. Maternal and neonatal morbidity after elective repeat cesarean delivery versus a trial of labor after previous cesarean delivery in a community teaching hospital. J Matern Fetal Neonatal Med. 2004;15:243–6.
21. McMahon MJ, Luther ER, Bowes WA Jr, Olshan AF. Comparison of a trial of labor with an elective second cesarean section. N Engl J Med. 1996;335:689–95.
22. Niino Y. The increasing cesarean rate globally and what we can do about it. Biosci Trends. 2011;5:139–50.
23. Petrou S, Khan K. An overview of the health economic implications of elective caesarean section. Appl Health Econ Health Policy. 2013;11:561–76.
24. OptiBIRTH. The OptiBIRTH project. www.optibirth.eu. Accessed 14 Jan 2014.
25. ISRCTN registry. Improving the organisation of maternal health service delivery, and optimising childbirth, by increasing vaginal birth after caesarean section (VBAC) through enhanced women-centred care. ISRCTN10612254. http://www.isrctn.com/ISRCTN10612254. Accessed 23 July 2015.
26. National Institute for Health Care and Excellence. Intrapartum care: Care of healthy women and their babies during childbirth. https://www.nice.org.uk/guidance/cg190. Accessed 24 July 2014.
27. Burrows LJ, Meyn LA, Weber AM. Maternal morbidity associated with vaginal versus cesarean delivery. Obstet Gynecol. 2004;103:907–12.
28. Caughey AB, Shipp TD, Repke JT, Zelop CM, Cohen A, Lieberman E. Rate of uterine rupture during a trial of labor in women with one or two prior cesarean deliveries. Am J Obstet Gynecol. 1999;181:872–6.
29. Cowan RK, Kinch RA, Ellis B, Anderson R. Trial of labor following cesarean delivery. Obstet Gynecol. 1994;83:933–6.
30. Flamm BL, Newman LA, Thomas SJ, Fallon D, Yoshida MM. Vaginal birth after cesarean delivery: results of a 5-year multicenter collaborative study. Obstet Gynecol. 1990;76:750–4.
31. Badawi N, Kurinczuk JJ, Keogh JM, Alessandri LM, O'Sullivan F, Burton PR, et al. Intrapartum risk factors for newborn encephalopathy: the western Australian case-control study. BMJ. 1998;317:1554–8.
32. Landon MB, Spong CY, Thom E, Hauth JC, Bloom SL, Varner MW, et al. Risk of uterine rupture with a trial of labor in women with multiple and single prior cesarean delivery. Obstet Gynecol. 2006;108:12–20.
33. Murphy DJ, Liebling RE, Patel R, Verity L, Swingler R. Cohort study of operative delivery in the second stage of labour and standard of obstetric care. BJOG. 2003;110:610–5.
34. Richardson BS, Czikk MJ, daSilva O, Natale R. The impact of labor at term on measures of neonatal outcome. Am J Obstet Gynecol. 2005;192:219–26.
35. Glinianaia SV, Rankin J, Colver A. Cerebral palsy rates by birth weight, gestation and severity in north of England, 1991-2000 singleton births. Arch Dis Child. 2011;96:180–5.
36. Leung AS, Leung EK, Paul RH. Uterine rupture after previous cesarean delivery: maternal and fetal consequences. Am J Obstet Gynecol. 1993;169:945–50.
37. Moster D, Lie RT, Markestad T. Long-term medical and social consequences of preterm birth. N Engl J Med. 2008;359:262–73.
38. Petrini JR, Dias T, McCormick MC, Massolo ML, Green NS, Escobar GJ. Increased risk of adverse neurological development for late preterm infants. J Pediatr. 2009;154:169–76.
39. Badawi N, Felix JF, Kurinczuk JJ, Dixon G, Watson L, Keogh JM, et al. Cerebral palsy following term newborn encephalopathy: a population-based study. Dev Med Child Neurol. 2005;47:293–8.
40. David M, Gross MM, Wiemer A, Pachaly J, Vetter K. Prior cesarean section–an acceptable risk for vaginal delivery at free-standing midwife-led birth centers? Results of the analysis of vaginal birth after cesarean section (VBAC) in German birth centers. Eur J Obstet Gynecol Reprod Biol. 2009;142:106–10.
41. Eden KB, Denman MA, Emeis CL, McDonagh MS, Fu R, Janik RK, et al. Trial of labor and vaginal delivery rates in women with a prior cesarean. J Obstet Gynecol Neonatal Nurs. 2012;41:583–98.
42. Fruscalzo A, Salmeri MG, Cendron A, Londero AP, Zanni G. Introducing routine trial of labour after caesarean section in a second level hospital setting. J Matern Fetal Neonatal Med. 2012;25:1442–6.
43. Kyvernitakis I, Reichelt J, Kyvernitakis A, Misselwitz B, Hadji P, Schmidt S, et al. Trends of vaginal birth after cesarean delivery in Germany from 1990 to 2012: a population-based study. Z Geburtshilfe Neonatol. 2014;218:203–9.
44. Yap OW, Kim ES, Laros RK Jr. Maternal and neonatal outcomes after uterine rupture in labor. Am J Obstet Gynecol. 2001;184:1576–81.
45. Capri SCA, Terranova L, Merlo F, Mantovani L, The members of the Italian group for pharmacoeconomic studies. Guidelines for economic evaluations in Italy: recommendations from the Italian group of pharmacoeconomic studies. Drug Inf J. 2001;35:189–201.
46. Graf von der Schulenburg JM, Greiner W, Jost F, Klusen N, Kubin M, Leidl R, et al. German recommendations on health economic evaluation: third and updated version of the Hanover consensus. Value Health. 2008;11:539–44.
47. Cleemput INM, Van de Sande S, Thiry N. Belgische richtlijnen voor economische evaluaties en budget impact analyses: tweede editie. Health technology assessment.. Report number. Brussel: Federaal Kenniscentrum voor de Gezondheidszorg (KCE; 2012.
48. Authority HIaQ. Guidelines for the Economic Evaluation of Health Technologies in ireland. Report number. Dublin: HIQA; 2014.
49. Eurostat. HICP - health 2016. http://ec.europa.eu/eurostat/en/web/products-datasets/-/TEICP060. Accessed 15 June 2016.
50. Szende AJB, Cabasés J. Self-reported population health: an international perspective based on EQ-5D. London: Springer; 2014.
51. Wetenschappelijk Instituut Volksgezondheid. HISIA: Belgian Health Interview Survey - Interactive Analysis 2015. https://hisia.wiv-isp.be/SitePages/Home.aspx. Accessed 15 July 2015.
52. Bennett JE, Sumner W 2nd, Downs SM, Jaffe DM. Parents' utilities for outcomes of occult bacteremia. Arch Pediatr Adolesc Med. 2000;154:43–8.
53. International Monetary Fund. Gross domestic product per capita, current prices 2016. https://www.imf.org/external/pubs/ft/weo/2016/01/weodata/weorept.aspx?sy=2016&ey=2016&scsm=1&ssd=1&sort=country&ds=.&br=1&pr1.x=80&pr1.y=9&c=124%2C134%2C178%2C136&s=NGDPPC&grp=0&a=. Accessed 18 June 2016.

Elective caesarean section at 38–39 weeks gestation compared to > 39 weeks on neonatal outcomes

Reihaneh Pirjani[1,2], Motahareh Afrakhteh[3], Mahdi Sepidarkish[4], Shahin Nariman[5], Mahboobeh Shirazi[6], Ashraf Moini[7,8] and Ladan Hosseini[9*]

Abstract

Background: This study was conducted to compare neonatal complications in scheduled cesarean sections (CS) between 38 and 39 gestational weeks with CS performed after 39 gestational weeks in Iranian low -risk pregnant women.

Methods: In this cohort study, 2086 patients were enrolled based on the inclusion and exclusion criteria. The neonates were evaluated in terms of the following items: transient tachypnea of the newborn (TTN), respiratory distress syndrome (RDS), sepsis, need for NICU hospitalization, birth weight, birth height, head circumference, and the first minute and fifth minute Apgar score. Several multiple logistic regression models were performed for each response variable (adverse outcome) separately.

Results: The incidence of NICU admission was significantly higher in neonates born at 38–39 gestational weeks than those who were born after 39 gestational weeks. No significant differences were found in the incidence of neonatal sepsis, TTN, and RDS between the two groups.

Conclusion: According to our study results, elective CS at 38–9 weeks' gestation is associated with a higher rate of TTN and NICU admission in comparison with elective CS performed after 39 completed gestational weeks.

Keywords: Caesarean section, Intensive care units, Neonate, Transient tachypnea of the newborn, Respiratory distress syndrome

Background

The appropriate gestational age for scheduled cesarean section (CS) has become a topic of interest in prenatal care [1]. For the past four decades, obstetricians and pediatricians, assuming that fetal maturity could be completed at the end of 37 gestational weeks, have defined "the term pregnancy" from that time onwards [2]. However, it has now become clear that even in "the term pregnancy" (37 gestational weeks), neonatal respiratory complications will decrease with an increase in the gestational age to 39 weeks. These findings have challenged the old definition of "theterm pregnancy" [3]. Recently, the definition of "the term pregnancy" has changed to cover three categories of premature term (37–38 weeks + 6 days), full term (39–40 weeks and 6 days), and late term (41-41 weeks + 6 days) [4].

Experts recommend that scheduled cesarean delivery be conducted from 39 weeks onwards [5], so that fetal maturity is complete. Some studies have shown discrepancies in respiratory complications according to the gestational age pattern between Asian and Caucasian ethnicities. The lowest complication rate was observed in 39–40 gestational weeks in the Caucasians and in 38 gestational weeks in Asians [1]. Accordingly, this study aimed to compare neonatal complications in scheduled CS between 38 and 39 gestational weeks with scheduled

* Correspondence: hosseiniladan@yahoo.com
[9]Research development center, Arash Women's Hospital, Tehran University of Medical Sciences, Tehran, Iran
Full list of author information is available at the end of the article

CS performed after 39 gestational weeks in Iranian pregnant women.

Method and materials

This prospective cohort study was conducted at a university hospital (Arash Hospital, Tehran, Iran) from April 2013 to April 2015. All term singleton pregnancies (≥38 gestational weeks) scheduled for elective CS were enrolled in this study. The research protocol of the study was approved by the Ethical Research Committee of Tehran University of Medical Sciences. The informed consent was obtained from all pregnant women. The inclusion criteria were singleton pregnancy and elective CS scheduled for 38 complete gestational weeks or later. The exclusion criteria were gestational age below 38 completed gestational weeks, multiple pregnancy, maternal chronic diseases, gestational diabetes, preeclampsia, CS due to fetal distress, intra uterine growth restriction, meconium defecation, placenta previa or accreta, fetal abnormalities, CS during the active phase of labor, repeated CS after beginning of uterine contracture, and any other cause of emergency CS.

All patients had two ultrasonography reports in the first trimester, one at 6–9 gestational weeks and the other at 11–14 gestational weeks. Gestational age was determined based on the date of the last menstrual period (LMP). If the difference was more than 5 days, gestational age was estimated based on ultrasound criterion at 6–9 gestational weeks provided that it was confirmed by ultrasound at 11–14 weeks. In our practice, at least two ultrasound examinations are routinely performed in the first trimester in all pregnant women, one at 6–9 gestational weeks and the other at 11–14 gestational weeks. All ultrasound examinations were performed by a perinatologist or radiologist experienced in obstetric sonography. Gestational age (GA) was determined by measuring of the fetal crown-rump-length (CRL) at 6–9 and 11–14 gestational weeks. The average CRL measurement in mm was derived from three satisfactory images. CRL was converted to the equivalent number of gestational days according to Hadlock *et al.* (1992). All pregnant women received their antenatal care at our hospital.

The collected data were maternal age, parity, neonatal weight, and neonatal complications. The following items were considered to evaluate the neonatal outcomes: transient tachypnea of the newborn (TTN) defined as the presence of tachypnea within hours after birth; respiratory distress syndrome (RDS) defined as the signs of respiratory distress (radiological features and oxygen therapy), sepsis, need for NICU hospitalization, and first minute and fifth minute Apgar scores.

Statistical analysis and sample size

The sample size was calculated on the assumption that the incidence of TTN would be 3% in women with a delivery time between 38 and 39 gestational weeks and 1% in women with a delivery time ≥ 39 gestational weeks. The estimated sample size was 866 women in each group ($\alpha = 0.05$; $1 - \beta = 0.80$).

Categorical and continuous variables are expressed as number (percentage) and mean ± (standard deviation), respectively. Chi-square test was applied to compare categorical variables. Student's t-test was used to compare parametric continuous variables. In order to control the potential confounders, a multiple logistic regression model was fitted for each dependent outcome variable (TTN, RDS, sepsis and need for NICU hospitalization). Explanatory variables were considered into the model for adjustment in the following order: maternal age, parity, neonatal weight, first minute Apgar, and fifth minute Apgar. The results are presented as odds ratios (OR) with 95% confidence intervals. Data analysis was undertaken using the Stata statistical software, released 13.0 (Stata Corp, College Station, Tex, USA).

Results

Totally, 4892 CS were performed in our hospital during the study period, and based on the inclusion and exclusion criteria, 2086 patients were enrolled. In our study, 1002 (48%) women delivered between 38 and 39 gestational weeks and 1084 (52%) women delivered after 39 gestational weeks. Indications for elective caesarean delivery were prior caesarean section in 54.5% (1137 women), breech presentation in 7.2% (150 women), suspected cephalopelvic disproportion in 4.6% (96 women), maternal requested CS in 28.8% (601 women), and other causes such as retinopathy or myopathy and a history of infertility in 4.9% (102 women).

The mean ± (SD) age of the mothers who delivered between 38 to 39 gestational weeks was 27.77 ± (5.29) years, which was significantly higher than the mean (SD) age of mothers who delivered at > 39 gestational weeks (27.27 ± 5.74 years) ($P = 0.041$) (Table 1).

As shown in Table 1, repeated caesarean was more frequent in mothers who delivered between 38 and 39 gestational weeks compared to mothers who delivered after 39 gestational weeks (64.7% vs. 45.1%, $P < 0.001$). Inversely, the frequency of breech presentation (10% vs. 4.2%), Cephalopelvic Disproportion (CPD) (5.4% vs. 3.8%), and maternal request (35.4% vs. 21.7%) were higher in mothers who delivered after 39 weeks' gestation compared to mothers who delivered between 38 and 39 gestational weeks (P < 0.001).

The weight of neonates born after 39 gestational weeks was significantly higher than neonates born between 38 and 39 gestational weeks (mean difference: 136.76, 95%

Table 1 Comparison of demographic characteristics of participants

Parameters	Elective caesarean delivery between 38 and 39 weeks gestation (n = 1002)	Elective caesarean delivery after 39 weeks gestation (n = 1084)	P-value
Maternal age (year)	27.77 ± (5.29)	27.27 ± (5.74)	0.041
Parity	1.89 ± (0.70)	1.90 ± (0.73)	0.675
Cause of cesarean			
Repeat cesarean	648(64.7)	489(45.1)	< 0.001
Breach and transverse presentation	42(4.2)	108(10)	
Cephalopelvic Disproportion (CPD)	38(3.8)	58(5.4)	
Maternal request	217(21.7)	384(35.4)	
Other reasons	57(5.7)	45(4.2)	
Birth weight of neonate	3190.77 ± (394.19)	3327.54 ± (377.70)	< 0.001
Height of neonate	49.57 ± (1.93)	50.17 ± (2.02)	< 0.001
Head circumference	34.47 ± (1.46)	34.59 ± (1.90)	0.113
Apgar min 1	8.97 ± (0.21)	8.99 ± (0.14)	0.033
Apgar min 5	9.99 ± (0.10)	10.00 ± (0.06)	0.529
NICU admission	22(2.2)	8(0.7)	0.004
Sepsis	6(0.6)	4(0.4)	0.329
Respiratory distress syndrome	7(0.7)	3(0.3)	0.141
TTN	15(1.5)	5(0.5)	0.013

Values given as mean ± SD(standard deviation), or number (percentage) unless otherwise indicated

CI: 103.61 to 169.91, P < 0.001). Also, the one-minute Apgar score was significantly different between the two groups (mean difference: 0.02, 95% CI: 0.002 to 0.04, P = 0.029). There was no statistical significant difference in other characteristics between the two groups .

No significant differences were found in the incidence of neonatal sepsis between the two groups (0.6 and 0.4% in neonates born between 38 and 39 and after 39 gestational weeks respectively, adjusted OR: 1.60, 95% CI: 0. 48 to 5.31, P = 0.440). The incidence of respiratory distress syndrome (RDS) was 0.7% (7 neonates) and 0.3% (3 neonates) in group 1 and 2, respectively. (Adjusted OR: 2.07, 95%CI: 0.56 to 7.56, P = 0.270).

The incidence of NICU admission was 2.2% (22 people) in neonates born between 38 and 39 gestational weeks and 0.7% (8 people) in those born after 39 gestational weeks. The difference was statistically significant (adjusted OR: 2.59, 95%CI: 1.16 to 5.79, P = 0.020).

The incidence of TTN was 1.5% (15 neonates) in neonates born between 38 and 39 gestational weeks (95% CI: 0.74 to 2.25) and 0.5% (5 people) in neonates born after 39 gestational weeks (95% CI: 0.05–0.08). The adjusted odds ratio of the association between TTN and time of delivery was 2.91 (95%CI: 1.09–7.76) (P = 0.032) using multiple logistic regression analysis, indicating that the minimal risk of TTN in neonates born between 38 and 39 gestational weeks was 9% higher compared to neonates born after 39 gestational weeks. Table 2 shows crude and adjusted odds ratio of the association between adverse outcomes and time of delivery.

Discussion

This study showed that elective CS delivery between 38 to 39 gestational weeks is associated with a higher rate of TTN and NICU admission in comparison with elective CS performed after 39 completed gestational weeks. Other major complications and more serious disorders such as respiratory distress syndrome (RDS) and sepsis were not significantly different between the two groups.

Matsuo et al. reported severe neonatal respiratory complications (RDS and TTN) that were similar in 415 Japanese pregnant women who underwent scheduled cesarean delivery in 38 and 39 gestational weeks [6]. In a study of 442,596 South Asian and Black women, Balchin et al. found that the rate of respiratory dysfunction was the lowest in white infants whose mothers underwent C-section after 39 gestational weeks and in South Asian infants whose mothers underwent C-section at 38 gestational weeks [7]. Moreover, Trata et al. examined 1951 cases of elective cesarean delivery in Japan and reported that elective cesarean should be performed at 38 weeks and two days or later in order to avoid respiratory complications [8].

A retrospective study of 1221 singleton pregnant women in Taiwan and Southeast Asia with scheduled cesarean delivery at 38 gestational weeks compared to

Table 2 Crude and adjusted odds ratio (OR) for relationship between adverse outcomes and time of delivery

Variables	Crude OR	95% CI for Crude OR	Adjusted[a] OR	95% CI for Adjusted OR
NICU admission	2.90	1.31–6.42	2.59	1.16–5.79
Respiratory distress syndrome	2.32	0.65–8.30	2.07	0.56–7.56
TTN	3.08	1.16–8.18	2.91	1.09–7.76
Sepsis	1.56	0.46–5.22	1.60	0.48–5.31

[a] Adjusted for age of mothers, parity, weight of neonate, Apgar 1 min, Apgar 5 min

39 weeks revealed no statistically significant difference in severe neonatal complications including TTNB, RDS and NICU admission [1]. In contrast, the rate of NICU admission was higher in our study at 38 gestational weeksthan 39 gestational weeks. This difference may be attributed to differences in the hospital strategy to admit infants to NICU or high frequency of TTN.

Furthermore, most studies on Caucasian and mainly white women have emphasized the improved neonatal outcome in scheduled cesarean deliveries at 39 gestational weeks [9, 10]. It has been suggested that difference in the prevalence of respiratory dysfunction at different gestational ages in white and Asian infants can be due to genetic differences when the fetus matures in the uterine [7, 11]. Black and Asian infants have mostly shown meconium-stained amniotic fluid, indicating prematurity [11].

On the other hand, a multicentre clinical trial in Denmark showed that NICU admission was higher in scheduled cesarean delivery at 38 gestational weeks than those born at 39 gestational weeks,even though the difference was not significant [5]. It can be concluded that race alone cannot determine neonatal complications at different pregnancy ages. The difference of these studies conducted in the Caucasian and Asian communities in terms of the gestational age at the time of scheduled cesarean delivery can be due to differences in the sample size, failure to control confounding variables, or race.

In this study, the main reason for NICU admission was TTN, not other serious complications including RDS and sepsis. NICU admissions may lead to a large financial burden. Christopher J. Robinson et al. reported that waiting until 39 gestational weeks to perform an elective CS is cost effective [12]. However, the likelihood of emergency cesarean delivery and its maternal complications should also be taken into account. As suggested by some studies, the mean gestational age in Asian and black populations is less than the whites, which can be due to fetal prematurity [11]. Emergency cesarean can be followed by complications for mothers and infants [13]. Thus, in our study, we cannot draw a definite conclusion that delivery should be performed after 39 gestational weeks. Further studies are required to compare the rate and complications of emergency and scheduled cesarean delivery in Iranian population at 38 and 39 gestational weeks.

One of the concerns that causes scheduled cesarean delivery at 38 gestational weeks is prevention of unexpected fetal death. In this study, we did not have any cases of stillbirth. The risk of unexplained stillbirth at 38 gestational weeks was reported to be about 0.05 per 1000 births among women with the history of cesarean delivery in a Scottish and a Canadian cohort study [14, 15]. To measure the prevalence of 0.01–1% with sufficient accuracy and confidence, as many as 20,000 cases are needed [16]. Therefore, a small size of the sample may be the reason.

In this study, the most common causes of cesarean delivery in the two groups were a previous history of CS and maternal request. However, the frequency of repeated cesarean delivery was higher at 38–39 gestational weeks than its frequency after 39 gestational weeks. Two-thirds of births were done at 38–39 gestational weeks for this reason. Moreover, 56% of all repeated cesarean deliveries were performed before 39 gestational weeks. A multicentric cohort in the United States showed that one-third of cesarean deliveries are performed before 39 gestational weeks. The rate is between 50 and 80% in some European countries. The reason for this concern is maternal complications in pregnancy associated with previous CS [17]. In this study, other reasons, including maternal request, breech presentation, and CPD, were more prevalent at 39 gestational weeks.

In our study, almost half of elective caesarean sections were performed before 39 gestational weeks. Wilmink et al. reported that more than 50% of the elective cesarean sections were done before 39 gestational weeksin the Netherlands (8.3% at 37 gestational weeks and 48.3% at 38 gestational weeks [10]. Zanardo V. et al. reported that about 60% of elective cesarean sections in their hospital were performed before 38 weeks and 6 days [18] It seems that physicians, regardless of the existing documents, perform a large percentage of CS deliveries before 39 gestational weeks. It may be due to the physician's opinion or practice patterns, maternal request for early CS, birth certificate data, or any other reason.

The strong points of this study were excluding the cases of emergency cesarean delivery and a large sample size. The limitations of this study were evaluating neonatal complications only up to 28 days after birth not beyond 28 days.

Conclusion

According to our study findings, scheduled CS delivery between 38 and 39 gestational weeks is associated with a higher rate of NICU admission in comparison with scheduled CS performed after 39 gestational weeks. The main reason for NICU admission was TTN, not other serious complications. Although no cases of intrauterine fetal death occurred in women who underwent CS delivery after 39 gestational weeks, we did not have any information on the incidence and complications of emergency CS in those who delivered after 39 weeks' gestation.Therefore, based on the results of this study, it cannot be concluded that scheduled caesarean section should be performed after 39 gestational weeks. We suggest that the above issue be examined in the future studies to determine the time of scheduled CS more accurately.

Abbreviations

CPD: Cephalopelvic Disproportion; CRL: Fetal crown-rump-length; CS: Cesarean sections; GA: Gestational age; LMP: The last menstrual period; OR: Odds ratios; RDS: Respiratory distress syndrome; TTN: Transient tachypnea of the newborn

Acknowledgements

We would like to thank the research development center of Arash women's hospital for their contributions in the process of preparing this article.

Authors' contributions

RP designed the study. RP,MA, SHN,AM, LH and MSH contributed in participants selection and data collection and revised the manuscript. RP and LH wrote the manuscript. MS helped in the analysis of the data. All authors read and approved the final manuscript.

Competing interests

The authors declare that they have no competing interests.

Author details

[1]Obstetrics and Gynecology Department, Arash Women's Hospital, Tehran University of Medical Sciences, Tehran, Iran. [2]Research development center, Arash Women's Hospital, Tehran University of Medical Sciences, Tehran, Iran. [3]School of medicine, Tehran University of Medical Sciences, Tehran, Iran. [4]Department of Epidemiology and Reproductive Health, Reproductive Epidemiology Research Center, Royan Institute for Reproductive Biomedicine, ACECR, Tehran, Iran. [5]Department of Pediatrics, Arash women's Hospital, Tehran University of Medical Sciences, Tehran, Iran. [6]Maternal, Fetal and Neonatal Research Center, Tehran University of Medical Sciences, Tehran, Iran. [7]Obstetrics and Gynecology Department, Arash Women's Hospital, Tehran University of Medical Sciences, Tehran, Iran. [8]Department of Endocrinology and Female Infertility, Reproductive Biomedicine Research Center, Royan Institute for Reproductive Biomedicine, ACECR., Tehran, Iran. [9]Research development center, Arash Women's Hospital, Tehran University of Medical Sciences, Tehran, Iran.

References

1. Phaloprakarn C, Tangjitgamol S, Manusirivithaya S. Timing *of elective cesarean delivery at term and its impact on maternal and neonatal outcomes among Thai and other Southeast Asian pregnant women.* J Obstet Gynaecol Res. 2016;42(8):936–43.
2. Glavind J, Uldbjerg N. Elective cesarean delivery at 38 and 39 weeks: neonatal and maternal risks. Curr Opin Obstet Gynecol. 2015;27(2):121–7.
3. Doan E, Gibbons K, Tudehope D. *The* timing *of elective caesarean deliveries and early neonatal outcomes in singleton infants born 37–41 weeks' gestation.* Aust N Z J Obstet Gynaecol. 2014;54(4):340–7.
4. Spong CY. Defining "term" pregnancy: recommendations from the defining "term" pregnancy workgroup. JAMA. 2013;309(23):2445–6.
5. Glavind J, et al. Elective caesarean section at 38 weeks versus 39 weeks: neonatal and maternal outcomes in a randomised controlled trial. BJOG Int J Obstet Gynaecol. 2013;120(9):1123–32.
6. Matsuo K, et al. Is 38 weeks late enough for elective cesarean delivery? Int J Gynecol Obstet. 2008;100(1):90–1.
7. Balchin I, et al. Timing *of planned cesarean delivery by racial group.* Obstet Gynecol. 2008;111(3):659–66.
8. Terada K, et al. Timing *of Elective Cesarean Singleton Delivery and Neonatal Respiratory Outcomes at a Japanese Perinatal Center.* Journal of Nippon Medical School. 2014;81(4):285–8.
9. Chiossi G, et al. Timing *of delivery and adverse outcomes in term singleton repeat cesarean deliveries.* Obstet Gynecol. 2013;121(3):561.
10. Wilmink FA, et al. Neonatal outcome following elective cesarean section beyond 37 weeks of gestation: a 7-year retrospective analysis of a national registry. American journal of obstetrics and gynecology. 2010;202(3):250. e1–8.
11. Patel RR, et al. Does gestation vary by ethnic group? A London-based study of over 122 000 pregnancies with spontaneous onset of labour. Int J Epidemiol. 2004;33(1):107–13.
12. Robinson CJ, et al. Timing of elective repeat cesarean delivery at term and neonatal outcomes: a cost analysis. American journal of obstetrics and gynecology. 2010;202(6):632. e1–6.
13. Daniel S, et al. Comparison of fetal outcomes of emergency and elective caesarean sections in a teaching hospital in Kerala. Academic medical journal of India. 2014;2(1):32–6.
14. Smith GC, Pell JP, Bobbie R. Caesarean section and risk of unexplained stillbirth in subsequent pregnancy. Lancet. 2003;362(9398):1779–84.
15. Wood S, et al. The risk of unexplained antepartum stillbirth in second pregnancies following caesarean section in the first pregnancy. BJOG Int J Obstet Gynaecol. 2008;115(6):726–31.
16. Tita AT, et al. Timing of elective repeat cesarean delivery at term and neonatal outcomes. N Engl J Med. 2009;360(2):111–20.
17. Tita AT, Lai Y, Landon MB, Spong CY, Leveno KJ, Varner MW, et al. Timing of elective repeat cesarean delivery at term and maternal perioperative outcomes. Obstet Gynecol. 2011;117(2 Pt 1):280–6.
18. Zanardo V, et al. *Neonatal respiratory morbidity risk and mode of delivery at term: influence of* timing *of elective caesarean delivery.* Acta Paediatr. 2004; 93(5):643–7.

7

Risk factors for Korean women to develop an isthmocele after a cesarean section

IY Park[1], MR Kim[1], HN Lee[2], Y Gen[2] and MJ Kim[2*]

Abstract

Background: The increase in number of cesarean section (CS) operations has resulted in an increase in cases of isthmocele development. The objective of this study is to determine the risk factors for isthmocele development after CS.

Methods: Isthmocele measurements were taken for 404 women with a history of at least one low transverse CS. The following potential risk factors were investigated: patient's age at CS, cause of CS, weeks of gestation at CS, premature rupture of membrane (PROM), phase of labor, type suture (single/double layer), operation time, uterine flexion (anteversion/retroversion), and blood transfusion during operation. A transvaginal ultrasound was carried out to examine the isthmocele in the uterus after CS, including the shape of the isthmocele, residual myometrial thickness, depth and width of isthmocele, cervical thickness, location of the isthmocele, and clinical characteristics.

Results: In our study population, the isthmocele had a prevalence of 73.8%. Most isthmocele had a triangular (65.4%) or semicircular shape (10.4%). The presence of an isthmocele was significantly associated with repeat CS, premature rupture of membrane (PROM), short operation time, and extent of cervix dilatation at CS. The risk of isthmocele was low in women who had placenta previa totalis (PPT), twin, a long operation time, or a transfusion during the operation.

Conclusions: In our study, isthmocele development was significantly associated with repeat CS, PROM, a short operation time, and the extent of cervix dilatation at CS. Therefore, PROM prevention and a more careful uterine closure are needed to reduce the risk of developing an isthmocele after CS.

Keywords: Cesarean section, Isthmocele, Transvaginal ultrasound, Residual myometrial thickness, Uterine flexion

Background

The number of cesarean section (CS) per 1000 live births in Korea was 380.3 in 2014, which was 1.4 times higher than the average number of CS (264.7 per per 1000 live births) in the Organization for Economic Cooperation and Development (OECD) member countries. It was lower only when compared to that in Turkey (511.3 cases per 1000 live births) [1].

A cesarean-induced isthmocele is a reservoir-like pouch defect on the anterior wall of the uterine isthmus located at the site of a previous cesarean delivery scar [2]. There is no consensus regarding the definition of an isthmocele or a standardized approach for its assessment. The prevalence of an isthmocele in a random population with a history of CS differs between 24 and 70% for transvaginal ultrasound (TVUS) [3]. Although an isthmocele is usually asymptomatic, symptoms related to this condition have been described, and it is a relatively new entity that needs further evaluation.

As the number of CS increases, the number of isthomocele cases has increased, and its associated complications are an important concern. Obstetric complications, such as scar tissue dehiscence, scar pregnancy, and abnormally adherent placenta are associated with this defect. Gynecologic complications due to isthmocele have only recently been identified and described, including abnormal uterine bleeding (postmenstrual spotting), dysmenorrhea, chronic pelvic pain, infertility, adenomyosis, endometriosis, and abscess formation [4]. Three methods exist to conduct a surgical excision of the isthmocele, including hysteroscopic resection, laparoscopic resection and repair with or without robotic assistance, or repair of the isthmocele through vaginal approach [5].

* Correspondence: poouh74@catholic.ac.kr
[2]Department of Obstetrics and Gynecology, College of Medicine, Bucheon St. Mary's Hospital, The Catholic University of Korea, 327 Sosa-ro, Bucheon, Gyeonggi-do 14647, Republic of Korea
Full list of author information is available at the end of the article

An isthmocele is the result of incomplete healing of the isthmic myometrium after a low transverse uterine incision for CS. However, risk factors to develop the isthmocele after CS are currently unknown. Therefore, this study intends to determine the risk factors for isthmocele in the caesarean scars of Korean women who have undergone caesarean section at a single university hospital.

Methods

A case control study was carried out with data collected from January 1, 2009 to November 30, 2016 for women with a history of cesarean section (CS) who were screened with transvaginal ultrasound (TVUS) for various gynecological indications. The exclusion criteria included vertical or inverted "T" uterine incision, congenital uterine malformations, fetal death, sepsis, and insertion of intrauterine device. This study was approved by the Ethics Committee of the Catholic University of Korea (approval number: HC17RESI0044). A sonographic assessment of the isthmocele was performed by a single experienced doctor (MJK) using an Accuvix V20 Prestige ultrasound machine (Samsung Medison Co Ltd. , Seoul, Korea) equipped with a 4–9 MHz transvaginal probe. The isthmocele was diagnosed when a hypoechogenic area (a filling defect) within the myometrium of the lower uterine segment was present at the site of a previous cesarean incision.

The CS operations had been performed by three doctors with more than 5 years of experience with the operation using a unified single or double layer closure technique with a continuous absorbable suture.

The patients' clinical information regarding the factors related to isthmocele were collected from medical records, including gestational and maternal age at CS, height, change of weight, BMI, comorbidity, obstetrical history, operation time, repair of uterine incision, duration of active labor, cervical dilatation at CS, type of uterine flexion, and blood transfusion.

The operation time was defined from the skin incision to baby out and from baby out to skin closure according to the anesthetic records. A repair of the uterine incision was performed as a single layer by two operators and a double layer by one operator.

The duration of active labor was classified as follows: without active labor; < 5 h; 5–9 h; and > 10 h. The extent of cervical dilatation was categorized as the following: cervical os was closed; ≤ 4 cm; 5–7 cm; and ≥ 8 cm.

In this study, the type of isthmocele was categorized into triangle (Fig. 1a), semicircle (Fig. 1b), rectangle (Fig. 1c), circle (Fig. 1d), droplet (Fig. 1e) and inclusion cysts (Fig. 1f), and these types had been used in a previously published study [3].

The isthmocele in the uterus was measured and saved in the longitudinal plane. The residual myometrial

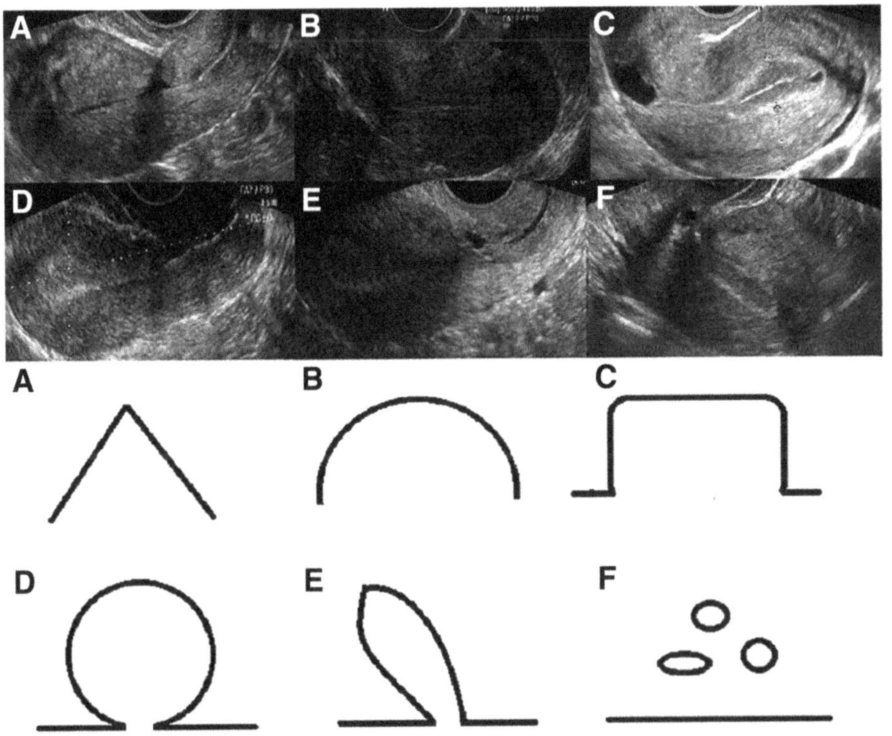

Fig. 1 Transvaginal ultrasonography and schematic diagram demonstrating classification used to assess isthmocele shape as **a** triangle, **b** semicircle, **c** rectangle, **d** circle, **e** droplet and **f** inclusion cysts

thickness (A), depth of the isthmocele (B), width of the isthmocele (C), cervical thickness (D), distance from the uterine fundus to the isthmocele (E), and distance from the isthmocele to the cervix (F) were measured in the sagittal plane (Fig. 2). The residual myometrial thickness (A) was defined as the shortest visible distance in a sagittal plane between the uterine serosal surface and the delineation of the endometrium at the level of the CS scar. TVUS was performed, and the following details of the uterus were recorded: position, length, width, endometrial thickness, and presence of intrauterine fluid.

Statistical analysis

The data are presented as means ± standard deviation or numbers including percentages based on variables characteristics. An independent t-test was performed for continuous variables while a Chi-square test or Fisher's exact test was performed for categorical variables. A multivariable analysis of the relationship between the risk of development of an isthmocele and the baseline characteristics was performed using a backward elimination method. Variables displaying $p < 0.10$ based on a univariable analysis were considered as candidates for inclusion in the multivariable logistic analysis. All statistical analyses were performed using SAS software, version 9.4 (SAS Institute Inc., Cary, NC, USA). A two-sided P value of less than 0.05 was considered to be statistically significant.

Results

The study group included 404 women with a mean age of 33.04 ± 1.63 years. The gestational age at CS varied from 28 to 41 weeks with a median value of 37 gestational weeks. A total of 298 (73.8%) women who underwent CS had an isthmocele (the isthmocele group), and 106 (26.2%) women had no isthmocele (without isthmocele group) with intact caesarean scars, including 231 (57.2%) who had underwent CS once, 138 (34.2%) who had underwent CS twice, 28 (6.9%) who underwent CS three times, and 7 (1.7%) who underwent CS four times.

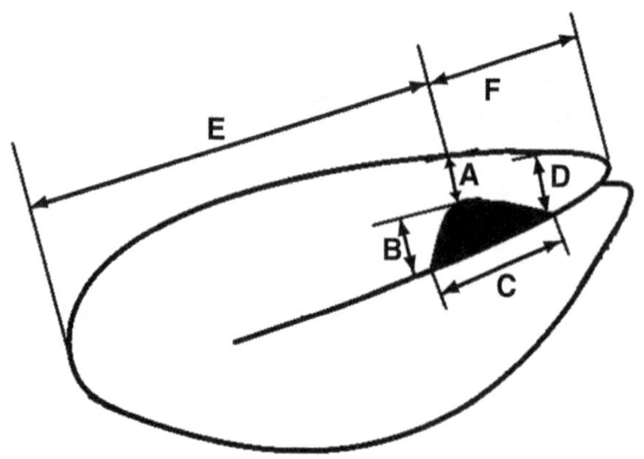

Fig. 2 Schematic diagram demonstrating measurement of isthmocele in the longitudinal plane. **a** Residual myometrial thickness; **b** Depth of isthmocele; **c** Width of isthmocele; **d** Cervical thickness; **e** Distance from uterine fundus to isthmocele; **f** Distance from isthmocele to cervix

Age, height, weight, BMI, ultrasonographic follow up period, and comorbidity were not significantly different between the two groups (isthmocele group and without isthmocele group). There were no significant differences in the number of CS, parity, abortion, or preterm delivery history between the two groups either. The most frequent gynecological symptoms for visiting the hospital after cesarean section were vaginal spotting and pelvic pain (Table 1).

The shape of isthmocele was categorized into the following 6 groups: triangle, 195 (65.4%); semicircular, 31 (10.4%); rectangle, 25 (8.4%); circle, 22 (7.4%); droplet, 13 (4.4%), inclusion cyst 12(4.0%).

The residual myometrial thickness in the group without isthmocele was 3.08 ± 2.67 mm, which was smaller than that in the group with isthmocele (4.87 ± 3.38 mm) without statistical significance ($P = 0.099$). There was no significant difference in the uterine size, endometrial thickness, or isthmocele location between the two groups. Intrauterine fluid was observed in 47% of patients with an isthmocele. The ratio of E/F (E: distance from uterine fundus to isthmocele; F: distance from isthmocele to cervix) was not significantly different according to the extent of the cervical dilatation or the duration of active labor. Therefore, the location of a cervical incision was not a significant factor to develop the isthmocele (Table 2).

Table 3 presents the results of a logistic regression analyzing the associations between isthmocele and the risk factors. The risk of the isthmocele increased with repeat CS (odds ratio/OR: 2.30, 95% CI: 1.26–4.23; $P = 0.007$), PROM (OR: 1.90, 95% CI: 1.08–3.34; $P = 0.027$), cervical dilatation (1–4 cm and 5–7 cm) at CS (OR: 3.04, 95% CI: 1.57–5.92; $P = 0.001$; OR: 13.11; 95% CI: 1.77–97.27; $P = 0.012$, respectively).

The risk of an isthmocele was low in those with placenta previa totalis (PPT) (OR: 0.46, 95% CI: 0.23–0.93; $P = 0.031$), twin (OR: 0.25, 95% CI: 0.11–0.59; $P = 0.001$), long operation time (OR: 0.97, 95% CI: 0.96–0.99; $P = 0.002$), and transfusion (OR: 0.33, 95% CI: 0.14–0.79; $P = 0.013$).

After CS, there was no correlation between the changes in the uterine direction (anterflexion/retroflexion) and the occurrence of an isthmocele (Table 4).

Discussion

An isthmocele is a common incidental finding on TVUS that is usually asymptomatic (the prevalence of a symptomatic isthmocele remains unknown). Morris first described cesarean-delivery scar defects, including utero

Table 1 Baseline characteristics and the risk factors for presence of an isthmocele

	Without Isthmocele	With Isthmocele	*P* value
Number	106	298	
Age (years)	32.64 ± 4.80	33.19 ± 4.19	0.269
Height (cm)	160.16 ± 4.60	160.24 ± 5.62	0.881
Weight (before pregnancy, kg)	56.74 ± 10.40	58.36 ± 11.66	0.207
Weight (during pregnancy, kg)	70.14 ± 11.18	70.61 ± 11.75	0.720
BMI (before pregnancy, kg/m^2)	22.12 ± 3.96	22.71 ± 4.23	0.215
BMI (during pregnancy, kg/m^2)	27.36 ± 4.33	27.47 ± 4.14	0.816
Number of CS (n)	1.43 ± 0.70	1.57 ± 0.70	0.094
Comorbidity (n, %)			
DM	9 (8.5)	30 (10.1)	0.637
Hypertension	14 (13.2)	44 (14.8)	0.695
Parity (n)	1.56 ± 0.74	1.69 ± 0.77	0.127
Preterm experience (n, %)	32 (30.2)	94 (31.5)	0.796
Reason for visiting (n, %)			
Routine examination	65 (61.3)	185 (62.1)	0.890
Vaginal spotting	13 (12.3)	48 (16.1)	0.343
Abnormal uterine bleeding	11 (10.4)	29 (9.7)	0.848
Dysmenorrhea	2 (1.9)	3 (1.0)	0.610
Pelvic pain	14 (13.2)	32 (10.7)	0.492
Sterility	3 (2.8)	1 (0.3)	0.057
Irregular menstruation	3 (2.8)	13 (4.4)	0.772
Follow up period of ultrasound (month)	17.72 ± 25.07	16.38 ± 24.53	0.631
Reason for CS (n, %)			
Repeat CS	34 (32.1)	135 (45.3)	0.018*
Fetal distress	14 (13.2)	41 (13.8)	0.887
PPT	15 (14.2)	21 (7.1)	0.028*
Preeclampsia	11 (10.4)	23 (7.7)	0.397
Breech	15 (14.2)	25 (8.4)	0.088
Twin	13 (12.3)	10 (3.4)	0.001*
Arrest of descent	5 (4.7)	19 (6.4)	0.535
Arrest of dilatation	1 (0.9)	5 (1.7)	1.000
PROM (n, %)	18 (17.0)	83 (28.0)	0.025*
Type of CS (n, %)			
Elective CS	59 (55.7)	137 (46.0)	0.087
Emergency CS	47 (44.3)	161 (54.0)	
Gestational weeks	36.72 ± 2.58	36.87 ± 2.74	0.626
Birth weight (g)	2861.9 ± 691.4	2895.2 ± 720.7	0.680
Operation time (total, min)	56.69 ± 18.27	51.88 ± 15.75	0.010*
From skin incision to baby out	7.91 ± 5.14	6.78 ± 4.43	0.032*
From baby out to skin closure	48.78 ± 15.42	45.10 ± 13.66	0.022*
Repair of uterine incision (n, %)			0.579
Single layer	68 (64.2)	200 (67.1)	
Double layer	38 (35.9)	98 (32.9)	

Table 1 Baseline characteristics and the risk factors for presence of an isthmocele *(Continued)*

	Without Isthmocele	With Isthmocele	*P* value
Induction of labor (n, %)	15 (14.2)	55 (18.5)	0.315
Oxytocin augmentation during labor (n, %)	12 (11.3)	56 (18.8)	0.077
Duration of active labor (n, %)			0.218
not in active labor	75 (70.8)	177 (59.6)	
< 5 h	15 (14.2)	62 (20.9)	
5–9	4 (3.8)	18 (6.1)	
≥10 h	12(11.3)	40(13.5)	
With uterine contractions (n, %)	38 (35.9)	137 (46.0)	0.071
Cervical dilatation at CS (n, %)			0.057
closed	72 (67.9)	163 (54.7)	
≤ 4 cm	25 (23.6)	95 (31.9)	
5–7 cm	2 (1.9)	20 (6.7)	
≥ 8 cm	7 (6.6)	20 (6.7)	
Interval of previous CS (years)	1.64 ± 3.14	1.81 ± 2.56	0.610
Uterine position at ultrasound (n, %)			0.205
anteversion	31 (29.3)	114 (38.3)	
retroversion	7 (6.6)	13 (4.4)	

Independent t test was performed for continuous variables, Chi-square test or Fisher's exact test was performed for categorical variables
BMI body mass index, *CS* cesarean section, *PPT* placenta previa totalis, *PROM* premature rupture of membrane
[*] $P < 0.05$ was considered statistically significant

peritoneal fistula, niche, and isthmocele in 1995 [5]. Ofili-Yebovi et al. [6] described this finding as a "detectable myometrial thinning at the site of the Cesarean section scar". This defect is also referred to as a "cesarean scar defect", "uterine scar defect", "uterine diverticulum", "niche", "isthmocele", "pouch", or "sacculation" [7].

When diagnosing an isthmocele, an important consideration is whether a radiologic identification correlates with clinical symptoms. Patients with an isthmocele often present spotting after menstruation due to the accumulation of blood in the defect of the uterus. The best time to perform TVUS is in the early follicular phase when the accumulation of blood within the defect enables its detection [8]. Some women with isthmocele also experience pelvic pain, vaginal discharge, dysmenorrhea, and dyspareunia.

Table 2 Characteristics of isthmocele shape

	Without Isthmocele	With Isthmocele	*P* value
Endometrial thickness (mm)	5.48 ± 3.26	5.90 ± 3.00	0.228
Uterine length (mm)	77.24 ± 13.16	77.91 ± 11.15	0.641
Uterine width (mm)	43.29 ± 8.29	43.33 ± 6.83	0.967
Isthmocele size (mm)			
A[a]	3.08 ± 2.67	4.87 ± 3.38	0.099
B[b]	2.72 ± 2.74	4.18 ± 2.41	0.093
C[c]	1.62 ± 1.70	6.24 ± 3.48	<.001[*]
D[d]	9.31 ± 2.98	9.95 ± 3.13	0.191
E[e]	50.06 ± 9.19	51.65 ± 9.68	0.145
F[f]	27.03 ± 6.76	26.83 ± 7.42	0.814
Ratio (E/F)	1.97 ± 0.63	2.11 ± 0.85	0.076

[a] Residual myometrial thickness
[b] Depth of isthmocele
[c] Width of isthmocele
[d] Cervical thickness
[e] Distance from uterine fundus to isthmocele
[f] Distance from isthmocele to cervix
[*] $P < 0.05$ was considered statistically significant

Table 3 Association between isthmocele and demographic background variables

	Univariable		Multivariable	
	Odds ratio (95% CI)	*P* value	OR (95% CI)	*P* value
Age (years)	1.03 (0.98–1.08)	0.268		
Number of CS	1.34 (0.95–1.88)	0.095		
BMI (before pregnancy)	1.04 (0.98–1.10)	0.216		
BMI (during pregnancy)	1.01 (0.95–1.06)	0.815		
Parity	1.27 (0.93–1.72)	0.128		
Preterm experience	1.07 (0.66–1.72)	0.796		
Reason for CS				
Repeat CS	1.75 (1.10–2.80)	0.019*	2.30 (1.26–4.23)	0.007*
Fetal distress	1.05 (0.55–2.01)	0.888		
PPT	0.46 (0.23–0.93)	0.031*		
Preeclampsia	0.72 (0.34–1.54)	0.399		
Breech	0.56 (0.28–1.10)	0.091		
Twin	0.25 (0.11–0.59)	0.001*	0.25 (0.11–0.59)	0.001*
Arrest of descent	1.38 (0.50–3.78)	0.537		
Arrest of dilatation	1.79 (0.21–15.52)	0.596		
PROM	1.90 (1.08–3.34)	0.027*		
Type of CS				
Elective CS	Reference		Reference	
Emergency CS	1.48 (0.95–2.30)	0.087		
Pregnancy (weeks)	1.02 (0.94–1.11)	0.625		
Birth weight	1.00 (1.00–1.00)	0.679		
Operation time (total, min)	0.98 (0.97–1.00)	0.011*	0.97 (0.96–0.99)	0.002*
From skin incision to baby out	0.95 (0.91–1.00)	0.037		
From baby out to skin closure	0.98 (0.97–1.00)	0.024		
Repair of uterine incision				
Single layer	Reference		Reference	
Double layer	0.88 (0.55–1.40)	0.579		
Induction of labor	1.37 (0.74–2.55)	0.316		
Oxytocin augmentation during labor	1.81 (0.93–3.53)	0.081		
Duration of active labor		0.224		
not in active labor	Reference		Reference	
< 5 h	1.75 (0.94–3.27)	0.079		
5–9 h	1.91 (0.62–5.82)	0.257		
≥ 10 h	1.41 (0.70–2.84)	0.333		
With uterine contractions	1.52 (0.96–2.41)	0.072		
Cervical dilatation at CS		0.072		0.002*
closed	Reference		Reference	
≤ 4 cm	1.68 (1.00–2.83)	0.051	3.04 (1.57–5.92)	0.001*
5–7 cm	4.41 (1.01–19.37)	0.049	13.11 (1.77–97.27)	0.012*
≥ 8 cm	1.26 (0.51–3.12)	0.614	2.04 (0.71–5.91)	0.188
Ratio (E/F)	1.27 (0.94–1.72)	0.124		
Blood transfusion	0.33 (0.14–0.79)	0.013*		

Multivariable logistic regression model was performed by backward elimination methods. Because of missing data, some isthmocele variables were not calculated
*$P < 0.05$ was considered statistically significant

Table 4 Relationship between the presence of isthmocele and change in uterine flexion from early pregnancy to post CS state

	Without Isthmocele ($n = 38$)	With Isthmocele ($n = 127$)	P value
Flexion changed	8 (21.1%)	37 (27.1%)	0.326
from A to P	8 (21.1%)	33 (26.0%)	0.537
from P to A	0 (0.0%)	4 (3.2%)	0.575
Flexion did not change	30 (79.0%)	90 (70.9%)	0.326
from A to A	23 (60.5%)	81 (63.8%)	0.716
from P to P	7 (18.4%)	9 (7.1%)	0.057

Comparisons of data were performed by Chi-squared test and significance was considered at $P < 0.05$
A Anteflexion
P Retroflexion

The most ischemic process change and slowest absorbable suture might be the worst combination, and they are more likely to produce isthmocele. The occurrence of a defective uterine scar after cesarean section depends on multiple factors, including the degree of cervical dilatation and possibly the contractile effort of the uterine musculature, resulting in thinning at the uterine incision site [2].

Between 2009 and 2014, the number of CS per 1000 births per 1000 OECD populations increased by 18.1. In Korea, there was an increase of 16.5 between 2009 and 2013 (OECD Health Statistics 2017, Ministry of Health and Welfare). As the number of cesarean deliveries increases, efforts are needed to reduce isthmocele-related complications after cesarean section.

The diagnosis of isthmocele is based on TVUS or hysteroscopy. The use of TVUS to diagnose a cesarean scar was reported in 1990, with the following four key sonographic findings: a wedge defect, inward protruding of the scar, outward protruding and hematoma, or retraction of the scar [9]. Others have described a cesarean scar on TVUS as a triangular anechoic area with the apex pointing anterior or a filling defect on the anterior isthmus [4, 8]. In our study, the type of isthmocele in TVUS was divided into triangle (65.4%), semicircle, rectangle, circle, and droplet and inclusion cysts.

The prevalence of isthmocele ranges from 24 to 70% when assessed by TVUS and from 56 to 84% when assessed by sonohysterography [10]. The frequency of the isthmocele on an ultrasonography was 73.8% in a random population of Korean women with a history of CS in the present study.

The occurrence of isthmocele was not associated with maternal age, change of BMI, parity, or preterm experience in our study. However, some studies reported that isthmocele development is associated with age, BMI, preeclampsia, post-operative anemia and WBC count [11, 12].

A history of multiple cesarean deliveries is associated with wider and larger isthmocele as the main risk factor for isthmocele development [4, 6, 11, 12]. However, our study showed different results. Although the risk of an isthmocele increased when repeated cesarean section was performed (OR: 2.30, 95% CI: 1.26–4.23, $P = 0.007$), the number of CS did not increase the risk of isthmocele (OR: 1.34, 95% CI: 0.95–1.88, $P = 0.095$). An isthmocele was more frequent in the group with repeated cesarean section than in that with its first CS operation, and it was not related to the increase in the number of cesarean section. Therefore, reducing CS incidence is an important factor to reduce the risk of isthmocele.

PROM is a major risk factor of infection and is known to weaken healing in uterus closure [12, 13]. PROM patients might have an immature lower segment of the uterus, which might be detrimental to uterine suture and wound healing. Hayakawa et al. [13] reported that premature rupture of the membranes increases the risk of isthmocele. Our study also showed that the risk of isthmocele increased by 1.9 (95% CI: 1.08–3.34) in those with PROM. Therefore, appropriate management should be taken to prevent infection and to facilitate proper healing and remodeling of the myometrial incision if PROM is accompanied during delivery.

Emergency CS and the presence of labor are not risk factors for the presence of an isthmocele [13, 14]. Our results also indicated that emergency surgery and coexisting uterine contractions did not increase the risk of isthmocele.

During cesarean section, a uterine suture can be performed using the single- or double-layer method. The relationship between the different types of uterine closure and the prevalence of cesarean scar defects is currently unclear. A prospective cohort study reported that large niches are more frequent in women with one-layer uterine closure (90.9%) when compared to those in a two-layer closure (9.1%) [15]. However, the difference was not statistically significant [15]. In our study, 268 cases (66.3%) were sutured in a single layer and 136 cases (33.7%) were performed in a double layer. The OR for isthmocele development was 0.88 (0.55–1.40) in the double-layer suture, which was not statistically significant.

A cesarean section during active labor with cervical dilatation over 5 cm is associated with a large cesarean scar defect [15]. The association between a low uterine incision and the development of a niche during active labor can be explained by a thin myometrium and impaired healing [10, 15, 16]. The risk of a large niche increases if the station of the presenting part of the fetus at CS is below the pelvic inlet, cervical dilatation is ≥5 cm, or duration of labor was ≥5 h [15]. Incomplete healing of the uterine scars in cases of CSs performed during advanced labor might be a result of the incision through cervical tissue because the cervix becomes incorporated into the lower uterine segment in the physiological process of cervical effacement [17]. In the present study, the risk of isthmocele increased when the uterine cervix was dilated to less than 7 cm. However, when the cervix was dilated to more than 8 cm, it did not increase the risk of isthmocele. The operator might have intentionally performed the incision at the upper side when the uterine cervix was completely dilated. Although those without a scar defect had a significantly higher scar location above the internal cervical os than those with a scar defect [18], the cause of this result is unclear. The effect of the location of the incision in the uterus might be difficult to study, so further research is needed to confirm the hypothesis that the cervical location of the uterine scar impairs wound healing.

For the first time, this study investigated the association between isthmocele risk and the operation time based on the anesthetic record. The operating time was divided into skin incision to baby out and baby out to skin closure. The multivariate logistic analysis showed that the isthmocele was less occurred with a longer operation time (OR: 0.97, 95% CI: 0.96–0.99, $P = 0.002$). Shortening the operation time seems to affect the occurrence of an isthmocele. Although a definite mechanism for this is uncertain, a more careful uterine closure and bleeding control may be important if the procedure is performed over a short period of time.

In our study, repeat CS, PROM, the extent of cervical dilatation at CS, and short operation time were factors associated with the occurrence of isthmocele whereas PPT, twin, and blood transfusion during operation did not increase the risk of isthmocele. Although PPT, cervical lacerations and extensive blood loss (blood transfusion) causing surgical difficulties could affect the healing process of the myometrial incision site, more careful attention (by the operator) during procedures could be performed. Manipulations such as uterine suture, bleeding control, and uterotonics (carbetocin, methergine, oxytocin etc.) decreased the incidence of an isthmocele. However, transfusions only occurred in 21 cases (small sample size), and this is a limitation of our study, so further study is needed.

The association between a retroverted uterus and isthmocele occurrence or extent was evaluated in other studies [4, 6, 11, 12]. A suggested explanation for this association is that the hysterotomy in a retroverted uterus might have greater tension during healing, leading to mechanical traction and impaired perfusion [6]. A change in the uterine flexion after CS could be due to surgery-related factors, such as a low (cervical) location of the uterine incision during CS, incomplete closure of the uterine wall due to single-layer suture, endometrial saving closure technique or the use of locking sutures, and surgical activities that may induce adhesion formation [18]. It is currently unclear whether a retroflexed uterus that causes the scar to heal improperly is a reason or the retroflection is the result of isthmocele itself due to the lack of support of the corpus by the incomplete closure of the uterine wall. Our results revealed no relationship between the flexion of the uterus and the occurrence of isthmocele in preoperative or postoperative changes.

It is not known whether an isthmocele during an ultrasound examination in nonpregnant women developed a greater risk for complications in subsequent pregnancies than intact scars, or whether large defects are related to greater risk compared to small defects.

Treatment of symptomatic women with an isthmocele ranges from hormonal treatment to hysterectomy, and a failure of hormonal treatment for abnormal uterine bleeding in women with isthmocele eventually required surgical treatment. However, there has been no evidence that surgical correction for an isthmocele improves obstetric outcomes [17].

Although the most important thing to reduce the incidence of isthmocele is to reduce the incidence of CS, it is important to know which factors impair proper wound healing in order to prevent the formation of an isthmocele when CS is needed. The results of this study could be used to guide future research to elucidate the etiology of isthmocele development. A standard definition of an isthmocele and an assessment method should be defined in the future to enable meta-analyses and further research on risk factors to prevent isthmocele development.

Conclusion

In conclusion, the presence of an isthmocele was significantly associated with repeat CS, PROM, short operation time, and extent of cervix dilatation at CS. However, the risk of isthmocele was low in women who had PPT, twin, long operation time, or transfusion during operation. Considering the increasing incidence of cesarean section, PROM prevention, longer operation time, and more careful uterine closure are needed to reduce the risk isthmocele development after CS.

Abbreviations

CS: Cesarean section; OR: Odds ratio; PPT: Placenta previa totalis; PROM: Premature rupture of membrane; TVUS: Transvaginal ultrasound

Funding
The statistical consultation (interpretation of data) was supported by a grant (HC14C1062) of the Korea Health Technology R&D Project through the Korea Health Industry Development Institute (KHIDI) funded by the Ministry of Health & Welfare, Republic of Korea.

Authors' contributions
IYP, MJK –designed the study concept and wrote the manuscript. MRK, HNL-interpreted data, statistical analysis of the results. MJK, YG contributed to data analysis. All authors read and approved the final manuscript.

Competing interests
The authors declare that they have no competing interests.

Author details
[1]Department of Obstetrics and Gynecology, College of Medicine, Seoul St. Mary's Hospital, The Catholic University of Korea, Seoul, Republic of Korea. [2]Department of Obstetrics and Gynecology, College of Medicine, Bucheon St. Mary's Hospital, The Catholic University of Korea, 327 Sosa-ro, Bucheon, Gyeonggi-do 14647, Republic of Korea.

References
1. OECD. Caesarean sections. 2017. https://data.oecd.org/healthcare/caesarean-sections.htm. Accessed 31 Oct 2017.
2. Florio P, Filippeschi M, Moncini I, Marra E, Franchini M, Gubbini G. Hysteroscopic treatment of the cesarean-induced isthmocele in restoring infertility. Curr Opin Obstet Gynecol. 2012;24:180–6.
3. Marjolein Bij de Vaate AJ, Linskens IH, van der Voet LF, Twisk JW, Brölmann HA, Huirne JA. Reproducibility of three-dimensional ultrasound for the measurement of a niche in a caesarean scar and assessment of its shape. Eur J Obstet Gynecol Reprod Biol. 2015;188:39–44.
4. Tower AM, Frishman GN. Cesarean scar defects: an underrecognized cause of abnormal uterine bleeding and other gynecologic complications. J Minim Invasive Gynecol. 2013;20:562–72.
5. Nezhat C, Falik R, Li A. Surgical management of niche, isthmocele, uteroperitoneal fistula, or cesarean scar defect: a critical rebirth in the medical literature. Fertil Steril. 2017;107:69–71.
6. Ofili-Yebovi D, Ben-Nagi J, Sawyer E, Yazbek J, Lee C, Gonzalez J, et al. Deficient lower-segment cesarean section scars: prevalence and risk factors. Ultrasound Obstet Gynecol. 2008;31:72–7.
7. Raimondo G, Grifone G, Raimondo D, Seracchioli R, Scambia G, Masciullo V. Hysteroscopic treatment of symptomatic cesarean-induced isthmocele: a prospective study. J Minim Invasive Gynecol. 2015;22:297–301.
8. Fabres C, Aviles G, De La Jara C, Escalona J, Munoz JF, Mackenna A, et al. The cesarean delivery scar pouch: clinical implications and diagnostic correlation between transvaginal sonography and hysteroscopy. J Ultrasound Med. 2003;22:695–700. quiz 1-2
9. Chen HY, Chen SJ, Hsieh FJ. Observation of cesarean section scar by transvaginal ultrasonography. Ultrasound Med Biol. 1990;16:443–7.
10. Bij de Vaate AJ, van der Voet LF, Naji O, Witmer M, Veersema S, Brolmann HA, et al. Prevalence, potential risk factors for development and symptoms related to the presence of uterine niches following cesarean section: systematic review. Ultrasound Obstet Gynecol. 2014;43:372–82.
11. Osser OV, Jokubkiene L, Valentin L. High prevalence of defects in cesarean section scars at transvaginal ultrasound examination. Ultrasound Obstet Gynecol. 2009;34:90–7.
12. Chen Y, Han P, Wang YJ, Li YX. Risk factors for incomplete healing of the uterine incision after cesarean section. Arch Gynecol Obstet. 2017;296:355–61.
13. Hayakawa H, Itakura A, Mitsui T, Okada M, Suzuki M, Tamakoshi K, et al. Methods for myometrium closure and other factors impacting effects on cesarean section scars of the uterine segment detected by the ultrasonography. Acta Obstet Gynecol Scand. 2006;85:429–34.
14. Yazicioglu F, Gokdogan A, Kelekci S, Aygun M, Savan K. Incomplete healing of the uterine incision after caesarean section: is it preventable? Eur J Obstet Gynecol Reprod Biol. 2006;124:32–6.
15. Vikhareva Osser O, Valentin L. Risk factors for incomplete healing of the uterine incision after caesarean section. BJOG. 2010;117:1119–26.
16. Tulandi T, Cohen A. Emerging manifestations of cesarean scar defect in reproductive-aged women. J Minim Invasive Gynecol. 2016;23:893–902.
17. Vervoort AJ, Uittenbogaard LB, Hehenkamp WJ, Brölmann HA, Mol BW, Huirne JA. Why do niches develop in caesarean uterine scars? Hypotheses on the aetiology of niche development. Hum Reprod. 2015;30:2695–702.
18. Pomorski M, Fuchs T, Rosner-Tenerowicz A, Zimmer M. Morphology of the cesarean section scar in the non-pregnant uterus after one elective cesarean section. Ginekol Pol. 2017;88:174–9.

Association between first caesarean delivery and adverse outcomes in subsequent pregnancy

Hong-Tao Hu[1†], Jing-Jing Xu[1†], Jing Lin[1], Cheng Li[1], Yan-Ting Wu[2], Jian-Zhong Sheng[3], Xin-Mei Liu[4,5*] and He-Feng Huang[2,4,5*]

Abstract

Background: Few studies have explored the association between a previous caesarean section (CS) and adverse perinatal outcomes in a subsequent pregnancy, especially in women who underwent a non-indicated CS in their first delivery. We designed this study to compare the perinatal outcomes of a subsequent pregnancy in women who underwent spontaneous vaginal delivery (SVD) or CS in their first delivery.

Methods: This retrospective cohort study included women who underwent singleton deliveries at the International Peace Maternity and Child Health Hospital from January 2013 to December 2016. Data on the perinatal outcomes of all the women were extracted from the medical records. Multivariate logistic regression was conducted to assessed the association between CS in the first delivery and adverse perinatal outcomes in the subsequent pregnancy.

Results: CS delivery in the subsequent pregnancy was more likely for women who underwent CS in their first birth than for women with previous SVD (97.3% versus 13.2%). CS in the first birth was also associated with a significantly increased risk of adverse outcomes in the subsequent pregnancy, especially in women who underwent a non-indicated CS. Adverse perinatal outcomes included pregnancy-induced hypertension [adjusted odds ratio (OR), 95% confidence interval (CI): 2.20, 1.59–3.05], gestational diabetes mellitus (1.82, 1.57–2.11), gestational anaemia (1.27, 1.05–1.55), placenta previa (3.18, 2.15–4.71), placenta accreta (2.75, 1.75–4.31), and polyhydramnios (2.60, 1.57–4.31) in the mother and preterm delivery (1.37, 1.06–1.78), low birth weight (3.78, 2.07–6.90), macrosomia (5.04, 3.95–6.44), and neonatal jaundice (1.72, 1.39–2.14) in the baby.

Conclusions: CS in the first delivery markedly increases the risk of repeated CS and maternal-fetal complications in the subsequent pregnancy, especially in women with a non-indicated CS.

Keywords: Cohort, Pregnancy outcomes, Caesarean delivery, Subsequent pregnancy

* Correspondence: nanlilac@hotmail.com; huanghefg@sjtu.edu.cn

[†]Hong-Tao Hu and Jing-Jing Xu contributed equally to this work.

[4]Institute of Embryo-Fetal Original Adult Disease, Shanghai Key Laboratory for Reproductive Medicine, School of Medicine, Shanghai Jiao Tong University, Shanghai, China

[2]Department of Reproductive Medicine, International Peace Maternity and Child Health Hospital, School of Medicine, Shanghai Jiao Tong University, Shanghai, China

Full list of author information is available at the end of the article

Background

The high prevalence of caesarean section (CS) is a global public health issue. According to a WHO statement in 1985, regional CS rates should not exceed 10–15% [1, 2]. However, the rate of CS has markedly increased from approximately 6 to 40% in low, medium and high income countries in the past three decades [3–6]. China has a high rate of CS as well as CS without medical indication [4, 6]. Between 1988 and 2010, caesarean rates in all of China rose from 3.4 to 52.5%, while urban rates increased from 10 to 57% [7, 8]. Maternal request and previous CS are the most common indications for CS in mainland China [9]. According to a large, cross-sectional study of 496,054 caesarean deliveries, the prevalence of primary non-indicated CS increased from 0.6% in 1993–1995 to 21.3% in 2006–2010 [10]. Other studies have reported national rates of non-indicated CS ranging from 28.43 to 38.1% in China [9, 11]. Prior CS is an important factor in the determination of a subsequent CS, which has led to overall high CS rates [6]. As implementation of China's 'two-child policy' has triggered the next baby boom, many women with a previous CS might require repeated CS in their subsequent deliveries [9, 12]. Thus, the adverse outcomes in subsequent pregnancies for Chinese women with a previous CS must be further surveyed.

Although CS is accepted as a fairly safe procedure, and the overall rates of CS complications have decreased during the last decade [13], CS is still associated with an increased risk of maternal complications. According to recent data up to 2015, the WHO announced that CS rates higher than 10% were not associated with reductions in maternal and newborn mortality rates at the population level [2, 14, 15]. The WHO global survey indicated that caesarean delivery was positively associated with an increased risk of postpartum antibiotic use, maternal morbidity and mortality, and fetal and neonatal morbidity [3, 4]. Furthermore, prior CS was significantly associated with a deficit in subsequent fertility [16–19] and an increased risk of unexplained stillbirth in the subsequent pregnancy [20, 21]. Repeated CS was reported to increase maternal morbidity, including placenta accreta, reduced fetal growth, preterm delivery, pelvic pain, and adverse reproductive effects [22, 23]. However, few studies [24–27] of the Chinese population have explored the association between previous CS and adverse perinatal outcomes in a subsequent pregnancy, especially in women with a first non-indicated CS. Thus, we designed this study to compare the perinatal outcomes of subsequent pregnancies in women with a first spontaneous vaginal delivery to those with a CS.

Methods

Data source

The data for this study were obtained from the databases of the International Peace Maternity and Child Health Hospital. The perinatal database contains pregnancy, delivery, and pregnancy outcome data for all births submitted as paper copies of the delivery record or through an electronic extract in this hospital. Validation was performed on the data to check for errors and inconsistencies in documentation and coding. This study was performed in accordance with the declaration of Helsinki. Complications related to pregnancy and delivery, as well as related co-morbidities, were coded using criteria taken from the 9th and 10th revisions of the International Classification of Diseases (ICD-9 and -10).

Study population

In this retrospective study, we included all parous women who underwent a singleton delivery at the International Peace Maternity and Child Health Hospital from January 2013 to December 2016. Subjects with missing information on the previous mode of delivery, with multiple pregnancies in the first birth, or with parity over twice were excluded. To reduce heterogeneity of the study population, women were respectively excluded due to their foreign nationality and first instrumental vaginal delivery. We ultimately included women with spontaneous vaginal delivery (SVD group) and those with CS (CS group) in the first delivery into the analysis.

Study design and definitions

A retrospective cohort study design was used, and there were two groups according to the first mode of delivery in the cohorts. In consideration of the effects of indications for first CS on the next pregnancy, a subgroup analysis was performed between the previous SVD group and previous non-indicated CS group. Potential confounders were extracted, including birth place, nationality, insurance, marital status, age at second delivery, height, body mass index (BMI), education level, gravidity, and interpregnancy interval. Age was given in completed years at the time of delivery and was further subgrouped into < 25, 25–29, 30–34, 35–39, and ≥ 40 years. Height was classified into < 155, 155–164.9, 165–174.9, and ≥ 175 cm. BMI was calculated by dividing antenatal booking weight (kg) by height squared (m) and was then recoded into the following five categories: < 18.5, 18.5 to 24.9, 25 to 29.9, and ≥ 30 kg/m^2. Educational level was given as the higher level of the couple, which was divided into five groups (≤9, 10–12, 13–15, and ≥ 16 years). Interpregnancy interval (< 1, 1–3, 3–5, 5–10, and ≥ 10 years) was defined as the time elapsed from the date of the first delivery to the date of subsequent conception adjusted by ultrasound with the unit of measurement recorded in years. In terms of outcomes at first birth, women with pregnancy-induced hypertension (PIH), preeclampsia (PE), gestational diabetes mellitus (GDM), preterm delivery, low birth weight (LBW), macrosomia, or stillbirths in the first birth were compared in groups to assess differences.

In the second pregnancy, the following outcomes were assessed: PIH (diastolic blood pressure > 90 mmHg on two occasions 4 h apart or a single reading of > 110 mmHg from 20 weeks gestation), PE (PIH and proteinuria 0.3 g/24 h) [28, 29], GDM (diagnosed using a 2-h, 75 g oral glucose tolerance test) [30], gestational anaemia (anaemia occurred in subsequent pregnancy, excluding haematological diseases and history of anaemia), gestational thyroid dysfunction (thyroid dysfunction existed during the subsequent pregnancy, excluding surgery history of the thyroid, prior diagnosis of thyroid diseases, and taking medicines that influence thyroid function), intrahepatic cholestasis of pregnancy (ICP), premature rupture of membranes (PROM, defined as rupture of fetal membranes at least 1 h prior to the onset of labour) [31], fetal distress, meconium-staining of the amniotic fluid, amniotic fluid volume (AFV), placental abruption and placenta previa (placental abruption was defined as premature separation of a normally implanted placenta from the uterus, while placenta previa was defined as implantation of the placenta over or near the internal opening of the cervix), placenta accreta (placenta accreta refers to the entire spectrum of conditions, including accreta, increta, and percreta, as well as to cases of clinically apparent morbidly adherent placenta) [32, 33], rupture of the uterus, antepartum haemorrhage (APH), fetal growth restriction (FGR), abnormal fetal position, dystocia, antepartum fever, mode of delivery (spontaneous vaginal, instrumental, or CS) in subsequent pregnancy, postpartum haemorrhage (PPH; blood loss > 500 ml for vaginal delivery, > 1000 ml for caesarean), and puerperal infection. Neonatal outcomes included stillbirth (delivery of a dead baby at or after 24^{+0} weeks gestation), preterm (24^{+0} to 36^{+6} weeks of gestation), LBW (< 2500 g), macrosomia (> 4000 g), Apgar score at 1 min, neonatal infection, neonatal death (death of a liveborn infant in the first 4 weeks of life), admission to a neonatal intensive care unit, neonatal respiratory distress syndrome (NRDS), transient tachypnea of newborn (TTN), neonatal jaundice, and birth injury.

The primary indications for CS were divided into 3 categories: maternal indications, fetal indications, and maternal request with no obstetric reasons. To clarify these indications, we divided caesarean deliveries into 2 categories, medically indicated or non-medically indicated [11]. Medically indicated CS included fetal distress; prolonged labour (dystocia); cephalopelvic disproportion; malpresentation; PE or eclampsia; haemolysis, elevated liver enzyme, and low platelets syndrome (HELLP); ICP; placental abruption; placenta praevia; scarred uterus; oligohydramnios; intrauterine infection; and suspected macrosomia. Non-medically indicated CS was defined as a primary CS done on maternal request without medical indication (CDMR) or a physician documented "social influence". These included: elderly primigravida as the only indication, a "precious" infant-defined as in vitro pregnancy or poor obstetric history, severe myopia, isolated PROM without fetal heart rate (FHR) abnormalities, request for concomitant myomectomy or ovarian cystectomy, or other factors (isolated chronic hypertension; gestational hypertension; diabetes mellitus without macrosomia).

Statistical analyses

Statistical analyses were performed using SPSS version 20 software (IBM, SPSS Statistics, Armonk, NY, USA). Descriptive statistics were reported as the means and standard deviations for continuous variables and percentages for categorical variables. Differences in demographics and first birth outcomes in the cohorts were assessed using the Pearson Chi-square test or Fisher's exact test. Odds ratios (ORs) with their 95% confidence intervals (CIs) were calculated to evaluate the association between CS in the first delivery and perinatal outcomes in the subsequent pregnancy via univariate (unadjusted for covariates) and multivariate statistical methods (adjusted for potential confounders to ascertain that relationships were due to demographic characteristics or adverse obstetric events). Variables found to be statistically significant in univariate analysis and confirmed as a risk factor by published literature were entered into the multivariate logistic regression model. Statistical significance was set at $P < 0.05$.

Results

In total, 59,831 singleton births were recorded in the International Peace Maternity and Child Health Hospital between January 2013 and December 2016, and 12,390 who had a delivery history were treated as potential subjects. After excluding 49 women with missing information on the previous mode of delivery, 21 women with multiple pregnancies in the first birth, 329 women with parity over twice, 136 women with foreign nationality, and 187 women with instrumental vaginal delivery in the first birth, 11,662 subjects were included into the final analysis (6240 in the SVD group and 5422 in the CS group). Among the 5422 women in the CS group, 3595 (66.3%) women had medical indications for CS, and 1827 (33.7%) women had no medical indications for CS in their first birth (Fig. 1).

The demographic characteristics among the groups are compared in Table 1. Significant differences were

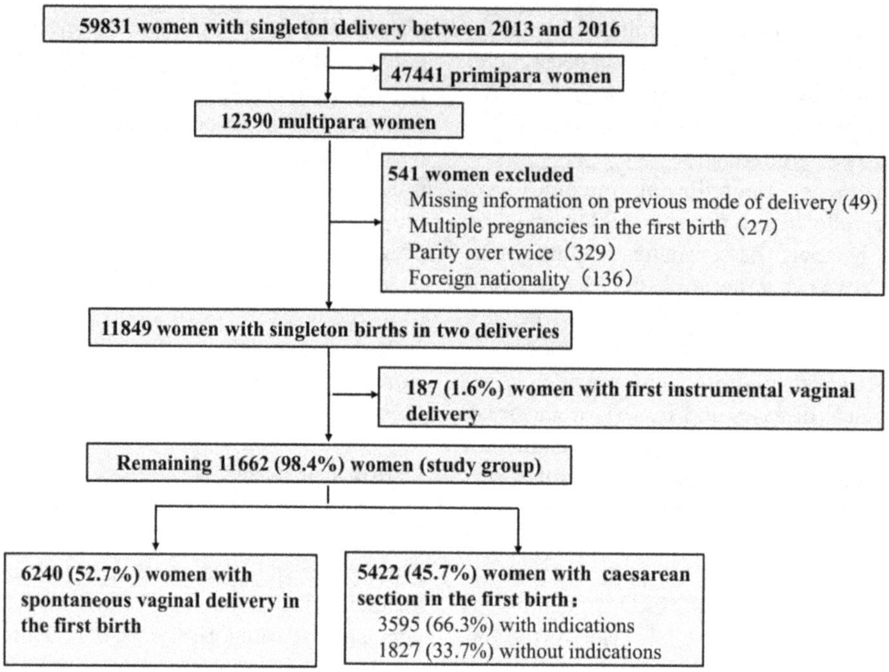

Fig. 1 Flow chart showing study population in cohorts

detected when comparing the CS group with the SVD group, including insurance, age at the subsequent delivery, height, maternal BMI, educational level, gravidity, and interpregnancy interval, while no differences in race were observed.

A comparison of the characteristics of the first birth is presented in Table 1. Women with an initial caesarean delivery were significantly more likely to have macrosomia (first CS group vs. first SVD group: 10.5% vs. 4.5%; $P < 0.001$) in the first birth than those in the SVD group. In contrast, women with an initial CS were less likely to have preterm delivery (first CS group vs. first SVD group: 3.5% vs. 4.3%; $P = 0.027$) and stillbirths (first CS group vs. first SVD group: 0.2% vs 1.0%; $P < 0.001$) in the first birth than those in the SVD group. There were no differences between the two groups in PIH, PE, GDM, or LBW in the first birth. However, there were significant differences in all first birth outcomes when comparing previous non-indicated CS to previous SVD.

Table 2 displays the associations between caesarean delivery in the first birth and maternal outcomes in the subsequent pregnancy, and the percentages of maternal outcomes are presented in Fig. 2a. After adjusting for potential confounders, women with previous CS were 1.38 times more likely to have PIH (95% CI: 1.04–1.82), 1.15 times more likely to have GDM (95% CI: 1.02–1.29), 1.72 times more likely to have ICP (95% CI: 1.04–2.84), 2.50 times more likely to have polyhydramnios (95% CI: 1.69–3.69), 2.11 times more likely to have placenta previa (95% CI: 1.52–2.94), 2.11 times more likely to have placenta accreta (95% CI: 1.47–3.04), 364.21 times more likely to choose caesarean delivery (95% CI: 294.74–450.06), and 8.3 times more likely to suffer instrumental vaginal delivery (95% CI: 4.41–15.6) in the next pregnancy. In contrast, the previous CS women were 66% less likely to have PROM (95% CI: 0.30–0.39), 67% less likely to suffer from fetal distress (95% CI: 0.27–0.40), 51 and 85% less likely to have moderate or severe meconium-staining of the amniotic fluid (95% CI: 0.39–0.62 and 0.11–0.19, respectively), respectively, and 46% less likely to have antepartum fever (95% CI: 0.33–0.89) in the next pregnancy. Given the risk of the first CS with medical indications in the subsequent pregnancy, we performed a subgroup analysis of pregnancy outcomes in women who did not have indications in the first delivery. In this subgroup, women with previous non-indication CS were more likely to experience PIH (adjusted OR: 2.20; 95% CI: 1.59–3.05), GDM (adjusted OR: 1.82; 95% CI: 1.57–2.11), gestational anaemia (adjusted OR: 1.27; 95% CI: 1.05–1.55), polyhydramnios (adjusted OR: 2.60; 95% CI: 1.57–4.31), placenta previa (adjusted OR: 3.18; 95% CI: 2.15–4.71), placenta accreta (adjusted OR: 2.75; 95% CI: 1.75–4.31), and CS (adjusted OR: 694.16; 95% CI: 468.45–1028.62). Seven women had uterine rupture in a subsequent pregnancy in the CS group, four of whom had a non-indicated CS in the first birth, but none of the women in the SVD group had uterine rupture.

Table 3 shows the association between previous caesarean delivery and neonatal outcomes in the subsequent

Table 1 Maternal baseline characteristics and the first birth characteristics among women with previous SVD and those with previous CS and non-indicated CS

	previous SVD (n = 6240)		previous CS (n = 5422)		P- value[a]	previous non-indicated CS (n = 1827)		P- value[b]
	N	%	N	%		N	%	
Baseline characteristics								
Birth place								
Shanghai	4753	76.2%	3991	73.6%	0.001	1413	77.3%	0.300
Out of Shanghai	1487	23.8%	1431	26.4%		414	22.7%	
Race								
Han	6164	98.8%	5353	98.7%	0.791	1812	99.2%	0.158
Minority	76	1.2%	69	1.3%		15	0.8%	
Insurance								
Public	4239	67.9%	3376	62.3%	< 0.001	1099	60.2%	< 0.001
Self-pay	2001	32.1%	2046	37.7%		728	39.8%	
Marital status								
Married/cohabitating	6158	99.7%	5366	99.5%	0.093	1802	99.3%	0.007
Not married/cohabitating	17	0.3%	25	0.5%		13	0.7%	
Age at the second delivery								
<25 years	73	1.2%	39	0.8%	< 0.001	10	0.5%	< 0.001
25–29 years	1152	18.5%	739	13.6%		228	12.5%	
30–34 years	3055	48.9%	2727	50.3%		917	50.2%	
35–39 years	1702	27.3%	1693	31.2%		585	32.0%	
≥ 40 years	258	4.1%	224	4.1%		87	4.8%	
Height (cm)								
<155	222	3.6%	317	5.8%	< 0.001	91	5.0%	0.001
155–164.9	4013	64.3%	3651	67.4%		1206	66.0%	
165–174.9	1935	31.0%	1419	26.2%		520	28.5%	
≥ 175	70	1.1%	35	0.6%		10	0.5%	
Maternal BMI (Kg/m2)								
<18.5	550	8.8%	405	7.5%	< 0.001	139	7.6%	< 0.001
18.5–24.9	5313	85.2%	4530	83.5%		1507	82.5%	
25–29.9	338	5.4%	423	7.8%		155	8.5%	
≥ 30	39	0.6%	64	1.2%		26	1.4%	
Educational level (years)								
≤ 9	266	4.4%	205	3.9%	0.042	35	2.0%	< 0.001
10–12	494	8.2%	469	9.0%		130	7.4%	
13–15	1205	20.1%	1119	21.6%		398	22.5%	
≥ 16	4049	67.3%	3399	65.5%		1203	68.1%	
Gravidity								
≤ 2	2984	47.8%	2366	43.6%	< 0.001	825	45.2%	0.045
≥ 3	3256	52.2%	3056	56.4%		1002	54.8%	
Interpregnancy interval (years)								
<1	431	7.0%	88	1.6%	< 0.001	29	1.6%	< 0.001
1–3	1935	31.2%	1350	25.0%		446	24.5%	
3–5	1357	21.9%	1521	28.2%		540	29.6%	

Table 1 Maternal baseline characteristics and the first birth characteristics among women with previous SVD and those with previous CS and non-indicated CS *(Continued)*

	previous SVD (n = 6240)		previous CS (n = 5422)		P- value[a]	previous non-indicated CS (n = 1827)		P-value[b]
	N	%	N	%		N	%	
5–10	1816	29.3%	1957	36.2%		665	36.5%	
≥ 10	657	10.6%	485	9.0%		142	7.8%	
First birth characteristics								
PIH								
Yes	109	1.7%	103	1.9%	0.538	65	3.6%	< 0.001
No	6131	98.3%	5319	98.1%		1762	96.4%	
PE								
Yes	81	1.3%	90	1.7%	0.105	40	2.2%	0.006
No	6159	98.7%	5332	98.3%		1787	97.8%	
GDM								
Yes	415	6.7%	378	7.0%	0.492	159	8.7%	0.003
No	5825	93.3%	5044	93.0%		1668	91.3%	
Stillbirths								
Yes	61	1.0%	10	0.2%	< 0.001	0	0.0%	< 0.001
No	6179	99.0%	5412	99.8%		1827	100.0%	
LBW								
Yes	144	2.3%	144	2.7%	0.227	26	1.4%	0.021
No	6096	97.7%	5278	97.3%		1801	98.6%	
Macrosomia								
Yes	279	4.5%	572	10.5%	< 0.001	211	11.5%	< 0.001
No	5961	95.5%	4850	89.5%		1616	88.5%	
Preterm delivery								
Yes	266	4.3%	188	3.5%	0.027	16	0.9%	< 0.001
No	5974	95.7%	5234	96.5%		1811	99.1%	

SVD spontaneous vaginal delivery, *CS* caesarean section, *BMI* body mass index, *PIH* pregnancy-induced hypertension, *PE* preeclampsia, *GDM* gestational diabetes mellitus, *LBW* low birth weight
[a]Comparison between previous CS and previous SVD
[b]Comparison between previous non-indicated CS and previous SVD

pregnancy, and the percentages of neonatal outcomes are displayed in Fig. 2b. After adjusting for potential confounders, previous CS women were 1.37 times more likely to have preterm delivery (95% CI: 1.14–1.66), 4.25 times more likely to have a baby with LBW (95% CI: 2.73–6.62), 4.79 times more likely to have macrosomia (95% CI: 3.94–5.83), and 1.39 times more likely to have their baby admitted to a neonatal unit (95% CI: 1.16–1.65) compared with women who had a first SVD. Babies with TTN (adjusted OR: 1.93; 95% CI: 1.33–2.81) were more common in women with a first CS, as were neonatal jaundice (adjusted OR: 1.72; 95% CI: 1.39–2.14). However, there were no differences in stillbirth or neonatal death in the subsequent pregnancy between the previous CS and SVD groups (95% CI: 0.27–2.18 and 0.34–13.74, respectively). Given the risk of the first CS with medical indications in the subsequent pregnancy, we performed a subgroup analysis of neonatal outcomes in women who did not have indications in the first delivery. In this subgroup, women with previous non-indication CS were 1.37 times more likely to have preterm delivery (95% CI: 1.06–1.78), 3.78 times more likely to have a baby with LBW (95% CI: 2.07–6.90), 5.04 times more likely to have macrosomia (95% CI: 3.95–6.44), and 1.58 times more likely to have a baby with neonatal jaundice (95% CI: 1.17–2.13) than women in the SVD group.

Discussion

Main findings

Our results indicate that having a CS in the first singleton pregnancy is associated with an increased risk of adverse maternal and neonatal outcomes in subsequent singleton pregnancy in comparison to an initial SVD. The outcomes included a higher risk of PIH, GDM, ICP, polyhydramnios, placental previa, placental accreta,

Table 2 Association between previous caesarean delivery and maternal outcomes in the subsequent pregnancy

Maternal outcomes	previous SVD(n = 6240)		previous CS(n = 5422)		Crude OR1 (95% CI)	Model 1 Adjusted OR1 (95% CI)	previous nonindicated CS(n = 1827)		Crude OR2 (95% CI)	Model 2 Adjusted OR2 (95% CI)
	N	%	N	%			N	%		
PIH	99	1.6%	131	2.4%	1.54 (1.18–2.00)	1.38 (1.04–1.82)[a]	75	4.1%	2.66 (1.96–3.60)	2.20 (1.59–3.05)[d]
PE	84	1.3%	90	1.7%	1.24 (0.92–1.67)	1.22 (0.88–1.69)[a]	34	1.9%	1.39 (0.93–2.08)	1.24 (0.79–1.94)[d]
GDM	705	11.3%	736	13.6%	1.23 (1.10–1.38)	1.15 (1.02–1.29)[a]	371	20.3%	2.00 (1.74–2.30)	1.82 (1.57–2.11)[d]
Gestational anaemia	455	7.3%	458	8.4%	1.17 (1.03–1.34)	1.13 (0.98–1.30)	166	9.1%	1.27 (1.06–1.53)	1.27 (1.05–1.55)[d]
Gestational thyroid disease	256	4.1%	223	4.1%	1.01 (0.84–1.20)	1.03 (0.85–1.24)	64	3.5%	0.85 (0.64–1.12)	0.86 (0.65–1.16)[d]
ICP	29	0.5%	43	0.8%	1.71 (1.07–2.75)	1.72 (1.04–2.84)	14	0.8%	1.65 (0.87–3.14)	1.65 (0.84–3.23)[d]
PROM	1217	19.5%	445	8.2%	0.37 (0.33–0.41)	0.34 (0.30–0.39)	140	7.7%	0.34 (0.29–0.41)	0.32 (0.26–0.39)[d]
fetal distress	493	7.9%	159	2.9%	0.35 (0.29–0.42)	0.33 (0.27–0.40)	55	3.0%	0.36 (0.27–0.48)	0.34 (0.25–0.46)[d]
meconium-staining of the amniotic fluid										
I degree	58	0.9%	50	0.9%	0.91 (0.62–1.33)	0.94 (0.63–1.40)	17	0.9%	0.91 (0.53–1.57)	0.97 (0.56–1.70)[d]
II degree	236	3.8%	114	2.1%	0.51 (0.41–0.64)	0.49 (0.39–0.62)	33	1.8%	0.44 (0.30–0.63)	0.39 (0.26–0.57)[d]
III degree	472	7.6%	67	1.2%	0.15 (0.12–0.19)	0.15 (0.11–0.19)	17	0.9%	0.11 (0.07–0.18)	0.11 (0.07–0.18)[d]
AFV										
Oligohydramnios	65	1.0%	67	1.2%	1.20 (0.85–1.69)	1.15 (0.81–1.64)	25	1.4%	1.33 (0.84–2.12)	1.37 (0.85–2.21)[d]
Polyhydramnios	39	0.6%	82	1.5%	2.45 (1.67–3.59)	2.50 (1.69–3.69)	27	1.5%	2.39 (1.46–3.92)	2.60 (1.57–4.31)[d]
Placental abruption	19	0.3%	7	0.1%	0.42 (0.18–1.01)	0.51 (0.21–1.25)	4	0.2%	0.72 (0.24–2.11)	0.92 (0.30–2.80)[d]
Placenta previa	66	1.1%	124	2.3%	2.19 (1.62–2.96)	2.11 (1.52–2.94)	62	3.4%	3.29 (2.31–4.67)	3.18 (2.15–4.71)[d]
Placenta accreta	53	0.8%	104	1.9%	2.28 (1.64–3.18)	2.11 (1.47–3.04)	45	2.5%	2.95 (1.97–4.40)	2.75 (1.75–4.31)[d]
Rupture of uterus	0	0.0%	7	0.1%	/	/	4	0.2%	/	/
APH	61	1.0%	59	1.1%	1.11 (0.78–1.60)	0.96 (0.64–1.43)	25	1.4%	1.41 (0.88–2.25)	1.13 (0.66–1.93)[d]
FGR	82	1.3%	70	1.3%	0.98 (0.71–1.35)	0.93 (0.65–1.33)	22	1.2%	0.92 (0.57–1.47)	0.89 (0.53–1.51)[d]
Abnormal fetal position	193	3.1%	194	3.6%	1.16 (0.95–1.42)	1.09 (0.88–1.35)	47	2.6%	0.83 (0.60–1.14)	0.77 (0.55–1.09)[d]
Dystocia	197	3.2%	196	3.6%	1.15 (0.94–1.41)	1.09 (0.88–1.34)	46	2.5%	0.79 (0.57–1.10)	0.73 (0.52–1.04)[d]
Antepartum fever	55	0.9%	27	0.5%	0.56 (0.36–0.89)	0.54 (0.33–0.89)	9	0.5%	0.56 (0.28–1.13)	0.60 (0.29–1.24)[d]
Mode of delivery										
Caesarean section	823	13.2%	5278	97.3%	263.28 (217.98–318.01)	364.21 (294.74–450.06)[b]	1795	98.2%	375.49 (261.30–539.58)	694.16 (468.45–1028.62)[e]
Instrumental delivery	80	1.3%	14	0.3%	7.18 (3.97–13.01)	8.30 (4.41–15.60)[b]	1	0.1%	2.15 (0.29–15.96)	6.40 (0.84–48.80)[e]
PPH	119	1.9%	107	2.0%	1.04 (0.80–1.35)	0.69 (0.42–1.14)[c]	43	2.4%	1.24 (0.87–1.76)	0.54 (0.30–0.97)[f]
Puerperal infection	16	0.3%	15	0.3%	1.08 (0.53–2.19)	0.99 (0.35–2.83)[c]	4	0.2%	0.85 (0.29–2.56)	0.50 (0.12–2.19)[f]

SVD spontaneous vaginal delivery, *CS* caesarean section, *PIH* pregnancy-induced hypertension, *PE* preeclampsia, *GDM* gestational diabetes mellitus, *ICP* intrahepatic cholestasis of pregnancy, *PROM* prelabour rupture of membranes, *AFV* amniotic fluid volume, *APH* antepartum haemorrhage, *PPH* postpartum haemorrhage, *FGR* fetal growth restriction, *OR* odds radio, *CI* confidence interval

Model 1: all ORs adjusted for birth place, insurance, age at the second delivery, height, maternal BMI, educational level, gravidity, interpregnancy interval

[a]ORs further adjusted for PIH, PE and GDM in first birth

[b]ORs further adjusted for PIH, GDM, ICP, gestational anaemia, PROM and meconium-staining of the amniotic fluid, AFV, fetal distress, placental abruption, placenta previa, placenta accreta, rupture of uterus and antepartum fever

[c]ORs further adjusted for PIH, GDM, ICP, gestational anaemia, PROM and meconium-staining of the amniotic fluid, AFV, fetal distress, placental abruption, placenta previa, placenta accreta, rupture of uterus, antepartum fever and mode of delivery

Model 2: all ORs adjusted for insurance, marital status, age at the second delivery, height, maternal BMI, educational level, gravidity, interpregnancy interval

[d]ORs further adjusted for PIH, PE and GDM in first birth

[e]ORs further adjusted for PIH, GDM, gestational anaemia, PROM, meconium-staining of the amniotic fluid, AFV, fetal distress, placenta previa, placenta accreta, rupture of uterus

[f]ORs further adjusted for PIH, GDM, gestational anaemia, PROM and meconium-staining of the amniotic fluid, AFV, fetal distress, placenta previa, placenta accreta, rupture of uterus and mode of delivery

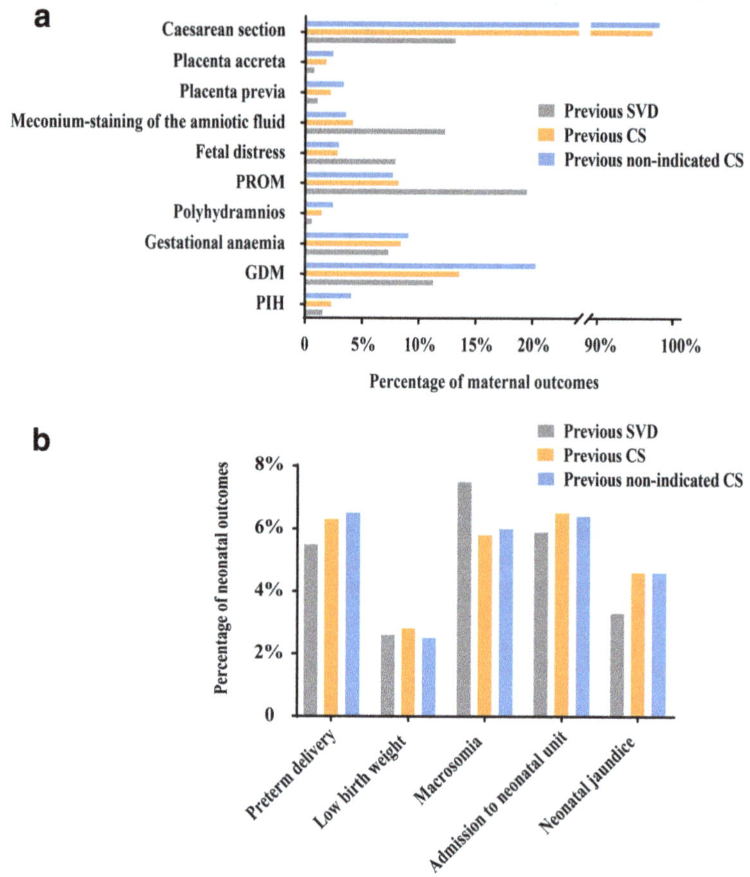

Fig. 2 Incidences of the main perinatal outcomes of the second births. **a** Percentages of the main maternal outcomes of the second births among the three groups. **b** Percentages of the main neonatal outcomes of second births among the three groups. SVD: spontaneous vaginal delivery; CS: caesarean section; PIH: pregnancy-induced hypertension; PE: preeclampsia; GDM: gestational diabetes mellitus; PROM: premature rupture of membranes

repeated caesarean delivery in the mother and preterm delivery, LBW, macrosomia, admission to a neonatal unit, TTN, and jaundice in the baby. Notably, in women without indications for CS in the first birth, there was still a significantly increased risk of PIH, GDM, polyhydramnios, placental previa, placental accrete, repeated caesarean delivery, and preterm, LBW, macrosomia, and neonatal jaundice.

Strengths and limitations

To the best of our knowledge, this is one of the few epidemiological studies exploring the association between CS in the first birth and perinatal complications in the subsequent pregnancy. There are several advantages to our study. First, the data analysed were taken from a geographically stable population and collected at the time of delivery from case notes, thereby minimizing selection and recall bias. Second, changes in clinical practice are unlikely to influence the findings, as the data of the two groups were recorded during the same period. Last but not least, we restricted our analyses to women with a second singleton birth, which eliminated potential confounding effects of parity and multiple gestations, and we also performed a subgroup analysis between previous non-indicated CS and previous SVD to avoid the risk of CS indications in the next pregnancy. Still, we should note that the presence of missing values and the retrospective nature of data collection may have biased the results to some extent. Briefly, the lack of adverse maternal outcomes in the first birth, such as PROM, placenta previa, and APH, which may be risk factors that need to be adjusted to adverse outcomes in the next pregnancy, may have influenced the results. It was difficult to confirm the indications for CS from the retrospective data. Further prospective studies are required to reduce the information bias. Additionally, as the study was restricted to a single centre in Shanghai, the results may only be generalizable to that local area in China.

Interpretation

In our study population, 45.7% of the subjects experienced CS in the first singleton birth, and 33.7% of them

Table 3 Association between previous caesarean delivery and neonatal outcomes in the subsequent pregnancy

Neonatal outcomes	previous SVD(*n* = 6240)		previous CS(*n* = 5422)		Crude OR1 (95% CI)	Model 1 Adjusted OR1 (95% CI)	previous nonindicated CS(*n* = 1827)		Crude OR2 (95% CI)	Model 2 Adjusted OR2 (95% CI)
	N	%	N	%			N	%		
Stillbirths	13	0.2%	11	0.2%	0.97 (0.44–2.18)	0.76 (0.27–2.18)[a]	4	0.2%	1.05 (0.34–3.23)	0.68 (0.13–3.55)[a]
Preterm delivery	341	5.5%	343	6.3%	1.17 (1.01–1.36)	1.37 (1.14–1.66)[b]	119	6.5%	1.21 (0.97–1.50)	1.37 (1.06–1.78)[b]
LBW	162	2.6%	151	2.8%	1.08 (0.86–1.35)	4.25 (2.73–6.62)[c]	46	2.5%	0.97 (0.70–1.35)	3.78 (2.07–6.90)[c]
Macrosomia	466	7.5%	317	5.8%	0.77 (0.66–0.89)	4.79 (3.94–5.83)[d]	110	6.0%	0.79 (0.64–0.98)	5.04 (3.95–6.44)[d]
Apgar at 1 min<8	79	1.3%	74	1.4%	1.08 (0.78–1.49)	1.13 (0.77–1.66)	25	1.4%	1.08 (0.69–1.70)	1.18 (0.69–2.01)
Neonatal infection	83	1.3%	46	0.8%	0.64 (0.44–0.91)	0.81 (0.54–1.23)	12	0.7%	0.49 (0.27–0.90)	0.51 (0.26–1.03)
Neonatal death	4	0.1%	4	0.1%	1.15 (0.29–4.60)	2.17 (0.34–13.74)	1	0.1%	0.85 (0.10–7.64)	0.70 (0.02–34.51)
Admission to neonatal unit	366	5.9%	355	6.5%	1.12 (0.97–1.31)	1.39 (1.16–1.65)	117	6.4%	1.10 (0.89–1.36)	1.20 (0.94–1.54)
NRDS	13	0.2%	21	0.4%	1.86 (0.93–3.72)	1.88 (0.83–4.24)	7	0.4%	1.84 (0.73–4.62)	1.49 (0.48–4.61)
TTN	71	1.1%	91	1.7%	1.48 (1.09–2.03)	1.93 (1.33–2.81)	28	1.5%	1.35 (0.87–2.10)	1.55 (0.93–2.58)
Neonatal jaundice	206	3.3%	249	4.6%	1.41 (1.17–1.70)	1.72 (1.39–2.14)	84	4.6%	1.41 (1.09–1.83)	1.58 (1.17–2.13)
Birth injury	16	0.3%	9	0.2%	0.65 (0.29–1.49)	0.85 (0.35–2.06)	4	0.2%	0.85 (0.29–2.56)	0.85 (0.25–2.85)

LBW low birth weight, *NRDS* neonatal respiratory distress syndrome, *TTN* transient tachypnea of newborn(TTN)
Model 1: all ORs adjusted for birth place, insurance, age at the second delivery, height, maternal BMI, educational level, gravidity, interpregnancy interval, PIH, GDM, ICP, gestational anaemia, PROM and meconium-staining of the amniotic fluid, AFV, fetal distress, placental abruption, placenta previa, placenta accreta, rupture of uterus, antepartum fever
Model 2: all ORs adjusted for insurance, marital status, age at the second delivery, height, maternal BMI, educational level, gravidity, interpregnancy interval, PIH, GDM, gestational anaemia, PROM and meconium-staining of the amniotic fluid, AFV, fetal distress, placenta previa, placenta accreta, rupture of uterus
[a]ORs further adjusted for stillbirth at the first birth
[b]ORs further adjusted for preterm delivery at the first birth
[c]ORs further adjusted for LBW at the first birth
[d]ORs further adjusted for macrosomia at the first birth

were non-indicated. The main reason for the high rate of CS and non-indicated CS may be attributed to the One Child Policy of the Chinese government during the period from 1978 to 2015. In the second singleton birth, the CS rate reached 52.3%, which was approximately three times the proportion recommended by the WHO. This finding is consistent with studies reported previously in China [9, 34]. We confirmed that some of the known baseline characteristics were associated with delivery mode, including maternal age, height, maternal BMI, educational level of the couples, gravidity, and interpregnancy interval, but these factors are not specific and were associated with a few of the adverse obstetric outcomes. Our present study findings suggest that CS in the first birth is linked with adverse maternal and neonatal outcomes in the next pregnancy. The effects of previous CS on the risk of placenta previa and placenta accreta are consistent with previous studies [24, 26, 27, 35–39]. These papers confirmed the association between placenta previa and previous CS and found that the ORs for placenta previa with one or more previous caesarean deliveries were 1.47–1.66, but the pooled OR of 2.2 from a meta-analysis [37] is consistent with the OR of 2.11 in our findings. Additionally, the risk of placenta accreta in our study was similar to results from previous research [27, 38]. Possible mechanisms for placenta previa and accreta following previous CS suggested by previous researchers have included failure of placental apparent migration, impaired differential growth of the lower uterine segment, and deficient decidua basalis in the presence of previous surgery injury [24, 40–42]. In the present study, we focused on the adverse outcomes in second births, and our study represents a homogeneous sample affected by previous CS, which ruled out the influence of parity. Although there is disagreement on the association of previous CS with a higher risk of placenta abruption in the second pregnancy in prior studies [24, 26, 27, 36, 38, 39], our study shows that previous CS does not increase the risk of placental abruption. Additionally, the incidence of uterine rupture (0.1%) in the previous CS cohort in our study was less than that reported in prior studies [26, 27, 43–46], which may be attributed to the lower rate of trial of labour in women with a first CS in our country. The risks of APH and PPH in our study were not associated with the initial caesarean delivery, which is not consistent with previous studies [26, 47]. Even in the subgroup analysis, there were no statistically significant differences for APH. However, the ORs were greater than one in the univariate analysis. There are several possible factors contributing to this finding: first, the missing information in the first birth may be confounding factors, and we cannot be certain whether they caused outcomes in the second birth; second, placental abruption, which is a primary cause of APH, was not increased in the first CS women in our study; third, the repeated CS reduced the occurrence of PPH.

Our study seems to be the first to document the associations between previous CS history and increased risk of PIH, GDM, ICP, and polyhydramnios in the next pregnancy. Especially in women without indications for a previous CS, the risks were much higher for PIH, GDM, and polyhydramnios. Similar research has shown the association between the first CS and the increased risk of PE [27, 48, 49], but no differences were found in our study. Prior CS has been shown to be an important risk factor for subsequent complications, including placental vasculopathies [50], which may lead to a high risk of PIH. Pregnant women with PIH and/or GDM in the first pregnancy are highly susceptible to recurrence in the next pregnancy [51, 52]. Thus, in our study, the high proportion of PIH and GDM in the first birth in the CS group may be a reason for the increased risk of PIH and GDM in the next pregnancy. Interestingly, when we regarded PIH and GDM in the first birth as confounding factors and adjusted for them, a high risk of PIH and GDM still existed in the next pregnancy for women with a first CS, especially in women without indications for the first CS. Moreover, uterine changes induced by prior CS may interfere with normal trophoblastic invasion and uteroplacental blood flow in subsequent pregnancies, resulting in abnormal placental function and subsequent gestational complications, including PIH and GDM [53, 54].

Compared to women with a prior SVD, the risks of PROM, fetal distress, meconium-staining of the amniotic fluid, and antepartum fever in the next birth were lower in women with an initial CS, which may be due to a missing confounding factor (PROM) in the first birth. Women with PROM were more likely to choose vaginal delivery in the first birth. Studies in the UK [31] and USA [55] showed that a PROM history was associated with a 6.6- to 20.6-fold increase in the risk of recurrent PROM. Furthermore, the decreased risk of fetal distress, meconium-staining of the amniotic fluid, and antepartum fever in women with primary CS in the second birth may also be related to the risks of these factors in the first birth.

The stillbirth rates were 2.0/1000 in both the previous CS group and previous SVD group, which was in accordance with preceding reports [26, 56], but there were no differences between the two groups in our research. Our findings on the effects of the first CS on the risk of preterm, LBW, macrosomia, admission to a neonatal unit, TTN of babies, and neonatal jaundice in the second pregnancy are consistent with previous studies [26, 43, 57, 58]. There are few published studies providing evidence to support our findings; therefore, it is difficult to interpret the risk of caesarean delivery on these outcomes. Although there was a higher risk of admission to a neonatal unit for babies of first CS women in the next pregnancy, it did not increase their neonatal death rate. Additionally, in the subgroup analysis, there was no difference in admission to a neonatal unit and TTN in the two groups.

With implementation of the "two-child policy" in China, an increasing number of families will choose to raise two children. To control the overall CS rate, it is important to decrease the occurrence of primary CS, especially elective CS with no medical indications. These study findings will help women and clinical doctors in making choices and balancing the risks and benefits of a caesarean delivery in the first and subsequent births. The decision for an elective primary caesarean delivery should be carefully considered for its impact on future births.

Conclusions

CS in the first birth is associated with an increased risk of repeated caesarean delivery and adverse obstetric and perinatal outcomes in the following delivery, especially in women without CS indications. Clinicians might consider this information valuable when counselling women during pregnancy.

Abbreviations

AFV: Amniotic fluid volume; APH: Antepartum haemorrhage; BMI: Body mass index; CI: Confidence interval; CS: Caesarean section; FGR: Fetal growth restriction; GDM: Gestational diabetes mellitus; HELLP: Haemolysis, elevated liver enzymes, and low platelets syndrome; ICP: Intrahepatic cholestasis of pregnancy; LBW: Low birth weight; NRDS: Neonatal respiratory distress syndrome; OR: Odds radio; PE: Preeclampsia; PIH: Pregnancy-induced hypertension; PPH: Postpartum haemorrhage; PROM: Premature rupture of membranes; SVD: Spontaneous vaginal delivery; TTN: Transient tachypnea of newborn

Acknowledgements

The authors would like to thank Lei Chen in International Peace Maternity and Child Health Hospital for his efforts in data collection and abstraction. The authors are also grateful to Han Liu for helping with data analysis.

Funding

This work was supported by the International Cooperation Project of China and Canada NSFC (81661128010), The National Key Research and Development Program of China (No. 2017YFC1001303), National Natural Science Foundation of China (31471405), and Medical Crossover Foundation of Shanghai Jiao Tong University (YG2015MS42). The funding agencies had no role in study design, data collection and analysis, and decision to submit the article for publication.

Authors' contributions
The study was conceived and designed by HFH XML and HTH. HHF had full access to all data in the study and take responsibility for the integrity of the data and accuracy of the data analysis. Validation was performed on the data to check for errors and inconsistencies in documentation and coding by HTH, JL and JJX. HTH and JJX performed the statistical analysis and wrote the manuscript. HFH, JZS, XML, YTW and CL revised the manuscript. All authors discussed the results and commented on the article. All authors read and approved the final manuscript.

Consent for publication
Not applicable.

Competing interests
The authors declare that they have no competing interests.

Author details
[1]Department of Obstetrics and Gynecology, International Peace Maternity and Child Health Hospital, School of Medicine, Shanghai Jiao Tong University, Shanghai, China. [2]Department of Reproductive Medicine, International Peace Maternity and Child Health Hospital, School of Medicine, Shanghai Jiao Tong University, Shanghai, China. [3]Department of Pathology and Pathophysiology, School of Medicine, Zhejiang University, Zhejiang, China. [4]Institute of Embryo-Fetal Original Adult Disease, Shanghai Key Laboratory for Reproductive Medicine, School of Medicine, Shanghai Jiao Tong University, Shanghai, China. [5]International Peace Maternity and Child Health Hospital, School of Medicine, Shanghai Jiao Tong University, 910 Hengshan Road, Shanghai 200030, China.

References
1. Appropriate technology for birth. Lancet (London, England). 1985;2(8452):436–7.
2. Betran AP, Torloni MR, Zhang JJ, Gulmezoglu AM, Section WHOWGC. WHO statement on caesarean section rates. BJOG. 2016;123(5):667–70.
3. Villar J, Valladares E, Wojdyla D, Zavaleta N, Carroli G, Velazco A, Shah A, Campodonico L, Bataglia V, Faundes A, et al. Caesarean delivery rates and pregnancy outcomes: the 2005 WHO global survey on maternal and perinatal health in Latin America. Lancet (London, England). 2006; 367(9525):1819–29.
4. Lumbiganon P, Laopaiboon M, Gulmezoglu AM, Souza JP, Taneepanichskul S, Ruyan P, Attygalle DE, Shrestha N, Mori R, Nguyen DH, et al. Method of delivery and pregnancy outcomes in Asia: the WHO global survey on maternal and perinatal health 2007-08. Lancet (London, England). 2010; 375(9713):490–9.
5. Betran AP, Ye J, Moller AB, Zhang J, Gulmezoglu AM, Torloni MR. The increasing trend in caesarean section rates: global, regional and National Estimates: 1990-2014. PLoS One. 2016;11(2):e0148343.
6. Vogel JP, Betrán AP, Vindevoghel N, Souza JP, Torloni MR, Zhang J, Tunçalp Ö, Mori R, Morisaki N, Ortiz-Panozo E, et al. Use of the Robson classification to assess caesarean section trends in 21 countries: a secondary analysis of two WHO multicountry surveys. Lancet Glob Health. 2015;3(5):e260-e270.
7. Feng XL, Xu L, Guo Y, Ronsmans C. Factors influencing rising caesarean section rates in China between 1988 and 2008. Bull World Health Organ. 2012;90(1):30–9. 39A
8. Hellerstein S, Feldman S, Duan T. China's 50% caesarean delivery rate: is it too high? Bjog. 2015;122(2):160–4.
9. Liu Y, Li G, Chen Y, Wang X, Ruan Y, Zou L, Zhang W. A descriptive analysis of the indications for caesarean section in mainland China. BMC Pregnancy Childbirth. 2014;14:410.
10. Zhu YB, Li HT, Zhang YL, Li ZW, Zhang L, Liu JM. Secular trends of cesarean delivery and cesarean delivery on maternal request among primiparous women with singleton pregnancy in southern and northern China during 1993-2010. Zhonghua Yi Xue Za Zhi. 2012;92(25):1734–7.
11. Hou L, Hellerstein S, Vitonis A, Zou L, Ruan Y, Wang X, Zhang W. Cross sectional study of mode of delivery and maternal and perinatal outcomes in mainland China. PLoS One. 2017;12(2):e0171779.
12. Wang L, Xu X, Baker P, Tong C, Zhang L, Qi H, Zhao Y. Patterns and associated factors of caesarean delivery intention among expectant mothers in China: implications from the implementation of China's new National two-Child Policy. Int J Environ Res Public Health. 2016;13(7):686. https://doi.org/10.3390/ijerph13070686.
13. Creanga AA, Bateman BT, Butwick AJ, Raleigh L, Maeda A, Kuklina E, Callaghan WM. Morbidity associated with cesarean delivery in the United States: is placenta accreta an increasingly important contributor? Am J Obstet Gynecol. 2015;213((3):384):e381–11.
14. WHO Statement on caesarean section rates. Reprod Health Matters. 2015; 23(45):149–50.
15. Ye J, Zhang J, Mikolajczyk R, Torloni MR, Gulmezoglu AM, Betran AP. Association between rates of caesarean section and maternal and neonatal mortality in the 21st century: a worldwide population-based ecological study with longitudinal data. Bjog. 2016;123(5):745–53.
16. O'Neill SM, Khashan AS, Kenny LC, Kearney PM, Mortensen PB, Greene RA, Agerbo E, Uldbjerg N, Henriksen TB. Time to subsequent live birth according to mode of delivery in the first birth. BJOG. 2015;122(9):1207–15.
17. Kjerulff KH, Zhu J, Weisman CS, Ananth CV. First birth caesarean section and subsequent fertility: a population-based study in the USA, 2000-2008. Hum Reprod. 2013;28(12):3349–57.
18. Gurol-Urganci I, Bou-Antoun S, Lim CP, Cromwell DA, Mahmood TA, Templeton A, van der Meulen JH. Impact of caesarean section on subsequent fertility: a systematic review and meta-analysis. Hum Reprod. 2013;28(7):1943–52.
19. Gurol-Urganci I, Cromwell DA, Mahmood TA, van der Meulen JH, Templeton A. A population-based cohort study of the effect of caesarean section on subsequent fertility. Hum Reprod. 2014;29(6):1320–6.
20. Smith GCS, Pell JP, Bobbie R. Caesarean section and risk of unexplained stillbirth in subsequent pregnancy. Lancet. 2003;362(9398):1779–84.
21. AA Moraitis CO-W, AM Wood M, Fleming JP, Pell GCS. Smith: previous caesarean delivery and the risk of unexplained stillbirth: retrospective cohort study and meta-analysis. BJOG. 2015;122(11):1475.
22. Clark EA, Silver RM. Long-term maternal morbidity associated with repeat cesarean delivery. Am J Obstet Gynecol. 2011;205(6 Suppl):S2–10.
23. Cahill AG, Stamilio DM, Odibo AO, Peipert JF, Ratcliffe SJ, Stevens EJ, Sammel MD, Macones GA. Is vaginal birth after cesarean (VBAC) or elective repeat cesarean safer in women with a prior vaginal delivery? Am J Obstet Gynecol. 2006;195(4):1143–7.
24. Yang Q, Wen SW, Oppenheimer L, Chen XK, Black D, Gao J, Walker MC. Association of caesarean delivery for first birth with placenta praevia and placental abruption in second pregnancy. BJOG. 2007;114(5):609–13.
25. Colmorn LB, Krebs L, Klungsoyr K, Jakobsson M, Tapper AM, Gissler M, Lindqvist PG, Kallen K, Gottvall K, Bordahl PE, et al. Mode of first delivery and severe maternal complications in the subsequent pregnancy. Acta Obstet Gynecol Scand. 2017;96(9):1053–62.
26. Kennare R, Tucker G, Heard A, Chan A. Risks of adverse outcomes in the next birth after a first cesarean delivery. Obstet Gynecol. 2007;109(2 Pt 1):270–6.
27. Daltveit AK, Tollanes MC, Pihlstrom H, Irgens LM. Cesarean delivery and subsequent pregnancies. Obstet Gynecol. 2008;111(6):1327–34.
28. Ayorinde AA, Bhattacharya S. Inherited predisposition to preeclampsia: analysis of the Aberdeen intergenerational cohort. Pregnancy Hypertens. 2017;8:37–41.
29. Davey DA, MacGillivray I. The classification and definition of the hypertensive disorders of pregnancy. Am J Obstet Gynecol. 1988;158(4):892–8.
30. Yang S, Shi FT, Leung PC, Huang HF, Fan J. Low thyroid hormone in early pregnancy is associated with an increased risk of gestational diabetes mellitus. J Clin Endocrinol Metab. 2016;101(11):4237–43.
31. Aris IM, Logan S, Lim C, Choolani M, Biswas A, Bhattacharya S. Preterm prelabour rupture of membranes: a retrospective cohort study of association with adverse outcome in subsequent pregnancy. BJOG. 2017; 124(11):1698–707.
32. Silver RM. Abnormal Placentation: Placenta Previa, Vasa Previa, and Placenta Accreta. Obstet Gynecol. 2015;126(3):654–68.
33. Fitzpatrick KE, Sellers S, Spark P, Kurinczuk JJ, Brocklehurst P, Knight M. The management and outcomes of placenta accreta, increta, and percreta in the UK: a population-based descriptive study. BJOG. 2014;121(1):62–70. discussion 70-61
34. Liu Y, Wang X, Zou L, Ruan Y, Zhang W. An analysis of variations of indications and maternal-fetal prognosis for caesarean section in a tertiary hospital of Beijing: a population-based retrospective cohort study. Medicine (Baltimore). 2017;96(7):e5509.

35. Taylor VM, Kramer MD, Vaughan TL, Peacock S. Placenta previa and prior cesarean delivery: how strong is the association? Obstet Gynecol. 1994;84(1):55–7.
36. Getahun D, Oyelese Y, Salihu HM, Ananth CV. Previous cesarean delivery and risks of placenta previa and placental abruption. Obstet Gynecol. 2006;107(4):771–8.
37. Gurol-Urganci I, Cromwell DA, Edozien LC, Smith GC, Onwere C, Mahmood TA, Templeton A, van der Meulen JH. Risk of placenta previa in second birth after first birth cesarean section: a population-based study and meta-analysis. BMC Pregnancy Childbirth. 2011;11:95.
38. Klar M, Michels KB. Cesarean section and placental disorders in subsequent pregnancies–a meta-analysis. J Perinat Med. 2014;42(5):571–83.
39. Lydon-Rochelle M, Holt VL, Easterling TR, Martin DP. First-birth cesarean and placental abruption or previa at second birth(1). Obstet Gynecol. 2001;97(5 Pt 1):765–9.
40. Sholapurkar SL. Increased incidence of placenta praevia and accreta with previous caesareans–a hypothesis for causation. J Obstet Gynaecol. 2013;33(8):806–9.
41. Clark SL, Koonings PP, Phelan JP. Placenta previa/accreta and prior cesarean section. Obstet Gynecol. 1985;66(1):89–92.
42. Paterson-Brown S, Singh C. Developing a care bundle for the management of suspected placenta accreta. Obstetrician Gynaecologist. 2010;12(1):21–7.
43. Taylor LK, Simpson JM, Roberts CL, Olive EC, Henderson-Smart DJ. Risk of complications in a second pregnancy following caesarean section in the first pregnancy: a population-based study. Med J Aust. 2005;183(10):515–9.
44. Guise JM, McDonagh MS, Osterweil P, Nygren P, Chan BK, Helfand M. Systematic review of the incidence and consequences of uterine rupture in women with previous caesarean section. BMJ (Clin Res ed). 2004;329(7456):19–25.
45. Spong CY, Landon MB, Gilbert S, Rouse DJ, Leveno KJ, Varner MW, Moawad AH, Simhan HN, Harper M, Wapner RJ, et al. Risk of uterine rupture and adverse perinatal outcome at term after cesarean delivery. Obstet Gynecol. 2007;110(4):801–7.
46. Motomura K, Ganchimeg T, Nagata C, Ota E, Vogel JP, Betran AP, Torloni MR, Jayaratne K, Jwa SC, Mittal S, et al. Incidence and outcomes of uterine rupture among women with prior caesarean section: WHO multicountry survey on maternal and newborn health. Sci Rep. 2017;7:44093.
47. Iyoke CA, Ugwu GO, Ezugwu FO, Lawani OL, Onah HE. Risks associated with subsequent pregnancy after one caesarean section: a prospective cohort study in a Nigerian obstetric population. Niger J Clin Pract. 2014;17(4):442–8.
48. Mbah AK, Sharma PP, Alio AP, Fombo DW, Bruder K, Salihu HM. Previous cesarean section, gestational age at first delivery and subsequent risk of pre-eclampsia in obese mothers. Arch Gynecol Obstet. 2012;285(5):1375–81.
49. Ventura Laveriano WR, Redondo CE. Obstetric outcomes in the second birth of women with a previous caesarean delivery: a retrospective cohort study from Peru. Rev Bras Ginecol Obstet. 2013;35(4):148–52.
50. Hemminki E, Merilainen BJ. Long-term effects of cesarean sections: ectopic pregnancies and placental problems. Am J Obstet Gynecol. 1996;174(5):1569–74.
51. van Oostwaard MF, Langenveld J, Schuit E, Papatsonis DN, Brown MA, Byaruhanga RN, Bhattacharya S, Campbell DM, Chappell LC, Chiaffarino F, et al. Recurrence of hypertensive disorders of pregnancy: an individual patient data metaanalysis. Am J Obstet Gynecol. 2015;212(5):624.e621–17.
52. Kim C, Berger DK, Chamany S. Recurrence of gestational diabetes mellitus: a systematic review. Diabetes Care. 2007;30(5):1314–9.
53. Cho GJ, Kim LY, Min KJ, Sung YN, Hong SC, Oh MJ, Seo HS, Kim HJ. Prior cesarean section is associated with increased preeclampsia risk in a subsequent pregnancy. BMC Pregnancy Childbirth. 2015;15:24.
54. Gauster M, Desoye G, Totsch M, Hiden U. The placenta and gestational diabetes mellitus. Curr Diab Rep. 2012;12(1):16–23.
55. Lee T, Carpenter MW, Heber WW, Silver HM. Preterm premature rupture of membranes: risks of recurrent complications in the next pregnancy among a population-based sample of gravid women. Am J Obstet Gynecol. 2003;188(1):209–13.
56. Wood SL, Chen S, Ross S, Sauve R. The risk of unexplained antepartum stillbirth in second pregnancies following caesarean section in the first pregnancy. BJOG. 2008;115(6):726–31.
57. Hemminki E, Shelley J, Gissler M. Mode of delivery and problems in subsequent births: a register-based study from Finland. Am J Obstet Gynecol. 2005;193(1):169–77.
58. Abenhaim HA, Benjamin A. Effect of prior cesarean delivery on neonatal outcomes. J Perinat Med. 2011;39(3):241–4.

9

The effect of uterine artery ligation in patients with central placenta pevia

Ahmad Sameer Sanad*, Ahmad E. Mahran, Mahmoud Elmorsi Aboulfotouh, Hany Hassan Kamel, Hashem Fares Mohammed, Haitham A. Bahaa, Reham R. Elkateeb, Alaa Gamal Abdelazim, Mohamed Ahmed Zeen El-Din and Hossam El-Din Shawki

Abstract

Background: Placenta previa is major obstetric surgical risk as it is associated with higher percentage of intraoperative and postpartum hemorrhage (PPH), increased requirement of blood transfusion and further surgical procedures. The current study aimed to evaluate uterine artery ligation prior to uterine incision as a procedure to minimize blood loss during cesarean section in patients with central placenta previa.

Methods: One hundred and four patients diagnosed with central placenta previa antenatally and planned to have elective caesarean section were recruited from the antenatal clinic at Minia Maternity University hospital. Patients were randomly allocated into either ligation group or control group.

Results: Both groups were similar regarding demographic features and preoperative risk factors for bleeding. The intraoperative blood loss was significantly lower in the ligation group as compared with the control group (569.3 ± 202.1 mL vs. 805.1 ± 224.5 mL respectively, $p = 0.002$). There was a significant increase in the requirement for blood transfusion in the control group as compared with the ligation group (786 ± 83 mL vs. 755 ± 56 mL respectively, $p = 0.03$) Three cases in the control group required further surgical interventions to control intraoperative bleeding, while no cases in the ligation required further surgical techniques and that was statistically significant ($p = 0.001$).

Conclusion: Uterine artery ligation prior to uterine incision may be a helpful procedure to minimize intraoperative and postpartum blood loss in cases with central placenta previa.

Keywords: Central placenta previa, Uterine artery ligation, Cesarean section

Background

Placenta previa is a potentially serious obstetric complication where the placental tissue abnormally lies within the lower uterine segment [1, 2]. The exact pathophysiology of this serious condition is not exactly known. However uterine scaring is a potential risk factor. Other risk factors for placenta previa include advanced maternal age, high parity, history of placenta previa and congenital uterine malformations [3–6].

The prevalence of placenta previa is estimated to be 5.2 per 1000 pregnancies. However, there is evidence of regional variation [7]. In Minia maternity University hospital where the study was conducted, data from labor ward registry showed that 5% of caesarean deliveries were performed due to placenta previa and its variants. This rate is expected to rise in the coming years due to high rate of caesarean deliveries and subsequently more pregnancies with uterine scarring.

Placenta previa is associated with higher incidence of intraoperative bleeding and postpartum hemorrhage (PPH), need for blood transfusion and further surgical procedures like devascularization and emergency hysterectomy

* Correspondence: ahmed.sameer@mu.edu.eg
Obstetrics and Gynecology, Faculty of Medicine, Minia Maternity University Hospital, Minia University, PO Box 61111, Minia, Egypt

[8, 9]. In addition, women with placenta previa are at higher risk of delivering premature babies with lower Apgar scores and with higher rates of neonatal intensive care (NICU) admission, stillbirth and neonatal death [10, 11].

In 2014, the total number of deliveries in Minia Maternity University Hospital was 10,854. There were 332 cases with antepartum hemorrhage, 224 of them were diagnosed as placenta previa.

In this study, we introduced uterine artery ligation prior to uterine incision as a novel technique to reduce intraoperative blood loss in patients with central placenta previa. It is proposed that the procedure is associated with reduction of the blood flow to the lower uterine segment and consequently leads to reduction of blood loss during placental separation.

The aim of this study was to evaluate the effect of uterine artery ligation prior to uterine incision in patients with central placenta previa on blood loss during caesarean section.

Methods

Project no.: MUH201310127

The study protocol was approved by scientific ethical committee of the Department of Obstetrics and Gynecology, Faculty of Medicine, Minia University in September 2013. The study procedure was explained to all eligible patients. All patients signed informed consent that include their agreement to participate in the study.

This study is a randomized controlled study including 104 patients diagnosed with central placenta previa antenatally and were planned to have elective cesarean section. Patients were recruited from attendees of the antenatal clinic at Minia Maternity University Hospital in the period between January 2014 and December 2016.

Patients were randomly allocated into study or control group. The random allocation was based on computer-generated random numbers sealed in consecutively numbered opaque envelopes that were picked up by the patients outside the operating theatre. As major outcomes were not patient-dependent or patient-reported, the patients and the surgeons were not blind to group allocation.

We included patients diagnosed with central placenta previa diagnosed with two-dimensional ultrasound scan at 28 weeks' gestation and remained so till the time of planned cesarean delivery. Central placenta previa was defined as placental localization in the lower uterine segment either anteriorly or posteriorly. Laterally situated placenta was not considered "central". We excluded patients with; a) known bleeding disorder, b) patients with hypertensive disorders or developed preeclampsia (PET) during the study, c) patients who had antepartum hemorrhage (APH) and delivered by emergency caesarean section, and d) patients with anterior placenta previa that were diagnosed antenatally with color Doppler ultrasound and MRI to have placenta accreta. These criteria were designed prior to initiation of the study.

Thorough assessment of the risk factors associated with each case was done. Patients were followed up with regular ultrasound scans every 2 weeks to ensure fetal wellbeing and placental localization till the time of planned delivery. Deliveries were planned to take place between 36 and 38 weeks according to each case situation. Preoperative hemoglobin (Hb) assessment was done and four to six blood units were cross matched for each case before planned cesarean section. Each cesarean section was performed by two consultant obstetricians with experience in operative management of placenta previa and placenta accreta. The two consultants were assisting each other in each case to ensure uniformity of the procedure in all patients. Postoperative hemoglobin level was checked 24 h after the CS (day 1) or after at least 6 h from the blood transfusion. We adhered to the CONSORT guidelines Fig. 1.

Sample size calculation

Sample size was calculated to prevent type II error. The average intraoperative blood loss in cases of central placenta previa at the hospital where the study was conducted was estimated to be 800 ml (figure obtained from the hospital audit report for the year preceding the trial). To be of clinical significance, it was assumed that uterine artery ligation prior to uterine incision should reduce intraoperative blood loss by 50%. Based on these data, we would need to study 27 patients in each arm to be able to reject the null hypothesis that the rates for study and control groups are equal in intraoperative blood loss at a probability of 80%. The type one error probability associated with this test for the null hypothesis is 0.05. To compensate for patients' withdrawal or cases in which the procedure cannot be performed, we recruited 35 patients in each arm.

Procedure

- Skin incision through Pfannenstiel approach and anterior abdominal wall layers were incised separately.
- The loose peritoneum covering the lower uterine segment is dissected to expose the lower uterine segment and mobilize the urinary bladder downwards.
- Uterine artery ligation was performed by grasping the broad ligament on each side with thumb anterior and the index finger posterior lifting the base below the site uterine incision; the uterine artery was singly ligated with No. 1 vicryl suture. Uterine vessels were ligated and not damaged through inclusion of myometrium. The procedure was then repeated on the other side.
- A curvilinear transverse lower uterine segment incision was performed as usual. Higher incisions

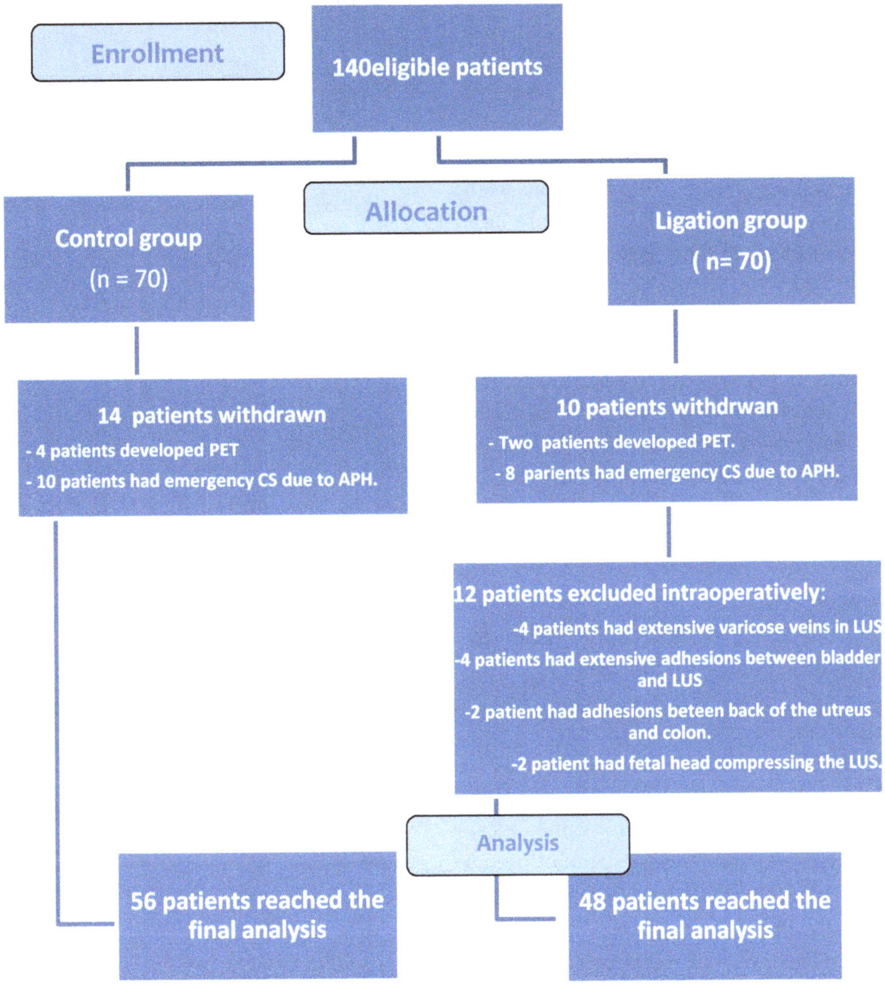

Fig. 1 Study flow chart. (PET: preeclampsia, LUS: lower uterine segment, CS: caesarean section, APH: antepartum hemorrhage)

were performed in cases where the traditional incision was expected to be directly through the placenta.

- Delivery of the baby and placenta.
- Closure of the uterine incision in 2 layers with no. 1 vicryl suture.
- Closure of the anterior abdominal wall in layers.

In the control group, lower segment caesarean section was performed in the classic way.

Assessment of intraoperative blood loss

The intraoperative blood loss was measured using the alkaline hematin method [12]. All the blood-stained swabs, diapers and pads and the contents in the drainage bottles were collected, put in a plastic bag and blended with 5% NaOH solution. The plastic bag was then transferred to the Stomacher Lab Blender (Model 3500, Seward Laboratories, London, UK) and processed for few minutes to extract hemoglobin. A portion of the fluid was collected and diluted with 5% NaOH solution. The concentration of alkaline hematin was obtained by assay in a spectrophotometer at 546 nm with the appropriate NaOH as a blank. The intra-assay coefficient for analyzing the concentration is 1%. The blood loss was then calculated using the patient's preoperative hemoglobin as a reference.

Outcome measures

The primary outcome measures of the study were:

- The amount of intra-operative blood loss.
- The change in pre and post-partum hemoglobin.

The secondary outcome measures were:

- The need for blood transfusion.
- The need for further surgical intervention to control intraoperative bleeding.
- The operative time.

Statistical methodology

Statistical analysis was performed using the Statistical Package for Social Science (SPSS Inc., NY) version 21 for Microsoft Windows. Data was described in terms of mean ± SD (standard deviation) for continuous variables and frequencies (number of cases) and percentages for categorical data. Independent Student's t-test was used to compare quantitative variables and Chi square test was used to compare categorical data. A p value < 0.05% was considered significant.

Results

We initially recruited 140 patients in this study. In the study group, 10 cases were withdrawn from the study (8 developed APH and had emergency CS and 2 developed PET). In the control group, 14 cases were withdrawn (10 cases developed APH and had emergency CS and 4 cases developed PET).

Difficulties during the procedure

In the study group, 12 cases were excluded intra-operatively due to difficulty in performing the procedure as:

1. Extensive varicosities over the lower uterine segment (LUS) in 6 cases
2. Extensive adhesions between the urinary bladder and LUS in cases with repeat cesarean sections in 3 cases,
3. Adhesions between the colon and the back of the uterus or the broad ligament in 2 cases,
4. Fetal head compressing over the lower uterine segment making fetal head injury possible during the procedure in one case,

In these cases, the procedure was not done, and patients were excluded from the final analysis. However, these cases were analyzed initially within the ligation group. Results remained significant by comparing 56 patients in the control group versus 60 patients in the ligation group (Additional file 1: Table S1, Additional file 2: Table S2, Additional file 3: Table S3 and Additional file 4: Table S4).

At the end, 104 patients reached the final analysis; 48 patients in the study (ligation) group and 56 patients in the control group. Study flow chart is shown in Fig. 1.

There was no statistically significant difference between the study and control groups regarding the demographic features and risk factors associated with placenta previa as shown in Table 1. The ultrasonographic features of the placentae in the study population are summarized in Table 2.

Patients in the ligation group had higher postoperative hemoglobin, which was statistically significant (p < 0.0001), shorter operative time that was not significant (p = 0.2). The intraoperative blood loss and requirements for blood transfusion were significantly lower in the ligation group compared with the control group

Table 1 Characteristics and risk factors in the study population

	ligation group (n = 48)	control group (n = 56)	p value
• Maternal age (years)	33.5 ± 4.8	34.1 ± 4.7	0.8
• BMI (kg/m2)	28.9.2 ± 4.7	29.2 ± 5.1	0.7
• Occupation:			
➢ housewife	28	38	0.6
➢ nonprofessional	14	12	
➢ professional	6	6	
• Residence:			
➢ Rural	34	42	0.6
➢ Urban	14	14	
• Smoking	1	0	0.5
• Parity	4.1 ± .0.9	4.3 ± 1.1	0.7
• Previous uterine surgery:			
➢ Caesarean section	20	23	0.6
➢ Dilatation and curettage	8	7	
➢ Myomectomy	2	1	
➢ Resection of septum	0	1	
➢ Resection of intrauterine adhesions	0	2	
➢ Repair of uterine rupture	2	2	
➢ B-lynch suture	0	1	
Previous placenta previa:			
➢ Minor	6	7	0.5
➢ Major	4	5	
• Manual removal of placenta	2	1	0.6
• Placenta previa and previous uterine surgery	8	12	0.7
• Pregnancy with assisted conception	2	4	0.5

Data are presented as mean ± SD or frequency and percentages

(569.3 ± 202.1 mL vs. 805.1 ± 224.5 mL, p < 0.0001 and 755 ± 56 mL vs. 786 ± 83 mL, p = 0.03 respectively) Three cases in the control group required further surgical interventions to control intraoperative bleeding; two cases of internal iliac artery (IIA) ligation and one case of supravaginal hysterectomy. In spite that patients with anterior placenta previa that were diagnosed antenatally with color Doppler and MRI to have placenta accrete were excluded from the study, one patient in the control group was discovered intra-operatively to have placenta accrete and that was the case in whom supravaginal hysterectomy was performed. No cases needed further surgical interventions in the study group. Two cases developed PPH in the control group compared to no cases in the ligation group (3.8% vs. 0%, p = 0.02). There were three cases of bladder injuries; one in the ligation group and two in the control group. Bleeding from varicosities over the bladder

Table 3 Outcome measures in the ligation and control groups

	Ligation group ($n = 48$)	Control group ($n = 56$)	p value
• Preoperative Hb (g/dL)	11.1 ± 0.61	11.2 ± 0.6	0.6
• Postoperative Hb (g/dL)	10.2 ± 0.34	9.3 ± 0.56	0.0001*
• Intraoperative blood loss (mL)	569.3 ± 202.1	805.1 ± 224.5	0.0001*
• Operative time (min)	54.2 ± 11.2	57 ± 10.9	0.2
• Amount of blood transfusion (mL)	755 ± 56	786 ± 83	0.03*
• Further surgical interventions:	0	3 (5.4%)	
➢ IIA ligation	0	2 (3.6%)	0.001*
➢ Supravaginal hysterectomy	0	1 (1.8%)	
• Urinary bladder injury	1 (2.1%)	2 (3.6%)	0.2
• Bleeding from varicosities over bladder surface	2 (4.2%)	3 (5.4%)	0.6
• Postpartum hemorrhage (n)	0	2 (3.6%)	0.02*

12 cases were excluded from ligation group in the final analysis due failure of the procedure. Results remained significant by comparing 56 patients in the control group versus 60 patients in the ligation group
Data is presented as mean ± SD or frequency and percentages
HB hemoglobin, *IIA* Internal iliac artery
*$p < 0.05$

surface was encountered in five cases; two in the ligation group and three cases in the control group. These differences were insignificant. Outcome measures in both groups are summarized in Table 3.

Regional anesthesia was used in all cases at the beginning. In the control group, six cases were converted to general anesthesia (GA) as spinal anesthesia worked off and additional surgical procedures were required and consumed longer time (two cases of internal iliac artery "IIA" ligation and one case of supravaginal hysterectomy). In these three cases, placenta was anterior. No cases in the study group required conversion to GA (0% vs. 23.1%, $p = 0.001$). There was no significant difference in the experience of anesthetist between the two groups. Anesthetic details are summarized in Table 4.

The mean gestational age at time of CS was 36.2 ± 1.1 weeks in the study group and 36.3 ± 0.9 weeks in the control group ($p = 0.7$). There was no significant difference between the two groups regarding the perinatal outcome difference as shown in Table 4.

Discussion

To our knowledge, it is the first study to assess the technique of uterine artery ligation in patients with central placenta previa. We recruited patients diagnosed with central placenta previa at 28 weeks' gestation by 2D ultrasound. We used the alkaline hematin test to allow objective assessment of the intraoperative blood loss.

The new procedure evaluated in this study was found to minimize the intraoperative blood loss and shorten the operative time. Patients in the study group had

Table 2 The ultra-sonographic criteria of the placenta in the study population

	Ligation group ($n = 48$)	Control group ($n = 56$)	p value
• Location:			
➢ Placenta previa anterior.	20(41.7%)	26(46.4%)	0.6
➢ Placenta previa posterior	28(58.3%)	30(53.6%)	0.8
Distance from internal os:			
➢ Incomplete Centralis	38(79.2%)	46(82.2%)	0.5
➢ Centralis	10(20.8%)	10(17.8%)	0.6
Color Doppler:			
➢ Normal	34(70.8%)	40(71.4%)	0.8
➢ Retro-placental hypervascularity	14(29.2%)	16(28.6%)	0.7
Clear zone:			
➢ Present	32(66.7%)	38(67.9%)	0.9
➢ Absent	16(33.3%)	18(32.1%)	0.7
Lacunae:			
➢ Present	8(16.7%)	10(17.9%)	0.8
➢ Absent	40(83.3%)	46(82.1%)	0.9

Data is presented as frequency and percentages

Table 4 Anesthetic details of CS and Perinatal outcome in the study population

	Ligation group ($n = 48$)	Control group ($n = 56$)	p value
• Type of anesthesia:			
➢ Spinal	38 (79.1%)	43 (76.8%)	
➢ Epidural	10 (20.9%)	13 (23.2%)	
➢ GA↑↑	0 (0%)	3 (5.3%)	
• Gestational age at time of CS (weeks)	36.2 ± 1.1	36.3 ± 0.9	0.7
• Birth weight (gram)	2875.6 ± 253.5	2976.5 ± 265.2	0.5
• Apgar score at 5 min:			
➢ 1–2	2(4.2%)	2(3.6%)	0.7
➢ 3–6	12(25%)	16(28.6%)	0.6
➢ ≥7	34(70.8%)	38(67.8%)	0.8
• Neonatal outcome:			
➢ Early neonatal death	1(2.1%)	1(1.8%)	0.88
➢ NICU admission	4(8.4%)	4(7.2%)	0.9
➢ Hospital discharge	44(91.6%)	51(91%)	0.91

Data is presented as frequency and percentages or mean ± SD
GA general anesthesia
↑↑: Conversion from spinal to general anesthesia as spinal worked off (2 cases of IIA ligation and 1 case of supravaginal hysterectomy)

higher postoperative hemoglobin and lower requirement for blood transfusion. In addition, none of the patients underwent the procedure needed further surgical interventions to control intraoperative bleeding, while three patients in the control group needed another surgical intervention; two IIA ligation and one case needed supravaginal hysterectomy.

The procedure was not easy in all cases and was not possible in some patients as those with extensive adhesions between the LUS and the urinary bladder, extensive varicose veins in the LUS. In these cases, the procedure was not done as we believed there would be a great risk of urinary bladder injury or severe bleeding from varicose veins. In some occasions, the fetal head was compressing LUS, and the ligation was not done.

Ligation of Internal iliac artery, used to be performed to overcome massive pelvic hemorrhage, is not the technique of choice for control of atonic PPH due to placenta previa. Apart from its efficacy it requires more time for dissection and effort for training [13]. In a comprehensive research for 30 years, O'Leary had suggested the procedure of uterine artery ligation as an efficient and alternate procedure to internal iliac artery ligation although in his trial, 10 out of 265 cases failed to respond [14]. In another excellent study concerning massive PPH due to uterine atony. The authors concluded that arterial embolization as effective as uterine artery ligation with success rate approaching 100%. Embolization can be performed after vaginal delivery in stable patients but it needs expertise and facilities [15].

The strengths of this study are the nature of the study (RCT) and reporting a novel technique in management of a serious obstetric condition as central placenta previa with potential for implication in clinical practice. The limitation of the study is the relatively small number of patients included.

Conclusion

Uterine artery ligation prior to uterine incision could be an effective method to reduce the intraoperative blood loss in patients with central placenta previa undergoing elective CS. Larger studies are required to reach a firm conclusion about the procedure.

Additional files

Additional file 1: Table S1. Characteristics and risk factors in the study population before exclusion. This table shows the socio-demographic and clinical data of all patients before exclusion.

Additional file 2: Table S2. The ultra-sonographic criteria of the placenta in the study population before exclusion. This table shows the ultrasound findings of all patients before enrollment.

Additional file 3: Table S3. Outcome measures in the ligation and control groups before exclusion. This tables shows postoperative outcome of all patients.

Additional file 4: Table S4. Anesthetic details of CS and Perinatal outcome in the study population before exclusion. This table shows the anesthetic and perinatal outcome.

Acknowledgements

The authors are grateful to the entire medical, nursing and laboratory staff at Minia Maternity University Hospital for their help and cooperation throughout the research work.

Authors' contributions

ASS: Design the study methodology, diagnosis of cases, operative management, data collection, results preparation, and manuscript writing. AEM: Design the study methodology, diagnosis of cases, operative management, data collection, results preparation, and manuscript writing. MEA: Design the study methodology data analysis, results preparation, and manuscript writing. HHK: Design the study methodology, operative management, diagnosis of clinical cases program, and data collection. HAB: Design the study methodology, operative management, diagnosis of cases. HFM: Design the study methodology, diagnosis of clinical cases program, and data collection. RRE: Design the study methodology, diagnosis of clinical cases program, and data collection. AGA: Design the study methodology, operative management, data collection, results preparation and manuscript writing. MAZ: Design the study methodology, diagnosis of cases, operative management, data collection, results preparation and manuscript writing. HES: Assist us in ethical consideration, help in reviewing the work, was involved in revising the manuscript and provide final approval of the version to be published. All authors read and approved the final manuscript.

Competing interests

The authors declare that they have no competing interests.

References

1. Getahun D, Oyelese Y, Salihu HM, Ananth CV. Previous cesarean delivery and risks of placenta previa and placental abruption. Obstet Gynecol. 2006;107(4):771–8.
2. Brace V, Kernaghan D, Penney G. Learning from adverse clinical outcomes: major obstetric haemorrhage in Scotland, 2003-05. BJOG. 2007;114(11):1388–96.
3. Olive EC, Roberts CL, Algert CS, Morris JM. Placenta praevia: maternal morbidity and place of birth. Aust N Z J Obstet Gynaecol. 2005;45(6):499–504.
4. Oyelese Y, Smulian JC. Placenta previa, placenta accreta, and vasa previa. Obstet Gynecol. 2006;107(4):927–41.
5. Gurol-Urganci I, Cromwell DA, Edozien LC, Smith GC, Onwere C, Mahmood TA, et al. Risk of placenta previa in second birth after first birth cesarean section: a population-based study and meta-analysis. BMC Pregnancy Childbirth. 2011;11:95.
6. Arlier S, Seyfettinoglu S, Yilmaz E, Nazik H, Adiguzel C, Eskimez E, et al. Incidence of adhesions and maternal and neonatal morbidity after repeat cesarean section. Arch Gynecol Obstet. 2017;295(2):303–11.
7. Cresswell JA, Ronsmans C, Calvert C, Filippi V. Prevalence of placenta praevia by world region: a systematic review and meta-analysis. Tropical Med Int Health. 2013;18(6):712–24.
8. Tuzovic L. Complete versus incomplete placenta previa and obstetric outcome. Int J Gynaecol Obstet. 2006;93(2):110–7.
9. Onwere C, Gurol-Urganci I, Cromwell DA, Mahmood TA, Templeton A, van der Meulen JH. Maternal morbidity associated with placenta praevia among women who had elective caesarean section. Eur J Obstet Gynecol Reprod Biol. 2011;159(1):62–6.
10. Rosenberg T, Pariente G, Sergienko R, Wiznitzer A, Sheiner E. Critical analysis of risk factors and outcome of placenta previa. Arch Gynecol Obstet. 2011; 284(1):47–51.
11. Schneiderman M, Balayla J. A comparative study of neonatal outcomes in placenta previa versus cesarean for other indication at term. J Matern Fetal Neonatal Med. 2013;26(11):1121–7.

12. Fraser IS, Warner P, Marantos PA. Estimating menstrual blood loss in women with normal and excessive menstrual fluid volume. Obstet Gynecol. 2001; 98(5 Pt 1):806–14.
13. Evans S, McShane P. The efficacy of internal iliac artery ligation in obstetric hemorrhage. Surg Gynecol Obstet. 1985;160(3):250–3.
14. O'Leary JA. Uterine artery ligation in the control of postcesarean hemorrhage. J Reprod Med. 1995;40(3):189–93.
15. Sergent F, Resch B, Verspyck E, Rachet B, Clavier E, Marpeau L. Intractable postpartum haemorrhages: where is the place of vascular ligations, emergency peripartum hysterectomy or arterial embolization? Gynecol Obstet Fertil. 2004;32(4):320–9.

10

A qualitative study to explore the attitudes of women and obstetricians towards caesarean delivery in rural Bangladesh

Tahmina Begum[1*], Cathryn Ellis[2], Malabika Sarker[3,4], Jean-Francois Rostoker[2], Aminur Rahman[1], Iqbal Anwar[1] and Laura Reichenbach[5]

Abstract

Background: Caesarean section is a lifesaving surgical intervention for women and their newborns, though overutilization is a public health concern. The caesarean rate in Bangladesh is approximately 23% overall, and in private facilities it is over 70%. It is essential to know both the supply side (obstetricians) and demand side (parturient women) views on caesarean birth in order to formulate specific interventions to address the escalating rate of caesareans.

Methods: This qualitative study took place in Matlab, a rural sub-district in Bangladesh. We interviewed women attending their 3rd antenatal visit, those with recent caesareans, and obstetricians from both public and private health facilities. In total there were twenty in-depth interviews and four focus group discussions. Study participants were asked about their preferences on birthing mode and knowledge of the caesarean section process. Thematic data analysis was done following a deductive approach.

Results: Women from this rural community had a strong preference for normal vaginal birth. However, they were willing to accept the attending health care provider's decision for caesarean birth. Antenatal care sessions did not provide information on the medical indications for caesarean section. Furthermore, some women had the misconception that episiotomy itself is a 'small caesarean.' Primary health care providers and clinic agents (brokers) had a strong influence on women's decision to choose a health facility for giving birth. However, obstetricians, having a preference for caesarean section, were receiving more patients from these brokers which may be an important reason for the high rate of clinically non-indicated caesareans at private hospitals in Bangladesh. Improper labour monitoring and inadequate staffing at health facilities were additional influences on the preference for caesarean section. However, critical knowledge gaps were also observed among study obstetricians, particularly with regards to the indications for and timing of elective caesarean sections.

Conclusion: There is a need to educate women about the advantages and disadvantages of different birthing modes to ensure their active participation in the decision making process. Strong policy regulations are needed to ensure legitimate decision making by obstetricians regarding mode of birthing.

Keywords: Caesarean delivery, Qualitative study, Perception, Attitude, Decision-making, Rural Bangladesh

* Correspondence: tbegum@icddrb.org
[1]Health Systems and Population Studies Division, International Centre for Diarrhoeal Disease Research Bangladesh (icddr,b), Dhaka, Bangladesh
Full list of author information is available at the end of the article

Background

Caesarean section is a life-saving surgical intervention for women and their newborns though its recent overutilization is a global public health concern [1, 2]. On average, there is a 4.4% annual rise in caesarean section rates worldwide, with Asian countries having the second highest annual increase during the period 1990–2014 [1]. In this context, the global recommendation of a 10–15% national caesarean rate has been critiqued and a revision urged [3]. A more recent multi-country survey conducted in 178 WHO member states has suggested that the population level caesarean section rate should not exceed 19%, as increased levels of neonatal and maternal mortality have been reported above this level [2]. Additionally, unnecessarily high caesarean rates have negative implications [4] at the individual, family, and national levels in terms of women's well-being, health expenditure, and efficient use of resources [1].

When considering the reasons for rapidly increasing caesarean section rates, non-clinical factors have emerged as equally important factors as clinical factors [5]. Lower fees for vaginal birth, fear of litigation, and patient's requests for the procedure are some of the non-clinical reasons for physicians to conduct caesarean sections [6]. Women who prefer caesarean birth consider vaginal birth to be a more painful and dangerous procedure, without considering the negative consequences of un-necessary surgical intervention [7]. Women with higher economic status and more formal education are more likely to make a self-request for caesarean section [8, 9]. Conversely, poor women with little education are presumed to have inadequate knowledge about caesarean section procedures [10] which is considered a significant barrier to involving women and their families in decision making related to the mode of birth [7]. As a result, service providers particularly the attending physicians are evolving as the solo decision makers regarding mode of birth, in low-income settings [6, 7].

However, physicians' decisions also differ based on the location of clinical practice. Doctors working in a public sector facility assess caesarean indications based on clinical guidelines, while private practitioners are more concerned with litigation issues and have a tendency to perform more caesarean sections for making more business out of this procedure [11, 12]. This attitude might explain the increasing caesarean rate in for-profit private health facilities. For example, in Brazil the caesarean rate was 72% in the private sector, compared to 31% in the public sector [13].

In Bangladesh, maternal health has evolved within an extensive national health care delivery system that includes peripheral level health posts (community clinics) and health centres (union health sub-centres and health and family welfare centres) supported by primary, secondary, and tertiary level hospitals situated at sub-districts, districts, and regional levels respectively. Different cadres of technical and lay community health workers are working for maternal health that include physicians, nurse-midwives; family welfare visitors (FWV) and community skilled birth attendants (CSBAs). At the most peripheral level, the CSBAs and FWVs are the main maternal healthcare caregivers who provide services both from health-posts and health centres, and through home-visits. At the government hospitals level nurses and midwives are the main caregivers for vaginal deliveries. Physicians work mostly at sub-district, district, and medical college hospitals and are responsible for managing complicated vaginal and caesarean births [14]. Until recently, there was no accredited midwifery professionals in Bangladesh educated to the standards of the International Confederation of Midwives (ICM) and WHO [14]. During the Millennium Development Goal (MDG) era, midwifery education drew special policy attention in Bangladesh and a new strategic direction was initiated resulting in a three-year diploma in midwifery program launched in 2013 by the Ministry of Health and Family Welfare with technical support from UNFPA and WHO. Six-month post-basic midwifery training for existing public sector nurses was also organized as an interim effort to produce a critical mass of ICM/WHO standard midwifery professionals [15]. To date, 800 midwives have been accredited at a diploma level, and the vast majority of them have been deployed in district and sub-district hospitals [15].

In line with health related Sustainable Development Goals (SDG) targets, the government of Bangladesh is committed to improve access to both basic and comprehensive emergency care services to reduce Maternal Mortality Ratio (MMR). However, progress is slow; the Bangladesh Demographic Health Survey (BDHS) 2014 shows that the majority of births (63%) still take place at home, mostly with unskilled birth attendants [16]. Despite poor progress in achieving high skilled attendance rate, the caesarean section rate increased from 4% in 2004 to 23% in 2014, contributed mainly by the for-profit private health sector [16].

Experience from high-income settings suggest that exploring obstetricians' and women's attitudes towards caesarean section might be a productive way to guide policy in reducing un-necessary caesarean sections [17]. However, such information is missing in a number of developing countries such as Bangladesh. To bridge the knowledge gap in this area, the present study attempts to explore the attitudes of both women and obstetricians towards caesarean section birth in a rural area of Bangladesh.

Methods

Study design, setting and participants

We conducted this qualitative study in 2012 in the rural setting of Matlab, a sub-district of Chandpur district in Bangladesh. Matlab was selected as the study site because the proportion of births taking place in health facilities (80%), as well as caesarean section rate (29%) in this area was much higher than the national average of 37% facility delivery rate and the 23% caesarean section rate [18]. We used in-depth interviews (IDIs) and focus group discussions (FGDs) to investigate both client and provider views on caesarean section as a mode of birth in a low-income over-medicalization contexts.

The study participants were currently pregnant women and recent post-caesarean mothers representing the demand side, and obstetricians working in public and private health facilities representing the supply side. Study participants were recruited from six health facilities, three public and three private. Public health facilities were chosen in such a way that covers a range of referral facilities that included one district hospital, one sub-district level Upazila Health Complex, and one union level Health and Family Welfare Centre (UHFWC). From the private sector two 'for-profit' private hospitals and one 'not-for-profit' maternity clinic were selected as study sites. All private facilities were situated in Maltab township area. Of the six study facilities, the public sector district hospital and two of the 'for profit' private facilities had capacity to perform caesarean sections while the remaining four were basic emergency obstetric care facilities where only vaginal births took place.

Data collection

Women's participation

To explore women's perspectives about caesarean section four focus group discussions (FGDs) and 14 in-depth interviews (IDIs) were conducted. FGDs were conducted with pregnant women during their third trimester of pregnancy while attending an antenatal care (ANC) visit in the study hospitals (public or private). In total 26 pregnant women participated in four FGDs. The third stage of pregnancy was chosen because women usually develop a birth plan by this time, as their expected date of delivery (EDD) is approaching [19]. The FGD sessions were conducted in a separate room in the study hospitals after completion of their scheduled ANC consultation.

A purposive sampling method was used to find the desired study participants from the targeted health facilities. Homogeneity of the participants in the focus groups was maintained in terms of education, socio-economic status, and area of residence. However, diversity in terms of parity, obstetric experience, and other socio-demographic characteristics was maintained while selecting FGD participants.

We also conducted fourteen IDIs with post-caesarean women, nine from private clinics and five from public sector health facilities. In private sector hospitals, we organized IDIs with post-caesarean women on their 4th postoperative day which took place in their hospital bed. Since no post-caesarean mothers were available in the public sector hospitals during the data collection period, women who had a caesarean in the Chandpur District Hospital within the last 42 days of the data collection period were tracked and sampled for interviews. We conducted IDIs with five such post-caesarean women and the interviews took place in the local health sub-centers where they came for scheduled postnatal checkups.

Obstetricians' participation

We conducted six IDIs with obstetricians, three in public facilities and three in private hospitals. Only currently practicing obstetricians with advanced post-graduate training in obstetrics and gynaecology (training for more than one year) from study hospitals were included. A convenience sampling method was used where obstetricians available in the study health facilities during data collection period were approached for an interview. The interview took place in the obstetrician's own visiting room in the hospital after regular office hours.

Each interview was forty-five to sixty minutes in length. Data collection was continued until saturation was reached. The data collection team comprised of the principal investigator (PI) and two experienced research assistants (RAs). All interviews were conducted by the PI while the RAs took notes. Each RA alternated with the other for each interview and did the same for data transcription and development of analytic memos.

We developed interview guidelines first in English and then translated them into Bangla which was finalized after field-testing in a similar rural setting to confirm the content and to identify any missing themes. Three separate guidelines were used to direct the interview session with the three different type of study participants. The interview guidelines are added as supplementary file (Additional file 1) with this manuscript.

All IDIs and FGDs were tape-recorded, with verbal informed consent, except one with an obstetrician from a private clinic who did not permit the audio recording. In that case, detailed notes were taken during the interview.

During the interview with women's, their perceptions and attitudes regarding caesareans, preferred mode of birth, source and level of knowledge, cultural beliefs, and factors influencing decision-making about mode of birthing were considered. When interviewing obstetricians, their medical knowledge on indications for caesarean section, pros and cons related to each mode of birthing, perceived non-medical reasons to choose caesareans by fellow colleagues, and fear of litigation, were explored.

Ethics approval and consent to participate

Ethical approval was obtained from the Ethical Review Committee of the James P Grant School of Public Health, BRAC University. Informed oral consent was obtained from all the participants and permission was obtained from hospital authorities for using the hospital premises for study data collection. The consent form that was used for taking permission from study participants is attached with the manuscript as Additional file 2. This consent form detailed out the interview procedure, risk and benefit of participating in the study in front of the interviewee. Ethical Review Committee of JPGSPH reviewed the consent form and gave permission for taking Verbal informed consent considering the rural culture and related constraints on taking written consent. However, the Relevance, Appropriateness, Transparency and Soundness review guidelines were used to check the completeness of all the required qualitative study activities while preparing this manuscript [20].

Data analysis

We undertook a thematic data analysis using a deductive approach developed by the National Centre for Social Research, Framework analysis [21]. Data collection, transcription, and analysis were undertaken on an iterative processes. Initial transcriptions were in Bengali which were then back translated to English before coding [22]. WHO recommended "onwards backwards technique" for qualitative data transcription in between two languages was followed [23]. A list of a-priori codes were developed based on research themes. (The definition of each code and sub-codes with the condition when to use and not to use is mentioned in the code book which is attached as Additional file 3). The study findings were arranged systematically in matrices using those A-priori codes, which helped to identify the recurrent themes between participants. The summarized findings were compared and contrasted under themes recorded in the matrices [24]. Women's attitude towards caesarean section was compared with obstetricians' views, and pregnant women's views towards caesarean section was compared with post-caesarean women's recent experiences. The same themes which were commonly being reflected across the participants were grouped together. However, divergent but relevant themes were also reported separately. Intra-coder reliability was reported as 80% when checked between one research assistant and the principal investigator's initial coding of two interviews and one focus group. Disagreement over coding was handled through re-reading interview data and further discussion between researchers.

Results

Study participants' background information

Women participating in FGDs (N = 26)

The average (mean) age of pregnant women who participated in the FGDs was 23 years. The education status ranged from below primary to completed higher secondary level and four of them were studying at the bachelor level. The majority of them were housewives. Regarding place and mode of last birth, ten births took place at home with TBAs, four were vaginal births at a health facility; and two were caesarean birth and the remaining ten were primigravidas.

Women participating in individual interviews (N = 14)

The ages of the 14 post-caesarean mothers ranged between 16 and 37 years. Of them, six had below higher secondary level, three had secondary level education, and five had no formal education. Two post-caesarean women in private hospitals received no ANC while the others received, on average, three ANC visits during their last pregnancies. All post-caesarean IDI participants were housewives. The average monthly family income of women having caesareans at a public hospital ranged from 77 USD to 192 USD, while those from private hospitals ranged from 128 USD to 384 USD. The direct cost for a caesarean ranged between 77 USD and 128 USD in public hospitals and between 282 USD and 320 USD in private clinics.

Obstetricians participating in individual interview (N = 6)

The work experience of obstetricians ranged from four and a half to twenty years. All public sector obstetricians interviewed were involved in private practice after office hours.

The summary of socio demographic characteristics of all three categories of study participants are mentioned in the Additional file 4.

The details of FGDs and *individual interviews* in terms of number of participants, and location of each event is presented in Table 1.

Study themes and findings

Perceptions and attitudes regarding caesarean birth among pregnant and post-caesarean women were explored using six major codes: preferred mode of delivery, preferred place of delivery, knowledge about caesarean section, influencing factors, difficulties faced, and cultural practices. The obstetricians' attitudes were investigated using three major codes: knowledge about caesareans, difficulties faced during vaginal birth, and women's preferences. (The summary of study findings under all different codes are presented in Additional file 5) Subsequently, all the study findings gathered under these nine different codes were merged into three common themes: **preferred mode and place of birth, knowledge about caesarean, and factors determining decisions to perform caesarean section**. Under the theme of 'preferred mode and place of birth,' *the codes* women's preference on place of birth, mode of birthing, and the reasons behind their attitudes were merged with obstetricians' experiences of talking with women about their wish for normal delivery. The theme 'knowledge about caesarean' was used to group the knowledge of both women and obstetricians regarding the

Table 1 Data collection methods and participants

Methodology	Participant type		Number of interview/ discussion session	Number of participants
Focus Group Discussion	Women	Pregnant women from private facilities	2	6
		Pregnant mothers from public facilities	2	7
Total			4	26
In depth Interview	Women	Post-caesarean mothers from public facilities	5	
		Post-caesarean mothers from private facilities	5	
			4	
	Obstetricians	Public health facilities	2	
			1	
			1	
		Private health facilities	1	
			1	
Total			20	

facts of caesarean births. Finally, the theme of 'factors determining decisions to perform caesarean sections' included the findings gathered under codes 'influencing factors' and 'difficulties faced' by the post-caesarean mothers and the obstetricians (Fig. 1).

Preferred mode and place of delivery

Both pregnant and post-caesarean women in this study expressed their preferences for vaginal birth at home where TBAs are the main delivery caregivers. Even if the cost of both normal vaginal and caesarean deliveries was assumed to be the same, they preferred a vaginal birth to a caesarean. The reasons included faster postpartum recovery and living in extended families where elderly members who were the main decision makers, had a strong preference for vaginal birth. Obstetricians also mentioned women's preference, including those working outside of their homes, for vaginal birth in this community. When asked about attitudes and preferred mode of birth among working and educated women, obstetricians mentioned that home birth is preferred among these women as they still rely on elder women's decisions in the family. A twenty-five year-old pregnant woman, during an FGD, commented on why having a caesarean is difficult and painful.

> *"We need to carry paddy [rice] bundle over our head and need to feed our cattle. If suddenly rain comes we have to take the cut [rice] paddy from the yard to inside the house. In that case if I would have caesarean section, I will not be able to run. Women's lives become really handicapped after having this operation" (Quote from pregnant woman)*

Perceived 'health hazards to the women and her baby due to caesarean section' were mentioned as another reason for preferring vaginal birth. Respondents expressed their views that caesarean babies are more prone to pneumonia and post-caesarean incisions remain painful for a long time. Obstetricians had similar views regarding incision pain; they mentioned that women who had caesarean sections visited their clinics with incision pain even six months post-surgery.

However, women in-general, were not rigid about their preferences but rather willing to accept physician's decision for a caesarean, if deemed necessary. A twenty five-year old post-caesarean woman from a private health facility expressed her concern,

> *"Before my case, none of my family members ever attended hospital for birthing purpose. As a part of the tradition, I also went to my natal home and they called our family 'daima' [traditional birth attendant]. When labour pain started, my baby defecated inside the uterus and instantly she referred me to this hospital. Consequently caesarean delivery saved my baby's life." (Post caesarean mother)*

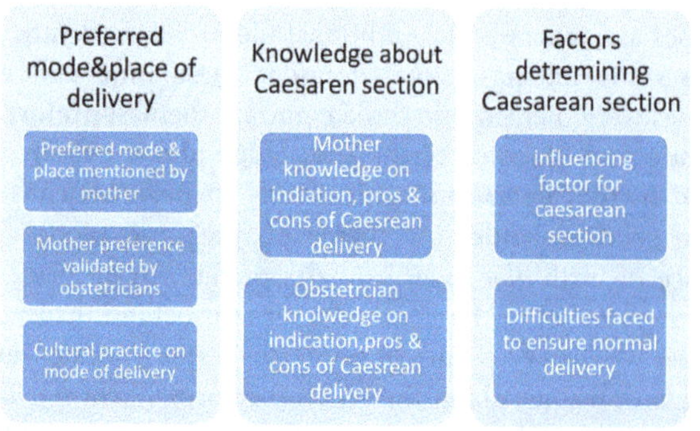

Fig 1. Study themes and sub-themes

Contrastingly, three of the twenty-six mothers participating in the FGDs showed a positive attitude toward caesarean section. One pregnant women mentioned:

> *"I prefer Caesarean delivery. I heard baby delivered by caesarean section had a healthier brain compared to normally delivered baby as it does not stay in the birth canal for a long time".(Quote from pregnant woman)*

One obstetrician from a public hospital mentioned that mothers demand caesarean sections for stillbirths. Considering it as unjustified on medical grounds, she commented:

> *"We never recommend caesarean section for fresh stillbirth. Rather we try to induce normal labour through medication. However, women often consider the dead fetus as a poison within the womb and request for caesarean section within the shortest possible time. I get surprised having similar request from multiple cases in the recent past where my counselling did not work" (Quote from Obstetrician)*

With regards to a health facility preference (public or a private)., the majority of the pregnant and post-caesarean women had no specific preference. Rather they relied completely on the attending health care provider's to choose the health facility.

Knowledge on caesarean section

Women had limited knowledge and several misconceptions about caesarean section. They perceived there to be two types of caesarean section: one, *'small caesarean'* where women deliver normally (vaginally) with a cut in the perineum (episiotomy), and the second, *'large caesarean'* where the abdomen is cut under anesthesia to extract the baby.

One multiparous, post-caesarean mother from a private hospital said:

> *"I am so happy that I have 'large caesarean' section this time. I had to suffer a lot ... such as pain & itching in my private parts ... even I had pain during sexual intercourse for a long time, since my last baby was delivered vaginally with 'small caesarean' section." (Quote from Post caesarean mother)*

However, none of the pregnant women received any information about the medical indications for caesarean section, nor its benefits and risks, although they were attending the third trimester antenatal checkup on the date of the FGD. They received information about caesarean section mostly from relatives and neighbors who had experienced a caesarean section in the past. They thought caesarean birth was becoming a common event as more and more private clinics and hospitals were being established in their neighborhood.

> *"The word caesarean section arose from the hospital. As, now-a-days number of hospitals has increased, caesarean birth has also increased. More mother and fetus used to die earlier but currently caesarean birth is saving lives of both, though sometime doctors do caesarean section unnecessarily for their financial interest." ... (Quote from Pregnant woman)*

When the pregnant women were asked to list the common clinical conditions for which their friends or relatives had undergone a caesarean, the top three causes were previous caesarean, less fluid, and baby defecating in the uterus.

On the other hand, obstetricians stated that they chose to not overburden the mothers with caesarean related information unless the current pregnancy had clear indications to deliver the baby surgically. All of them mentioned that although risks exist with operative procedures such as caesareans, it decreases maternal and neonatal deaths. Two (out of six) obstetricians in the study mentioned that having a vaginal birth attended by an inexperienced health care provider even in a hospital setting carries more health hazards than having a caesarean section.

When asked about common clinical reasons for performing caesareans, obstetricians mentioned two types: emergency and planned. Indications for emergency caesareans mentioned by all six obstetricians were similar. However, their responses for the cause of planned caesareans varied. While half of them mentioned that caesareans performed based on patient request are called 'elective', other obstetricians said that certain clinical conditions require a caesarean to be performed electively. However, while validating the obstetrician knowledge against the National Institute of Clinical Excellence (NICE) guideline recommended by the international expert committee, certain knowledge gap has observed. After excluding Cephalo Pelvic Disproportion (CPD), all the indications mentioned by obstetricians as planned C-section were in the contraindication list of NICE. The complete list of indications of planned Caesarean section mentioned by the study obstetricians are presented in the right column of Table 2 and the recommendation made by NICE on similar clinical conditions are presented in the left column of this table. For example, obstetrician believe women having breech pregnancy should be a case of caesarean delivery where birth order should not be a concern. On the other hand NICE guideline does not recommend planned caesarean section for breech pregnancy in higher order birth and for the first time mother without attempting to restore the fetal position through external cephalic version.

Table 2 Validation of obstetrician responses in contrast to National Institute of Clinical Excellence (NICE) guidelines on planned caesareans

Indication of planned caesarean section mentioned by obstetricians	Contraindication of planned caesarean section mentioned in NICE guidelines
• Previous caesarean • Breech presentation irrespective of parity • Twin pregnancy irrespective of parity and presentation • Preterm birth/ Small for gestational age • Cephalopelvic Disproportion (CPD) • Short stature of mother • Obese mother • Elective caesarean: to avoid conflict ✓ Hospital staff patients and well off family clients ✓ Patient with gestational diabetes ✓ Patient having bad obstetric history ✓ Primary/ secondary infertility ✓ Fear/can't tolerate labour pain • Pre-eclampsia • Postdates pregnancy	• Previous caesarean • Primigravida breech without attempt of external cephalic version and breech in multiparous women • Twin pregnancy in cephalic presentation • Preterm birth/ Small for gestational age • Suspected CPD (that means short stature women could not be an indication) • Obese women even with BMI ≥ 50 • Elective caesarean (without obstetrical or medical indication) [36]

There were also mixed findings regarding the timing of elective caesareans. With the exception of one respondent, all of them stated that an elective caesarean could be done any time after 37 gestational weeks. One obstetrician said that he would only perform an elective caesarean two to three days before the expected date of delivery. The reluctance of obstetricians to choose the time for elective caesarean was commented on by a post caesarean mother who had an elective caesarean fifteen days before the expected date of delivery. Although she had no risk factors for vaginal birth, her obstetrician met her directly at the operation theatre once she was admitted to hospital.

> *"I guess out of 100, only 10 lucky women could deliver normally. I wanted to deliver normally this time after having one 'Caesar' (caesarean section) five years back, but none of my doctors were willing to take the risk. Since there was no option other than caesarean, I came in this hospital 15 days prior to my given date of delivery and being delivered through C-section." – (Quote from post caesarean mother)*

Factors determining caesarean section

Community health care providers, from both the public and informal private sectors, played a significant role in the decision-making process regarding the mode of birth in this study. Being the first line health care provider; Community skilled birth attendants, Family welfare visitors, Traditional Birth Attendants and village doctors were the primary contact point for the pregnant women and their families at the community level. Almost all of the pregnant and post- caesarean mothers in the study mentioned visiting at least one of these community health providers before coming to the obstetrician.

The preference for a community health provider is shown in the following quote:

> *"I will contact with 'Apa' at the time of delivery, she will try her level best to deliver my baby here. If my luck would not be good enough to deliver my baby at her hand, she will refer me to appropriate health facility. I usually go to her to get the address of doctor when any of my family members or me fall sick" (Quote from pregnant woman)*

A similar comment was made by several pregnant women in different FGDs. However, obstetricians in the study expressed a different view about community health providers. They claimed these community healthcare providers were serving as brokers for local private clinics and receiving commissions from these clinics for referring obstetric patients. However, the referral fees given to them varied according to the procedure, get higher commission for caesarean birth. So that they refer patients to the obstetrician who does more number of caesarean sections. Two of the study obstetricians claimed that some doctors perform caesareans without valid indications to upsurge their practice.

> *"Here in this rural area patients are not choosing doctors based on academic degrees or experience, rather they choose doctors based on the recommendation from the referee (community health providers). Referrals were frequently for doctors who performed more caesareans instead of vaginal deliveries. I have heard that sometimes the tariff that they got is more than my operation charge."- (Quote from Obstetrician)*

Obstetricians claimed that private clinics were using their agents, known locally as *'dalals'* (brokers) to take the birthing women away from public hospitals. One study obstetrician mentioned that sometimes the service providers in the primary health facility refer birthing women to the higher facility without any valid medical indication and often with misleading clinical findings indicating the need for caesarean section.

> *"Once I received a referred patient with complaints of fetal distress and meconium for caesarean section, but on examination I found no evidence of such things. In contrast, the woman presented to me had progressive normal labour with normal fetal heart rate, maternal pulse and blood pressure was ok, and so she could be allowed to deliver normally. I allowed the woman to delivery by normal vaginal methods and that occurred successfully. But other doctors may not follow the same procedures, because most of the doctors meet patients in the operation theatre in the private clinic." (Quote from obstetrician)*

Poor quality of labour monitoring was also a concern for the private clinics. An obstetrician from a private clinic stated that:

> *"We usually do not take risks when there is 50/50 chance of vaginal delivery even in the private clinics, as nurses working there are reluctant to do regular follow up and are not competent to manage normal delivery. My whole career will be ruined for a single fetal death." (Quote from obstetrician)*

Similarly, obstetricians working in public hospitals claimed that inadequate numbers of skilled human resources was the main constraint for provision of high quality maternity care services. Although the health facility was well-equipped logistically, caesarean section services were not available after office hours (2 p.m.) due to unavailability of obstetricians and/or anaesthetists. Moreover, only one duty doctor was available after office hours to manage emergencies in both 50-bed UHC and in 250-bed district hospitals, and the duty nurses were not competent to manage normal vaginal deliveries. Obstetricians mentioned that they perform caesarean section in public hospitals only during office hours.

A lack of respectful treatment towards women in labour was reported to be a factor influencing the choice of delivery mode. One of the post-caesarean mothers complained about the attending nurse's unsupportive behavior as a cause of her self-request for a caesarean birth. A nineteen year-old post-caesarean mother from a private clinic expressed her frustration:

> *"I was admitted with labor pain in this hospital at 11 a.m. The nurse examined me there and said that it was not labor pain but I got sweating with that extreme pain. She did per vaginal examination several times, it was also much embarrassing and painful. I was losing my patience but they did not speak a single pleasant word to me. Then I left the hospital by giving 'risk bond' and went for caesarean section in a nearby clinic at 7 p.m." (Quote from post- caesarean mother)*

Discussion

This study identified three key factors affecting the mode of birth: client's attitude, obstetrician's attitude, and health facility influence. Client's attitude on Caesarean delivery was mostly influenced by the health care provider and the attending health facility type. Whereas obstetrician's attitude does not depend on their medical knowledge rather more subjective to financial interest of the clinics or brokers from whom they receive patients. In some instances Obstetricians knowledge on caesarean indications did not match with international guidelines and recommendations. On the other hand, public health facilities had certain challenges to provide 24/7 emergency obstetric services which creates more dependency to private health sector. However, private health facility's undue interest to do medically non- indicated caesarean section was also being critiqued by the study obstetricians.

In general, women in this rural community had strong preferences for normal vaginal birth. Financial access does not equate with autonomy around decision making for mode of birth among women who work for wages. They still rely on elderly women in the family as influential decision-makers. This custom has also been documented in a study about the reasons for using a TBA in Bangladesh [25]. Despite the strong cultural preference for vaginal birth, women did not demonstrate a negative attitudes towards caesareans; rather they perceived these surgeries as necessary to save lives. This attitude contradicts findings from an earlier qualitative study conducted in the same study area, which reported that women who had caesareans felt it was an insult to their identity as a mother [26]. Our study, on the contrary, suggests that non-supportive behavior of nurses in the health facility, fear of episiotomy during vaginal birth, and the risk of fetal death during labour were the main reasons for which participants made self-request for caesarean. Similar to this study, maternal request for caesarean delivery after having an episiotomy and subsequent experience of painful sexual intercourse in a previous pregnancy were mentioned by the women from Nigeria and Turkey [27, 28]. It has also been reported that obstetricians also believed that vaginal birth is associated with more perineal injury and sexual dysfunction [29]. Despite this, other research suggests that postpartum sexual functioning is not associated with the birthing mode [30]. In addition, episiotomy performed during vaginal birth as a means of protection against perineal injury has not been proven effective always. A recent study among a large cohort (22,800 births) confirmed that statistically significant amount of perineal injury occurred even with lower episiotomy rate (6.7% episiotomy rate) [31]. Given that episiotomy is not protective against perineal injury and in fact causes short and long term negative sequalae, birth attendants should refrain from this practice to avoid unnecessary fear of episiotomy among women willing to give birth vaginally.

Some women also mentioned the lack of kind, comforting, and respectful behavior towards them during labour. Since an individual's pain tolerance varies, it is recommended that health care workers be compassionate and supportive towards women in labour to increase confidence in their ability to give birth vaginally [32–34]. In our study, women were not knowledgeable regarding the medical indications for caesarean section. The antenatal care provided in the third trimester did not include information regarding risks and benefits of caesarean and normal vaginal delivery modes of childbirth. Friends and neighborhood women who had similar experiences remained the major source of information. Women's lack of health literacy about surgical birth was used by some peripheral level lay health workers and informal providers to convince women to have caesarean sections even in the absence of valid clinical indications. For example, meconium staining is not listed as an indication for caesarean in the NICE guidelines [35]. However, women in this study believed that caesareans done on the grounds of meconium stained liquor could save their baby and for that they were thankful to their physicians. This finding corresponds to one systematic review which determined that poor knowledge about caesarean section is the main reason for women requesting caesareans, and recommended the involvement of parturient women in informed decision making processes [34].

The obstetricians in the study were found to be more positive towards caesarean section compared to vaginal birth. Fear of litigation and their prior maternity experiences were of paramount importance in determining their attitudes. However, their knowledge of indications for caesarean delivery did not coincide with international recommendations as indicated by the recent NICE guideline [36] and the American College of Obstetricians and Gynecologists Guideline [37]. For example, other than primigravida breech and cephalopelvic disproportion, all other clinical indications provided as reasons for performing caesareans by the study obstetricians are not listed in either of these international guidelines [36, 37]. Additionally, the obstetricians were not certain of the recommended gestational age for planned caesarean sections. This study identified two women who were having an elective caesarean fifteen days prior to their expected date of delivery. In contrast, the NICE guideline has recommended the appropriate gestational age for elective caesarean section to be after 39 weeks. Elective caesareans performed at earlier gestational ages have been associated with adverse neonatal outcomes such as increased rate of infections, respiratory distress and more admissions to neonatal intensive care units [38]. In this study, physicians were reluctant to involve women in evidence-based informed decision making, and were unaware of internationally accepted guidelines. In this regard, some health experts mentioned that if the "ruling class" clinicians perform caesareans without valid clinical indications, this erroneous practice and corresponding attitude may be accepted as 'normal' among the general population [39]. Once a high caesarean section rate becomes 'normal' it is difficult to change provider attitudes and practices.

The attitudes of both women and obstetricians differ based on the type of facility - attending hospital, private, NGO, or public. Concerns about safety included lack of ability to monitor labour by hospital staff and inadequate staffing of the facility. Other than the NGO clinic, both the public and private hospitals' mothers and obstetricians did not have confidence on the nurse competency to monitor normal labour and their ability to handle any birthing emergency. In Bangladesh, normal childbirth in public hospitals is mostly attended by nurses and there is not yet a functioning midwifery profession. Poor quality of childbirth care has been reported in public health facilities [11, 40]. To address this gap, Bangladesh is in the process of adding newly trained midwives to the maternal and neonatal health care team, who will hopefully be proficient in attending normal childbirth, thus allaying some of the concerns voiced by mothers and obstetricians [15].

This study also highlighted the perception of inadequate human resources to provide basic and comprehensive emergency obstetric care after office hours in public facilities. Inadequate staffing and logistics has been documented as a barrier in public health facilities in the context of other developing countries as well [6, 11, 41]. To compensate for this constraint in resources, a defensive obstetric practice has been observed among the study obstetricians, who are performing elective caesareans during office hours. However, evidence suggests that a caesarean done without a valid medical indication increases the chance of maternal death 2.84 times in comparison to vaginal birth [1]. Women and obstetricians in this study appeared to be unaware of this evidence.

Financial motives and avoidance of possible lawsuits are documented as major influencing factors for caesarean births in private sector health facilities. Obstetricians interviewed from private clinics stated that they sometimes feel the need to perform unnecessary caesareans to meet the clinic's financial demands. In doing so, the community health care providers and clinic referral agents, performed 'patient counseling for caesareans' on behalf of clinic authorities and obstetricians in the private sector. Our study findings corroborate other study findings from rural Bangladesh that have also confirmed the presence of a broker or '*Dalal*' to move pregnant women from public health facilities to private facilities [11]. Our study findings depicts that women had to pay for caesarean section services in the public hospitals. This is a potential threat to the movement towards universal health coverage (UHC) as the poor may become poorer to meet maternity expenses; this is especially true in Bangladesh where the main mode of payment for health services is out-of-pocket [42].

Limitations and methodological considerations

It was definitely challenging to investigate both women's and obstetrician's views in the same study. While doing so, the strengths of the study include getting similar responses from both the caregivers and care receivers in regards to preferred birthing mode and quality of care in public facilities. Assumptions that most women choose caesarean sections is challenged, and the pain and fear that women experience after episiotomy was identified as a key reason for requests for caesarean birth.

While we are confident in the findings of this study, it was not without its limitations. The study setting and sampling strategy raise methodological issues. The study was conducted in Matlab, an area in Bangladesh known for its long history of public health interventions and research studies as well as the presence of icddr,b, an international health research organization well known to the community. It is possible that the presence of icddr,b researchers may introduce some response bias. Furthermore, it is possible that the study findings do not accurately represent women's and obstetrician's view from other areas in Bangladesh. While the objective of the study was not to produce nationally representative results, we did provide adequate contextual description allowing readers to determine whether the findings are relevant in other areas of Bangladesh and elsewhere in low and middle income countries [22].

Conclusion

The preference of women for vaginal birth in this study was not the major factor determining their attitude towards caesarean section birth. Women had inadequate information about caesarean birth and were mostly dependent on their provider's decision regarding mode of birth. The fear of episiotomy was strong among the study participants. The context and underlying reasons for this attitude and the methods and indications for performing episiotomies, require further investigation. The need for respectful behavior among health care providers, ethical clinical practice and education of women and their active participation in the decision making process have been highlighted in this study. Ensuring availability of 24-h obstetric services in public facilities and educating pregnant women about choices in the mode of childbirth, including indications for, and complications resulting from caesarean section, is a productive way to avert third party influence in promoting unnecessary surgical birth.

Additional files

Additional file 1: Code book. Description of A-priori codes and sub-codes. This file detail out the A-priori code and sub code-list that includes definition, when to use and when not use for each of the codes and sub codes.

Additional file 2: Consent form. Consent form in English. The consent form details out the interview procedure, risk and benefit of participating in the study.

Additional file 3: Interview guidelines. Guidelines to conduct In-depth interview and Focus Group Discussion. Three separate guidelines were used for in-depth interview with post caesarean women, obstetricians and Focus group discussions with pregnant women.

Additional file 4: Demography data. Demographic details of study participants. This excel sheet detail out the socio- demographic characteristics of all study participants including age in range, sex, education, religion, occupation, family income, cost of caesarean service etc..

Additional file 5: Data display. Summary of study findings. The study findings are grouped under different color codes.

Abbreviations

Caesarean section: Caesarean; FWV: Family Welfare Visitor; icddr,b: International Centre for Diarrhoeal Disease Research Bangladesh; JPGSPH: James P Grant School of Public Health; NGO: Non-Governmental Organization; NICE: National Institute for Health and Care Excellence; SBA: Skilled Birth Attendant; TBA: Traditional Birth Attendant; UHFWC: Union Health & Family Welfare Centre

Acknowledgements

We are thankful to all the study participants, hospital authorities, and research assistants. We also acknowledge James P Grant School of Public Health for their financial assistance, icddr,b Matlab hospital and HDSS officials for their support during data collection. Icddr,b is also grateful to the government of Bangladesh, Canada, Sweden and UK for providing core/ unrestricted support.

Funding

JPGSPH provided funding for this thesis research & some voluntary support was received from icddr,b Matlab hospital.

Authors' contributions

Conception and research design: TB, LR Data analysis: TB, LR Data interpretation: TB, LR, CE; JFR, IA, AR, MS. Drafting the manuscript: TB, LR, CE; JFR, IA, AR, MS. Language edit: LR, JFR. All authors read and approved the final manuscript.

Authors' information

All the authors listed in this article have many years of clinical and research experience in maternal health.

Consent for publication

The study participants gave the author permission to publish their research views regarding this specific research topic, provided that anonymity was maintained.

Competing interests

The authors declare that they have no competing interests.

Author details

[1]Health Systems and Population Studies Division, International Centre for Diarrhoeal Disease Research Bangladesh (icddr,b), Dhaka, Bangladesh. [2]Department of Family Practice, University of British Columbia, Vancouver, BC, Canada. [3]James P Grant School of Public Health, BRAC University, Dhaka, Bangladesh. [4]Institute of Public Health University, Heidelberg, Germany. [5]Population Council, Washington, DC, USA.

References

1. Betrán AP, Ye J, Moller A-B, Zhang J, Gülmezoglu AM, Torloni MR. The increasing trend in caesarean section rates: global, regional and national estimates: 1990-2014. PLoS One. 2016;11(2):e0148343.
2. Molina G, Weiser TG, Lipsitz SR, Esquivel MM, Uribe-Leitz T, Azad T, Shah N, Semrau K, Berry WR, Gawande AA. Relationship between cesarean delivery rate and maternal and neonatal mortality. JAMA. 2015;314(21):2263–70.
3. World Health Organisation: WHO Statement on Caesarean Section Rates. 2015.
4. Gibbons L, Belizán JM, Lauer JA, Betrán AP, Merialdi M, Althabe F. The global numbers and costs of additionally needed and unnecessary caesarean sections performed per year: overuse as a barrier to universal coverage. World Health Report. 2010;30:1–31.
5. Lo JC. Patients' attitudes vs. physicians' determination: implications for cesarean sections. Soc Sci Med. 2003;57(1):91–6.
6. Yazdizadeh B, Nedjat S, Mohammad K, Rashidian A, Changizi N, Majdzadeh R. Cesarean section rate in Iran, multidimensional approaches for behavioral change of providers: a qualitative study. BMC Health Serv Res. 2011;11(1):159.
7. Ajeet S, Jaydeep N, Nandkishore K, Nisha R. Women's knowledge, perceptions, and potential demand towards caesarean section. Natl J Community Med. 2011;2(2):244–8.
8. Anwar I, Nababan HY, Mostari S, Rahman A, Khan JA. Trends and inequities in use of maternal health Care Services in Bangladesh, 1991-2011. PLoS One. 2015;10(3):e0120309.
9. Feng XL, Xu L, Guo Y, Ronsmans C. Factors influencing rising caesarean section rates in China between 1988 and 2008. Bull World Health Organ. 2012;90(1):30–39A.
10. Stanton C, Ronsmans C. Caesarean birth as a component of surgical services in low-and middle-income countries. Bull World Health Organ. 2008;86(12):A-A.
11. Aminu M, Utz B, Halim A, Van Den Broek N. Reasons for performing a caesarean section in public hospitals in rural Bangladesh. BMC Pregnancy Childbirth. 2014;14(1):130.
12. Einarsdóttir K, Kemp A, Haggar FA, Moorin RE, Gunnell AS, Preen DB, Stanley FJ, Holman CAJ. Increase in caesarean deliveries after the Australian private health insurance incentive policy reforms. PLoS One. 2012;7(7):e41436.
13. Potter JE, Hopkins K, Faúndes A, Perpétuo I. Women's autonomy and scheduled cesarean sections in Brazil: a cautionary tale. Birth. 2008;35(1):33–40.
14. Bogren M, Begum F, Erlandsson K. The historical development of the midwifery profession in Bangladesh. J Asian Midwives. 2017;4(1):65–74.
15. Bogren M, Doriswamy S, Erlandsson K. Building a new generation of midwifery faculty members in Bangladesh. J Asian Midwives. 2017;4(2):52–8.
16. National Institute of Population Research and Training (NIPORT) MaA, and ICF International. 2015.: Bangladesh Demographic and Health Survey 2014: Key Indicators. 2014.
17. Keedle H, Schmied V, Burns E, Dahlen HG. The journey from pain to power: a meta-ethnography on women's experiences of vaginal birth after caesarean. Women Birth. 2018;31(1):69–79.
18. Rahman MM, Alam N, Razzaque A, Streatfield PK. Health and demographic surveillance system – MATLAB. JHPN. 2014;46(124):22.
19. Sanavi FS, Rakhshani F, Ansari-Moghaddam A, Edalatian M. Reasons for elective cesarean section amongst pregnant women; a qualitative study. J Reprod Infertility. 2012;13(4):237.
20. Wu S, Wyant DC, Fraser MW. Author guidelines for manuscripts reporting on qualitative research. J Soc Soc Work Res. 2016;7(2):000.
21. Ritchie J, Lewis J, Nicholls CM, Ormston R. Qualitative research practice: a guide for social science students and researchers. 2nd ed. Los Angeles: SAGE; 2014.
22. Shenton AK. Strategies for ensuring trustworthiness in qualitative research projects. Educ Inf. 2004;22(2):63–75.
23. World Health Organization: Process of translation and adaptation of instruments. http://www.who.int/substance_abuse/research_tools/translation/en/. 2009.
24. Liamputtong P. Qualitative data analysis: conceptual and practical considerations. Health Promot J Austr. 2009;20(2):133–9.
25. Sarker BK, Rahman M, Rahman T, Hossain J, Reichenbach L, Mitra DK. Reasons for preference of home delivery with traditional birth attendants (TBAs) in rural Bangladesh: a qualitative exploration. PLoS One. 2016;11(1):e0146161.
26. Khan R, Blum LS, Sultana M, Bilkis S, Koblinsky M. An examination of women experiencing obstetric complications requiring emergency care: perceptions and sociocultural consequences of caesarean sections in Bangladesh. J Health Popul Nutr. 2012;30(2):159.
27. Baksu B, Davas I, Agar E, Akyol A, Varolan A. The effect of mode of delivery on postpartum sexual functioning in primiparous women. Int Urogynecol J. 2007;18(4):401–6.
28. Serçekuş P, Okumuş H. Fears associated with childbirth among nulliparous women in Turkey. Midwifery. 2009;25(2):155–62.
29. Barrett G, Peacock J, Victor CR, Manyonda I. Cesarean section and postnatal sexual health. Birth. 2005;32(4):306–11.
30. Dabiri F, Yabandeh AP, Shahi A, Kamjoo A, Teshnizi SH. The effect of mode of delivery on postpartum sexual functioning in primiparous women. Oman Med J. 2014;29(4):276.
31. Yamasato K, Kimata C, Huegel B, Durbin M, Ashton M, Burlingame JM. Restricted episiotomy use and maternal and neonatal injuries: a retrospective cohort study. Arch Gynecol Obstet. 2016;294(6):1189–94.
32. Koblinsky M, Anwar I, Mridha MK, Chowdhury ME, Botlero R. Reducing maternal mortality and improving maternal health: Bangladesh and MDG 5. J Health Popul Nutr. 2008;26(3):280.
33. Wiklund I, Edman G, Andolf E. Cesarean section on maternal request: reasons for the request, self-estimated health, expectations, experience of birth and signs of depression among first-time mothers. Acta Obstet Gynecol Scand. 2007;86(4):451–6.
34. Gamble J, Creedy DK, McCourt C, Weaver J, Beake S. A critique of the literature on women's request for cesarean section. Birth. 2007;34(4):331–40.
35. Women's NCCf, Health Cs: Caesarean section. 2011.
36. Gholitabar M, Ullman R, James D, Griffiths M. Caesarean section: summary of updated NICE guidance. Bmj. 2011;343:d7108.
37. American College of Obstetricians Gynecologists. ACOG Practice bulletin no. 115: Vaginal birth after previous cesarean delivery. Obstet Gynecol. 2010; 116(2 Pt 1):450.
38. Minkoff H, Chervenak FA. Elective primary cesarean delivery. N Engl J Med. 2003;348(10):946–50.
39. Vivilaki V, Antoniou E. Caesarean section: the underpinning choice?Health Sci J. 2008;2(2):83–8.
40. Sikder SS, Labrique AB, Ali H, Hanif AA, Klemm RD, Mehra S, West KP, Christian P. Availability of emergency obstetric care (EmOC) among public and private health facilities in rural Northwest Bangladesh. BMC Public Health. 2015;15(1):36.
41. Ameh C, Msuya S, Hofman J, Raven J, Mathai M, van den Broek N. Status of emergency obstetric care in six developing countries five years before the MDG targets for maternal and newborn health. PLoS One. 2012;7(12):e49938.
42. World Health Organization. Bangladesh health system review. Manila: WHO Regional Office for the Western Pacific; 2015.

11

Factors influencing decision-making for caesarean section in Sweden

Sunita Panda[1*], Deirdre Daly[2], Cecily Begley[2,3], Annika Karlström[4], Birgitta Larsson[4], Lena Bäck[4] and Ingegerd Hildingsson[4,5]

Abstract

Background: Rising rates of caesarean section (CS) are a concern in many countries, yet Sweden has managed to maintain low CS rates. Exploring the multifactorial and complex reasons behind the rising trend in CS has become an important goal for health professionals. The aim of the study was to explore Swedish obstetricians' and midwives' perceptions of the factors influencing decision-making for CS in nulliparous women in Sweden.

Methods: A qualitative design was chosen to gain in-depth understanding of the factors influencing the decision-making process for CS. Purposive sampling was used to select the participants. Four audio-recorded focus group interviews (FGIs), using an interview guide with open ended questions, were conducted with eleven midwives and five obstetricians from two selected Swedish maternity hospitals after obtaining written consent from each participant. Data were managed using NVivo© and thematically analysed. Ethical approval was granted by Trinity College Dublin.

Results: The thematic analysis resulted in three main themes; 'Belief in normal birth – a cultural perspective'; 'Clarity and consistency – a system perspective' and 'Obstetrician makes the final decision, but...', and each theme contained a number of subthemes. However, 'Belief in normal birth' emerged as the core central theme, overarching the other two themes.

Conclusion: Findings suggest that believing that normal birth offers women and babies the best possible outcome contributes to having and maintaining a low CS rate. Both midwives and obstetricians agreed that having a shared belief (in normal birth), a common goal (of achieving normal birth) and providing mainly midwife-led care within a 'team approach' helped them achieve their goal and keep their CS rate low.

Keywords: Caesarean section, Decision-making, Midwives, Obstetricians, Normal birth, Nulliparous, Qualitative, Midwife-led care

Background

There are global concerns about the rising rate of caesarean section (CS) with wide variation in rates across countries [1] and no evidence of associated reductions in morbidities or mortalities [2]. Analysis of trends in CS rates from 121 countries indicates that rates increased from 6.7% in 1990 to 19.1% in 2014, representing an absolute increase of 12.4%. There is an increase in CS rates in developed countries (40% increase from 1993 to 2003, and an approximate 11% increase from 2003 to 2013), with the rates of CS remaining constantly higher than the World Health Organization's (WHO) recommendations [3]. A comparison of trends in rates between developed and underdeveloped countries shows that the increase was 14.6% (from 6.3% in 1990 to 20.9% in 2014) in underdeveloped, and 12.7% in developed countries (from 14.5% in 1990 to 27.2% in 2014) [1]. The concern surrounding this striking increase in CS rates is due to the documented morbidity caused by CS [4], including

* Correspondence: spanda@tcd.ie
[1]School of Nursing and Midwifery, Trinity College Dublin, 2 Clare Street, D02 CK80 Dublin, Ireland
Full list of author information is available at the end of the article

increased readmission rates [5] with their concomitant costs [6].

Analysis of European data indicated that CS rates ranged from 14.8% in Iceland to 52.2% in Cyprus [7]. Despite the rising trend in rates in many countries, Sweden's CS rate of 17% in 2010 remains among the lowest in Europe [8]. Birth choice UK (2002) has defined "normal birth" as one which starts naturally and does not involve any medical or technological intervention [9]. This working definition of normal birth thus includes spontaneous onset of labour, spontaneous progress of labour and spontaneous birth, and excludes induction of labour, epidural or spinal or general anaesthetic, forceps or ventouse, caesarean section, or episiotomy. In a concept analysis, Anderson (2003) defined normal birth as birth without intervention in an environment that enables choice and empowerment for the woman [10]. Traditionally, a culture of belief in normal birth has been evident in the Swedish maternity care system where birth is viewed as a natural process [11]. Factors that influence the decision to perform a CS are often complex and poorly explained in literature [12]. Understanding these complexities is one of many steps to help stop the rise of any unnecessary CSs or prevent its over-use. Exploring the multifactorial and complex reasons behind the rising trend in CS, and the declining rates in normal birth, has become an important goal for health professionals. Asking midwives and obstetricians about their perceptions of the factors that influence the decision to perform a CS is one way of exploring the decision-making process, and conducting this research in Sweden, a country with low CS rates, offered a unique research opportunity to achieve this goal.

Methods

Aim

The aim of the study was to explore Swedish obstetricians' and midwives' perceptions of the factors influencing decision-making for caesarean section (CS) in nulliparous women in Sweden.

Design

A qualitative design was chosen to gain in-depth understanding of the factors influencing the decision-making process for CS using focus group interviews (FGIs).

Setting

The study was conducted in two Swedish hospitals, each with approximately 1400 to 1600 births annually and CS rates of 14%. These are typical of Swedish maternity hospitals, and the average CS rate in the country is 17% [8], much lower than European averages. Women in these two settings and in Sweden generally, book for antenatal care with midwives. When complications exist or develop, women are referred to obstetricians. Women meet the same midwife during the antenatal visits; however, they do not have a known midwife at birth as the care is fragmented between pregnancy and birth, and belongs to two different health care systems. Antenatal care is provided within the primary health care sector and intrapartum care is hospital based (secondary health care) with no continuity with the same midwife [11].

Participants and participant recruitment

Purposive sampling, described as when researchers "intentionally select (or recruit) participants who have experienced the central phenomenon or the key concept being explored in the study" ([13] P.173), was used. So, all midwives working in the labour wards, and obstetricians involved in the decision-making process for CS, in the site hospitals, were eligible to take part. Midwifery students and obstetricians who were not involved in the decision-making process were excluded. The purposive sampling method thus selected the midwives and senior obstetricians who were directly involved in decision-making for CS on a day-to-day basis and therefore had a deep understanding of the factors influencing decision-making for CS.

A gatekeeper (research midwife) in each study site sent the study information to the clinicians (midwives and obstetricians) in the selected study sites one to two weeks before the FGIs, identified willing participants, and arranged the date, time and venues for the FGIs.

Data collection

After obtaining written consent from each clinician four FGIs were conducted, two with midwives (site 1, $n = 6$ and site 2 $n = 5$) and two with obstetricians (site 1 $n = 2$ and site 2 $n = 3$). The interview guide included open-ended questions; questions such as *'Tell me how CSs are defined in your hospital?'* and *'Tell me about your role in decision-making for CS in nulliparous women?'* were used to open the interviews, and probing questions such as *'Can you tell me more about that?'* or *'Can you explain that to me in a little more detail?'* were used to facilitate discussion. Terms such as *'fear of litigation'* or *'skills of clinicians'* were also used as prompts, when appropriate, to facilitate the flow of discussion. The FGIs lasted between 30 and 35 min, and were audio recorded. During the FGIs, participants discussed issues in the Swedish language occasionally, but immediately translated these into English. Notes were made on non-verbal cues immediately after each FGI [14].

The four audio recordings were transcribed by the first author. Participants' names, when used, were removed from the transcription and a numeric participant identification number was assigned.

Data analysis

Data from the interviews were managed and analysed using the NVivo© software package. Each step of data analysis (reading and re-reading the transcripts, coding, grouping the codes and deriving themes) was performed independently by SP and DD, and the coding and categories were compared and discussed to ensure accuracy of interpretation. To ensure reliability of the findings, all the authors discussed the interpretation of the results. The step-by-step process and stages of analysis were documented in an audit trail.

Results

The thematic analysis resulted in three main themes, each containing a number of subthemes. 'Belief in normal birth' emerged as the core central theme, overarching the other two themes (Fig. 1). The three themes and subthemes are described in the following section, using the clinicians' own words to illustrate.

Theme 1: Belief in normal birth – A cultural perspective

Participants regarded caesarean section as a procedure that should be performed only when absolutely necessary, and all agreed that this was the prevailing perspective of midwives and obstetricians in their respective hospitals, and in Sweden generally. Three subthemes were identified under this theme.

Subtheme 1.1. Promoting normal birth

Midwives and obstetricians shared the belief that normal birth is best for women and babies, and offers the best possible outcomes. Midwives also believed that vaginal birth is associated with a more positive experience (for women) than birth by CS. CS was performed only when there was a sound justifiable reason, usually in emergency situations, and only when normal birth was no longer a safe option. Midwives agreed that obstetricians always promote normal birth, and perform CSs only when all the other measures were unsafe or have failed. Midwives also believed that avoiding induction of labour was one way to reduce unnecessary CS.

"The culture in the hospital is normal birth." (FGI with Midwives, Site 2)

"Women with CS have a worse birth experience than women who give birth vaginally." (FGI with Midwives, Site 1)

Obstetricians stated that even the general public's opinion (in Sweden) is to promote normal birth, and midwives felt that they have a responsibility to ensure that this is explained to all pregnant women during antenatal visits.

"I think the main factor is public opinion about what is normal and what is abnormal delivery...Most people in Sweden, I think, promote normal delivery and they think that CS is not something normal." (FGI Obstetricians, Site 1)

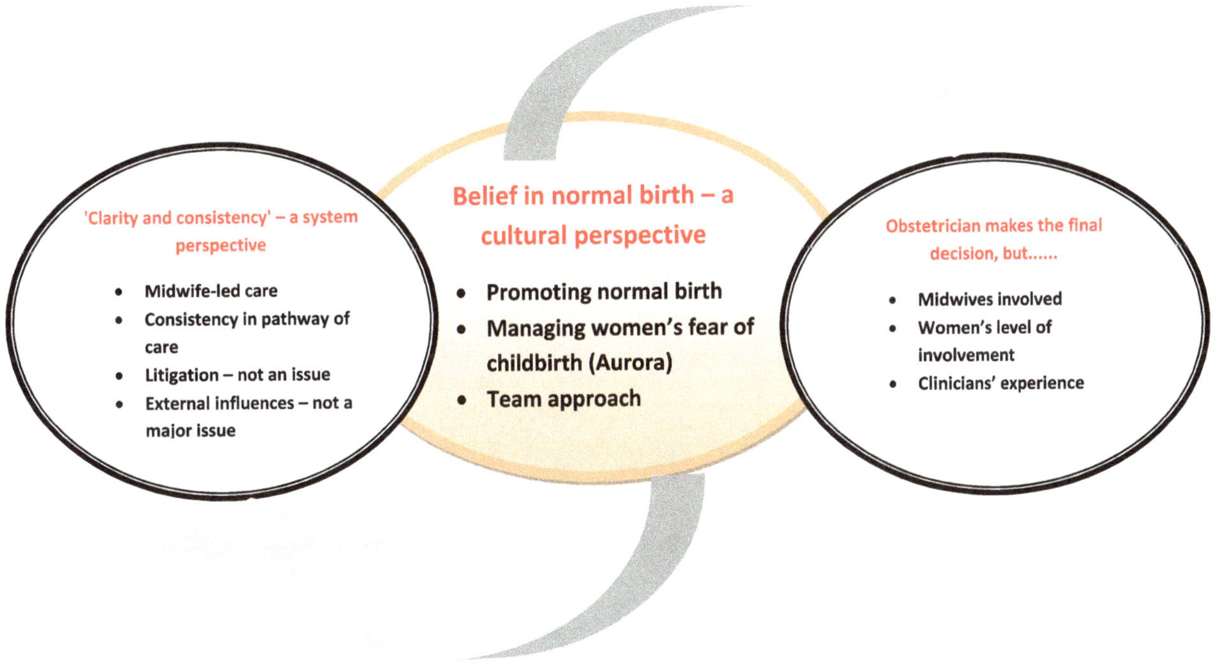

Fig. 1 Diagram representing Swedish clinicians' perspectives of factors influencing decision-making for CS in Sweden

Subtheme 1.2. Managing women's fear of childbirth (Aurora)

Although women's fear of childbirth, irrespective of parity, had some influence on the decision-making process, it was not considered to be a major influencing factor. Obstetricians stated that maternal request for CS was uncommon, especially in first-time mothers.

Midwives and obstetricians in both FGIs stated that Aurora, the team of midwives who counsels women with childbirth fear, played a significant role in helping women who request CS. Obstetricians confirmed that women who continue to request CS after adequate counselling are always seen by a senior obstetrician, never by junior obstetricians.

"We have Aurora, counselling team with midwives. [A] *woman who wish for a CS comes to this counselling programme and talks to a midwife, so we give them options like induction, pain relief, birth plan and ... a CS contract. Which means when... in labour* [if] *the woman feels that it's too traumatic or too painful... she can by herself request for CS... And when they have this contract they feel ... in control..."* (FGI with Midwives, Site 1)

Subtheme 1.3. Team approach

Obstetricians and midwives described a 'team approach' to improving outcomes in both site hospitals, and believed that group discussion and retrospective case analysis, without blaming any individual member of staff, have helped them learn from adverse outcomes and improve care.

"Every time it goes little bit wrong, we take it on......we talk about it and analyse...and talk about how can we do better about it next time... for example, [if] *you have an emergency CS ...we discuss afterwards...then you can learn something."* (FGI with Midwives, Site 1)

Theme 2 Clarity and consistency – A system perspective

Midwives and obstetricians described a consistent system of health care, with consistency in their beliefs and pathways of care, in both site hospitals. Four subthemes, which contributed to system clarity and consistency, were identified.

Subtheme 2.1. Midwife-led care

Women always book for antenatal care with midwives, and are referred to obstetricians only when complications exist or develop, with no access for booking privately under the care of a midwife or obstetrician.

"There is no private care here and women always go to the midwives. They book in with the midwives and the midwives refer them to the obstetricians, if and when required."(FGI with Midwives, Site 1)

Midwives said that midwifery staffing levels did not have an influence on the decision to perform CS; however, some obstetricians felt that the lack of experienced midwives in the labour ward did have some influence on the overall birth outcome.

"....never had issues with short staffs. Our goal is to have one-to-one care with midwife in the room as much as we can... to avoid...[any] *kind of distress with the woman or the couple to avoid a CS."* (FGI with Midwives, Site 1)

"Well, staffing might be a problem sometimes...you would like to have an experienced midwife with each woman to facilitate normal labour and maybe we can't offer that and ... it influences the results...." (FGI with Obstetricians, Site 1)

The midwife's level of experience also impacted on the outcome of labour.

"Of course... experienced midwives are the most important part of having a woman normally delivered and an experienced midwife in the room with a woman in labour ... who feels safe and confident, the woman will of course trust her..." (FGI with Obstetricians, Site 1)

Subtheme 2.2. Consistency in pathway of care

There was consistency in the care pathways and this approach was underpinned by clinicians' 'belief in normal birth' being the best option for women and babies.

Managing early labour and avoiding induction of labour were considered vital to achieving normal birth and reducing CSs.

"...[for] *women to be in labour ward they must be in active labour...Because if you have any women in latent* [phase or early labour], *there is a high risk to do something.... then a cesarean."* (FGI with Midwives, Site 1)

Antenatal education was believed to be of vital importance, especially for women with high Body Mass Index (BMI) who were at high risk for labour and birth complications.

"One of the reasons [for CS in first-time mothers] *is big women. So, we educate women during pregnancy...so that when they come to delivery it's not a big problem."* (FGI with Midwives, Site 2)

On most occasions, women whose babies are in the breech position (at term) have an elective CS. However, if women wished to have a vaginal breech birth, clear processes are followed, and all these women undergo pelvimetry prior to deciding on the mode of birth.

"...*for breech, everyone gets a CS, unless they absolutely want to give birth* [vaginally]. *But normally they don't. We only have few hospitals that perform breech births. You have to perform measurements,* [there] *can't be any complications in pregnancy...*" (FGI with Midwives, Site 1)

Subtheme 2.3. Litigation – Not an issue

Midwives and obstetricians did not have a fear of legal consequences or being blamed in cases of adverse outcomes. They believed this allows them to practise evidence-based care consistently.

"*We never had anything like that* [litigation issues] *in Sweden...The whole system is built on identifying systemic problems like education or treatment or routines...We try to see if we can educate the personnel or change routines...so that it will never happen again.*" (FGI with Obstetricians, Site 1)

"*... it's just that kind of system, where you don't get sued in a court. It makes it a little bit easier...*" (FGI with Midwives, Site 1)

"...*no fear of legal implications. You record everything in the journal* [women's clinical records] *about what you are doing. Of course we have to document and do everything right but no pressure that we are going to be accused... from patients...from doctors...It is not a routine that you will think 'I will be blamed'.*" (FGI with Midwives, Site 2)

Subtheme 2.4. External influences – Not a major issue

While other external influencing factors sometimes exist, most participants were of the view that these had very little or no influence on clinicians' decision-making to perform a CS.

Obstetricians in one of the study sites believed that the media can influence women's and their families' attitudes towards the high level of activities in hospitals and safety, but this did not impact their decision to perform CS.

"...*there might be an opinion in the society that there is a crisis at the hospital...But it does not influence our decisions about...CS.*" (FGI with Obstetrician, Site 1)

While shift times had no influence on the decision to perform CS, some midwives believed that the risk of complications increases on night shift and obstetricians believed, occasionally, that midwives' shift changes and handover times led to some actions or procedures being delayed.

"*Change of shift is the risk. We have not many, but some examples...*[where] *decision has not been made on time because doctors were reporting to the next shift and especially...midwives' shifts time...amniotomy gets delayed...start of oxytocin gets delayed...*" (FGI with Obstetrician, Site 1)

While availability of space in labour and birth rooms was never an issue, obstetricians in one of the study sites felt that the distance of the labour ward from the surgical theatre did, on occasions, have some influence on the timing of decision-making for CS, but not the decision to perform the CS per se.

"*Only the distance where we can perform the CS, it's in another building, that might influence* [the timing of decision to do a CS] *sometimes...*" (FGI with Obstetrician, Site 2)

Hospital policies were not perceived as influencing clinicians' decision-making processes; they were viewed as promoting vaginal birth.

"*The policy here is to increase...the number of normal deliveries among primipara. So it has a positive influence.*" (FGI with Obstetrician, Site 1)

Theme 3 Obstetrician makes the final decision, but

Obstetricians were regarded as the final decision-makers for CS, but both obstetricians and midwives stated that the decision was arrived at jointly. On occasion, women's level of involvement in the discussions, and clinicians' experience, exerted some influence.

Subtheme 3.1. Midwives involved

Although obstetricians make the final decision to perform a CS, midwives always played a vital role in the decision-making discussions.

"*When a woman comes to labour ward, we make a risk classification...and most of the cesareans are high risk, so* [it is] *team-work...but it's the doctor who makes the decision.*" (FGI with Midwives, Site 1)

"*In a case where the reason for CS is...dystocia...we would discuss it with the midwife more than when it's due to fetal distress. Even the junior colleagues may discuss it with the midwives...rather than calling...a senior consultant.*" (FGI with Obstetricians, Site 1)

Subtheme 3.2. Women's level of involvement

Women played very little role in decision-making when a CS was performed in an emergency. However, in non-emergency situations when it was clinically safe, it was common practice to discuss and consider women's preferred care pathway and mode of birth.

"Not if it is immediate [emergency]*...but otherwise* [the woman is] *definitely involved."* (FGI with Midwives, Site 1)

Subtheme 3.3. Clinicians' experience

Clinicians' experience had an influence in the process of decision-making, and midwives felt obstetricians with limited experience tended to perform a CS sooner than more experienced colleagues.

"...I think that some of the new doctors might not let people try for such a long time than really skilled ones." (FGI with Midwives, Site 2)

Consultant obstetricians stated that some senior obstetric registrars, depending on their level of experience, could make the final decision for CS, mainly in emergency situations. However, a consultant obstetrician's availability in the labour ward, mostly during day-time, was always perceived to make a difference to the decision-making process.

"If you are a resident [obstetric registrar], *and you are concerned, you will discuss with the senior. That depends on how experienced you are. If you are experienced, you make the decision by yourself."* (FGI with Obstetricians, Site 1)

"I think one advantage is that the consultants are always...in the labour ward... we are always available..." (FGI with Obstetricians, Site 2)

Discussion

A belief in normal birth, together with a multidisciplinary team approach, have been shown to have a positive impact on reducing CSs [15], including in the Swedish maternity system [11]. In this study, the main factor said to influence the mode of birth for first-time mothers was the culture of belief in normal birth.

A woman's first birth and her overall experience is crucial to her future reproductive health and, in Sweden fear of childbirth is one of the predominant causes of women requesting for CS [16] and most of these fears are attributed to previous negative birth experiences. In the Swedish maternity system, support and counselling services are offered to women who present with fear of childbirth. No differences in CS rates are reported for women with severe fear of child birth with no counselling service, but they are reported to have increased negative birth experiences [17] and, women who receive support and counselling for fear of childbirth have greater levels of satisfaction with the care they receive [18].

The reasons why women request a CS are complex [19] and are often influenced by previous birth experience, socio-cultural factors, media and body image [19–22]. In this study, maternal request for CS because of fear of childbirth was regarded as rare among nulliparous women. While attitudes to maternal request for CS differ among midwives and obstetricians in other countries [23, 24], in the absence of any medical indication, CS on maternal request is rarely an option in Sweden [11]. Clinicians in this study were clear and consistent about counselling women who request a CS.

Fear of adverse outcomes and subsequent litigation are frequently reported factors influencing the decision to perform a CS in many OECD [25–28] and non-OECD countries [21]. Clinicians in this study, however, described litigation as having no influence on their decision-making for CS. Litigation issues and complaints in Sweden are overseen by the Medical Responsibility Board; and most issues are investigated to improve future care [11].

Despite several studies that describe a lack of cooperation and professional disagreements among midwives and obstetricians on the decision-making process for CS [21, 24, 29], findings from these FGIs show that there is 'a team approach' with the midwifery and obstetric teams in these two sites that helps them maintain a low CS rate.

Avoiding induction of labour was viewed as a key element in reducing CS rates. Caring for women in the latent phase of labour outside the labour ward area was seen as essential, findings similar to those of a recent Irish study [30].

Midwives are the primary pregnancy care providers in Sweden [11], and have also been shown to play a pivotal role in ensuring a positive birth experience for women [31]. Clinicians in this study viewed 'one-to-one midwifery' and 'continuity of care' as vital elements for promoting normal birth and reducing CS, like other studies [25]. Swedish maternity care is acknowledged as having a culture that believes normal birth as the optimal birth mode for women, and maternity care models that emphasise continuity of care. Continuity of care with the same known midwife has been valued by all women, especially women with fear of childbirth, through facilitating normal birth and a positive birth experience [32]. Internationally, midwife-led care has been shown to reduce CS rates [33], and costs less than obstetrician-led care [34].

Attending obstetricians privately is frequently reported as contributing to the rising CS rate [12, 21, 35]. Private organisations providing antenatal care in Sweden, with midwives as primary care providers, have emerged in recent years, mostly in urban areas but there are no private labour wards [11]. However, the clinicians in the current study indicated that there was no privatisation of maternity care in their two sites, which has helped them retain uniformity and consistency in their care for women.

As findings from FGIs can be dominated by the opinions of one, or more, group participants [36], in this study, conducting separate FGIs with midwives and obstetricians was a strength and contributed to 'Clarity and consistency - a system perspective' emerging as one of three core themes. All clinicians volunteered to participate and actively contributed to the discussions. The two study sites (with approximately 1400 to 1600 births annually and CS rates of 14%) are typical of maternity hospitals outside the bigger cities in Sweden. Both offer care to all women above 28 weeks of pregnancy, and have successfully maintained low CS rates. However, while the hospitals are representative of Sweden, they may not be representative of other maternity hospitals throughout Europe in general, and this is a potential limitation.

Conclusion

Findings from the current study suggest that 'a belief in normal birth' offers the best possible outcome and contributes to maintaining a low rate of CS. Providing midwife-led care within a 'team approach,' with a common goal and shared belief in achieving normal birth, are some key elements to maintain a low CS rate. Findings from this study are highly applicable to maternity care in other countries. The implications are that, changing clinicians' attitudes to a common and shared 'belief in normal birth,' and acceptance of the core key issues may contribute to a reduction in CS rates and prevent the rates from rising further.

Abbreviations

CS: Caesarean Section; FGI: Focus Group Interview

Acknowledgements

Thanks to the Head of the Departments of Sundsvall and Ostersund Hospitals for granting permission to conduct this research.
Special thanks to the midwives and obstetricians in the two study sites for taking part in this research so willingly and enthusiastically, and for their hospitality.

Funding

Funding for this research was awarded as a Short Term Scientific Mission (STSM) through COST Action IS1405 which facilitated the visit to the two hospitals in Sweden, a COST country, and the conduct of the focus group interviews with Swedish clinicians.

Authors' contributions

SP (Corresponding and first author) developed and conducted the study as part of her research on *'Caesarean section in first-time mothers: factors influencing the decision-making process and outcomes for women'*. DD and CB developed the study with SP, conducted the data analysis and drafted the manuscript. IH advised on national ethical procedures, organised the focus group interviews and drafted the manuscript. AK organised the FGIs in Sundsvall Hospital, and contributed to the drafting and editing of the manuscript. BL and LB conducted the preparatory work at the site hospitals, gained access from the Heads of the Departments, identified and offered information to eligible participants, organised the FGIs, and contributed to the drafting and editing of the manuscript. All the authors read and approved the final manuscript.

Authors' information

SP is a PhD student, DD is an Assistant Professor of Midwifery and CB is the Chair of Nursing and Midwifery in School of Nursing and Midwifery, Trinity College Dublin. IH is a Professor of Midwifery, in Uppsala University and Mid Sweden University, Sundsvall, AK is a Senior Lecturer, LB and BL are PhD students at Mid Sweden University, Sundsvall, Sweden.

Competing interests

There are no competing interests associated with this article. Cecily Begley, a co-author in this manuscript is a member of the editorial board and a Section Editor of this journal.

Author details

[1]School of Nursing and Midwifery, Trinity College Dublin, 2 Clare Street, D02 CK80 Dublin, Ireland. [2]School of Nursing and Midwifery, Trinity College Dublin, 24 D'Olier Street, Dublin D02 T283, Ireland. [3]Sahlgrenska Academy, University of Gothenburg, Gothenburg, Sweden. [4]Department of Nursing, Mid Sweden University, 86170 Sundsvall, Sweden. [5]Department of Women's and Children's health, Uppsala University, Uppsala, Sweden.

References

1. Betran AP, Ye J, Moller AB, Zhang J, Gülmezoglu AM, Torloni MR. The increasing trend in caesarean section rates: global, regional and National Estimates: 1990-2014. PLoS One. 2016;11(2):e0148343.
2. Betran AP, Torloni MR, Zhang J, Ye J, Mikolajczyk R, Deneux-Tharaux C, Oladapo OT, et al. What is the optimal rate of cesarean section at population level? A systematic review of ecologic studies. Reprod Health. 2015;12:57.
3. Declercq E, Cabral H, Ecker J. The plateauing of cesarean rates in industrialized countries. Am J Obstet Gynecol. 2017 Mar 1;216(3):322–3.
4. Villar J, Carroli G, Zavaleta N, Donner A, Wojdyla D, Faundes A, et al. Maternal and neonatal individual risks and benefits associated with cesarean delivery: multicentre prospective study. Bmj. 2007;335:1025–9.
5. Panda S, Begley C, Daly D. Readmission following caesarean section: reasons for readmission and outcomes for women in one large Irish maternity hospital. Br J Midwifery. 2016;24(5):2–8.
6. Fobelets M, Beeckman K, Faron G, Daly D, Begley C, Putman K. Vaginal birth after cesarean versus elective repeat cesarean delivery after one previous cesarean section: a cost-effectiveness analysis in four European countries. BMC Pregnancy Childbirth. 2018;18:92. https://doi.org/10.1186/s12884-018-1720-6.
7. Macfarlane A, Blondel B, Mohangoo A, Cuttini M, Nijhuis J, Novak Z, et al. Wide differences in mode of delivery within Europe: risk-stratified analyses of aggregated routine data from the euro-Peristat study. BJOG. 2015;123(4):559–68. https://doi.org/10.1111/14710528.13284.
8. Swedish National Board of Health and Welfare. Birth Statistics 2016.www.socialstyrelsen.se. Retrived 11 Sept 2018.
9. Birth choice UK (2002).www.birthchoiceuk.com.http://bhpelopartonormal.pbh.gov.br/estudos_cientificos/arquivos/normal_birth_consensus.pdf.
10. Anderson G. A concept analysis of 'normal birth'. Evid Based Midwifery. 2003;1(2):48–54.
11. Thomas J, Hildingsson I. Sweden. In: Kennedy P, Kodate N. (Editors). Maternity services and policy in an international context – Risk, citizenship and welfare regimes. London: Routledge publication. 2015:258–79.
12. Brick A, Layte R. Exploring trends in the rate of Caesarean section in Ireland. Econ Soc Rev. 2011;42(4):383–406.
13. Creswell JW, Plano Clarke VL. Designing and conducting mixed methods research. London: SAGE Publication; 2011. p. 173.
14. Begley CM. Triangulation of communication skills in qualitative research interviews. J Adv Nurs. 1996;24(4):688–93.

15. Marshall JL, Spiby H, McCormick F. Evaluating the 'Focus on Normal birth and reducing cesarean section rates rapid improvement Programme': a mixed method study in England. Midwifery. 2015;31(2):332–40.
16. Wiklund I, Edman G, Ryding E, Andolf E. Expectation and experiences of childbirth in primiparae with caesarean section. BJOG. 2008;115:324–31.
17. Waldenstrom U, Hildingsson U, Ryding E. Antenatal fear of childbirth and its association with subsequent cesarean section and experience of childbirth. BJOG. 2006;113:638–46.
18. Larsson B, Karlström A, Rubertsson C, Hildingsson I. The effects of counselling on fear of childbirth. Acta Obstet Gynecol Scand. 2015;94(6): 629–36.
19. Karlstrom A, Engstrom-Olofsson R, Nystedt A, Thomas J, Hildingsson I. Swedish caregivers' attitudes towards caesarean section on maternal request. Women Birth. 2009;22(2):57–63.
20. Litorp H, Mgaya A, Mbekenga CK, et al. Fear, blame and transparency: obstetric caregivers' rationales for high caesarean section rates in a low-resource setting. Soc Sci Med. 2015;143:232–40.
21. Yazdizadeh B, Nedjat S, Mohammad K, et al. Cesarean section rate in Iran, multidimensional approaches for behavioral change of providers: a qualitative study. BMC Health Serv Res. 2011;11(159):1–14.
22. Weaver JJ, Statham H, Richards M. Are there 'unnecessary' cesarean sections? Perceptions of women and obstetricians about cesarean sections for nonclinical indications. Birth. 2007;34(1):32–41.
23. Cotzias CS, Paterson-Brown S, Fisk NM. Obstetricians say yes to maternal request for elective caesarean section: a survey of current opinion. Eur J Obstet Gynecol Reprod Biol. 2001;97(1):15–6.
24. Josefsson A, Gunnervik C, Sydsjö A, Sydsjö G. A comparison between Swedish midwives and obstetricians & gynecologists opinions on cesarean section. Matern Child Health J. 2011;15(5):555–60.
25. Foureur M, Turkmani S, Clack DC, Davis DL, Mollart L, Leiser B, et al. Caring for women wanting a vaginal birth after previous caesarean section: a qualitative study of the experiences of midwives and obstetricians. Women Birth. 2016;30(1):3-8.
26. Cox KJ. Providers' perspectives on the vaginal birth after cesarean guidelines in Florida, United States: a qualitative study. BMC Pregnancy Childbirth. 2011;11:72.
27. Fuglenes D, Oian P, Kristiansen IS. Obstetricians' choice of cesarean delivery in ambiguous cases: is it influenced by risk attitude or fear of complaints and litigation? Am J Obstet Gynecol. 2009;200(1):48.e1–8.
28. Kamal P, Dixon-Woods M, Kurinczuk JJ, et al. Factors influencing repeat caesarean section: qualitative exploratory study of obstetricians' and midwives' accounts. BJOG. 2005;112(8):1054–60.
29. Litorp H, Mgaya A, Kidanto HL, Johnsdotter S, Essen B. 'What about the mother?' Women's and caregiver's perspectives on caesarean birth in a low-resource setting with rising caesarean section rates. Midwifery. 2015;31(7):713–20.
30. Panda S, Begley C. 'Not in established labour': outcomes for women cared for in an Irish antenatal ward. Br J Midwifery. 2014;22(4):264–8.
31. Larkin P, Begley CM, Devane D. 'Not enough people to look after you': an exploration of women's experiences of childbirth in the Republic of Ireland. Midwifery. 2012;28(1):98–105.
32. Hildingsson I, Karlstrom A, Haines H, Johansson M. Swedish women's interest in models of midwifery care - time to consider the system? A prospective longitudinal survey. Sex Reprod Health. 2016;7:27–32.
33. Sandall J, Soltani H, Gates S, Shennan A, Devane D. Midwife-led continuity models versus other models of care for childbearing women. Cochrane Database of Systematic Reviews. 2016, Issue 4. Art. No.: CD004667. https://doi.org/10.1002/14651858.CD004667.pub5.
34. Kenny C, Devane D, Normand C, Clarke M, Howard A, Begley C. A cost-comparison of midwife-led compared with consultant-led maternity care in Ireland (the MidU study). Midwifery. 2015;31:1032–8.
35. Colomar M, Cafferata ML, Aleman A, et al. Mode of childbirth in low-risk pregnancies: Nicaraguan physicians' viewpoints. Matern Child Health J. 2014;18(10):2382–92.
36. Smithson J. Using and analysing focus groups: limitations and possibilities. Int J Social Research Methodology. 2000;3(2):103–19.

12

Adjunct clinical interventions that influence vaginal birth after cesarean rates

Aireen Wingert[1], Cydney Johnson[1], Robin Featherstone[1,2], Meghan Sebastianski[2], Lisa Hartling[1,2] and R. Douglas Wilson[3*]

Abstract

Background: Rates of cesarean deliveries have been increasing, and contributes to the rising number of elective cesarean deliveries in subsequent pregnancies with associated maternal and neonatal risks. Multiple guidelines recommend that women be offered a trial of labor after a cesarean (TOLAC). The objective of the study is to systematically review the literature on adjunct clinical interventions that influence vaginal birth after cesarean (VBAC) rates.

Methods: We searched Ovid Medline, Ovid Embase, Wiley Cochrane Library, CINAHL via EBSCOhost; and Ovid PsycINFO. Additional studies were identified by searching for clinical trial records, conference proceedings and dissertations. Limits were applied for language (English and French) and year of publication (1985 to present). Two reviewers independently screened comparative studies (randomized or non-randomized controlled trials, and observational designs) according to a priori eligibility criteria: women with prior cesarean sections; any adjunct clinical intervention or exposure intended to increase the VBAC rate; any comparator; and, outcomes reporting changes in TOLAC or VBAC rates. One reviewer extracted data and a second reviewer verified for accuracy. Two reviewers independently conducted methodological quality assessments using the Mixed Methods Appraisal Tool (MMAT).

Results: Twenty-three studies of overall moderate to good methodological quality examined adjunct clinical interventions affecting TOLAC and/or VBAC rates: system-level interventions (three studies), provider-level interventions (three studies), guidelines or information for providers (seven studies), provider characteristics (four studies), and patient-level interventions (six studies). Provider-level interventions (opinion leader education, laborist, and obstetrician second opinion for cesarean sections) and provider characteristics (midwifery antenatal care, physicians on night float call schedules, and deliveries by family physicians) were associated with increased rates of VBAC. Few studies employing heterogeneous designs, sample sizes, interventions and comparators limited confidence in the effects. Studies of system-level and patient-level interventions, and guidelines/information for providers reported mixed findings.

Conclusions: Limited evidence indicates some provider-level interventions and provider characteristics may increase rates of attempted and successful TOLACs and/or VBACs, whereas other adjunct clinical interventions such as system-level interventions, patient-level interventions, and guidelines/information for healthcare providers show mixed findings.

Keywords: Vaginal birth after cesarean, Trial of labor after cesarean, Systematic review

* Correspondence: doug.wilson@ahs.ca
[3]Department of Obstetrics and Gynecology, Cumming School of Medicine, University of Calgary, 1403 – 29 Street NW, Calgary, AB T2N 2T9, Canada
Full list of author information is available at the end of the article

Background

A cesarean delivery is the most common surgery in Canada, with one of the main contributors being an elective cesarean delivery in subsequent pregnancies [1, 2]. Canadian cesarean delivery rates have increased from 18.7% in 1997 to 27.5% in 2014 [3] and continue to increase globally, [4] the result of an interplay of multiple factors including, but not limited to, shifting clinical environments, provider and patient preferences, and changing maternal demographics (e.g., obesity, chronic disease prevalence and advanced age) [5–9]. These factors can lead to higher-risk and more complex pregnancies and deliveries and an increased likelihood of a cesarean delivery [10, 11].

Depending on the etiology or indication, a cesarean delivery contributes to short- and long-term risks for both mother and infant [12, 13]. The Society of Obstetricians and Gynaecologists of Canada (SOGC) recommends that a trial of labor be offered to women with one previous transverse low-segment cesarean section [12]. A woman's willingness to undergo a trial of labor after cesarean (TOLAC) may be influenced by a multitude of factors [14]. While a vaginal birth after a cesarean (VBAC) may be desired by some women, the patient-level benefits associated with a VBAC from avoiding major abdominal surgery and risk of complications in future pregnancies must be weighed against the potential for serious harms such as a failed TOLAC and subsequent maternal and neonatal morbidity including an unplanned repeat cesarean delivery [15]. For women with more than one previous cesarean delivery, a VBAC is likely to be successful, but with an estimated higher risk of uterine rupture (0.2 to 1.5% with a transverse uterine incision, 1.0 to 1.6% with a low-vertical uterine incision) [12]. This SOGC statement is consistent with recommendations from the American College of Obstetrics and Gynecology (ACOG) [16, 17].

This systematic review aimed to evaluate adjunct clinical interventions that could be directed at or used by patients, families, healthcare providers, and hospitals/health systems to influence the uptake and success of VBAC.

Methods

This summation followed the standardized methods and guidelines for systematic reviews, [18, 19] and used an 'a priori' protocol (available from authors).

Literature search

A research librarian searched the following databases in May 2017: Ovid Medline (1946-), Ovid Embase (1980-), Wiley Cochrane Library (inception-), CINAHL via EBSCOhost (1937-) and Ovid PsycINFO (1806-). Limits were applied for language (English and French) and publication year (1985). The search strategy used the Conference Proceedings Citation Indexes (Clarivate Analytics) and hand-searched meeting abstracts from the past 2 years from the following associations: The Society for Maternal-Fetal Medicine (SMFM), the Society of Obstetricians and Gynaecologists of Canada (SOGC), and the American Congress of Obstetricians and Gynecologists. Finally, we searched ClinicalTrials.gov and ProQuest Dissertations & Theses Global (1861-). Reference lists of relevant systematic reviews were reviewed for potentially eligible studies. The detailed search strategy is in Additional file 1: Appendix 1.

Eligibility criteria

The study population was women who had a previous cesarean delivery including women with more than one prior cesarean delivery. Births attended by any healthcare provider (e.g., family physician, midwife, obstetrician/gynecologist) were eligible. Any intervention or exposure that was intended to effect a change in the VBAC rate among women with a prior cesarean delivery was eligible for inclusion. To be eligible, studies had to report on at least one of the outcomes of interest to the review: the primary outcome was change(s) in VBAC rates; secondary outcomes included TOLAC rates, or where reported, rates of successful VBAC among women undergoing a TOLAC. Studies that examined deliveries in any setting (e.g., hospitals, primary care centers, birthing units, home births) were eligible. All study designs (randomized [RCT] and non-randomized controlled trials [NRCT], and observational studies) with a comparison group were eligible for inclusion.

Studies were not considered eligible if: all women had three or more prior cesareans; multiple births of three or more fetuses were explicitly included; there was an absence of an exposure or intervention, or an inappropriate exposure/intervention was used (e.g., ethnicity, socioeconomic status, insurance status, physician traits, malpractice premiums); there was absence of a comparator, or an inappropriate comparator was used (e.g., no data for comparison groups in before-after study designs, women without a previous cesarean delivery); VBAC rates or change were not reported; or, they were not primary research (e.g., letter, editorial, commentary). Systematic reviews were not included; reference lists therein were screened for potentially relevant studies.

Study selection

Two reviewers (CJ and AW) independently screened titles and abstracts using a priori eligibility criteria. Full texts of potentially relevant publications were retrieved and independently reviewed in duplicate for inclusion; disagreements were resolved through discussion or third-reviewer consultation.

Data extraction

One reviewer extracted data and another verified data from each included study using a pre-specified and piloted form. Data were extracted for relevant study characteristics (design features), population (number of previous cesarean deliveries, parity), intervention, comparator, outcome (TOLAC rate [the number of women with a previous cesarean delivery who attempt a vaginal delivery] and VBAC rate [the number of women with a previous cesarean delivery who undergo a successful vaginal delivery]), funding source, and setting.

Intention-to-treat results were extracted from individual studies whenever possible. For dichotomous data on rates of TOLAC and VBAC, we reported counts or proportions, and sample size, by study arm. Results of statistical tests (e.g., *p*-values) or summary statistics (e.g., odds ratio [OR], risk ratio [RR], with confidence intervals [CI]) were extracted whenever these were reported within the studies.

Assessment of methodological quality

Two reviewers independently assessed the methodological quality of included studies; disagreements were resolved via consensus. All studies were assessed using the Mixed Methods Appraisal Tool (MMAT [20]), a tool designed for systematic reviews that include multiple study designs.

Data synthesis

Due to heterogeneity of interventions and comparators, pooling of data across studies for a meta-analysis was not appropriate; therefore, results were described narratively.

Assessment of overall quality of evidence

Data from studies were not pooled for summary effect estimates; therefore, assessment of the quality of the body of evidence using the Grading of Recommendations Assessment, Development and Evaluation (GRADE [21]) was not conducted.

Results

The literature search identified 5269 unique records eligible for inclusion. After screening titles and abstracts, 305 potentially relevant articles were identified. Full text screening yielded 23 studies [22–44] included in the review. The screening process is illustrated in Fig. 1.

Studies published from 1987 to 2017 were conducted in the United States (13 studies; 57% [23–27, 30, 34, 35, 37–39, 42, 44]), Canada (three studies; 13% [28, 32, 36]), United Kingdom (three studies; 13% [33, 40, 41]), Australia (one study; 4% [29]), China (one study [43]), Portugal (one study; 4% [22]), and Taiwan (one study; 4% [31]). Funding was from non-industry sources (ten studies; 43% [25–28, 30, 32, 33, 36, 40, 42]), without funding (two studies; 9% [22, 43]), or was not reported (11 studies; 48% [23, 24, 29, 31, 34, 35, 37–39, 41, 44]). The sample size varied depending on unit of reporting, with a mean of 1276 women (14 studies; [23, 25–30, 32, 33, 36, 40–43] range 96 to 4732) or 306,097 deliveries (nine studies; [22, 24, 31, 34, 35, 37–39, 44] range 5308 to 1,260,186).

The majority of studies included women (or records of women) who delivered in hospital (20 studies; [23–25, 27–34, 36–44] 87%), health clinics (one study; [26] 4%), and in multiple settings including hospitals and at home (two studies; [22, 35] 9%). Of the 12 studies [23, 25, 26, 28, 29, 32, 36, 39, 40, 42–44] (52%) that reported maternal age, a wide range of women (18 years and younger to 40 years and older) were represented. Studies explicitly reported including women with 1 prior cesarean delivery (six studies [26, 28, 29, 40–42]), one or two prior cesarean deliveries (one study [37]), and at least one prior cesarean delivery (three studies [23, 33, 36]); the latter three included some women with three or more prior cesarean deliveries.

While all studies reported the proportion of women who had a VBAC, about half (13 studies; [25, 27–30, 32, 34, 36, 37, 40–42, 44] 57%) provided comparative proportions of women who had a TOLAC.

Most studies were cohorts (16 studies; one non-concurrent cohort contained 3-arms [22, 23, 25, 29–31, 34–42, 44]); a small proportion were RCTs (five studies; three trials contained three-arms [26, 28, 32, 33, 43]), before-after (one study [24]), and cross-sectional (one study [27]).

Table 1 summarizes the strategies/outcome themes among the studies. Tables 2, 3, 4, 5 and 6 summarize the included studies by categories of interventions. Additional file 1: Appendix 2 details characteristics of the individual studies.

Methodological quality of included studies

All of the studies received a score for having a clear research question or objective, and for collecting data that addressed the intended research question.

Of the five RCTs, four (80%) [26, 28, 32, 33] described the randomization process clearly, but only one (20%) [33] clearly described allocation concealment or blinding. Four (80%) RCTs [28, 32, 33, 43] had complete outcome data for at least 80% of the participants. Three (60%) RCTs [26, 28, 33] had a withdrawal or drop-out rate of less than 20%. Overall, one (25%) RCT [33] met all of the criteria (four out of four stars).

The majority (16 studies; 89%) [22–24, 27, 29–31, 35–42, 44] of the non-randomized controlled studies recruited participants or organizations in a way that minimized selection bias. Most (17 studies; 94%) [22–

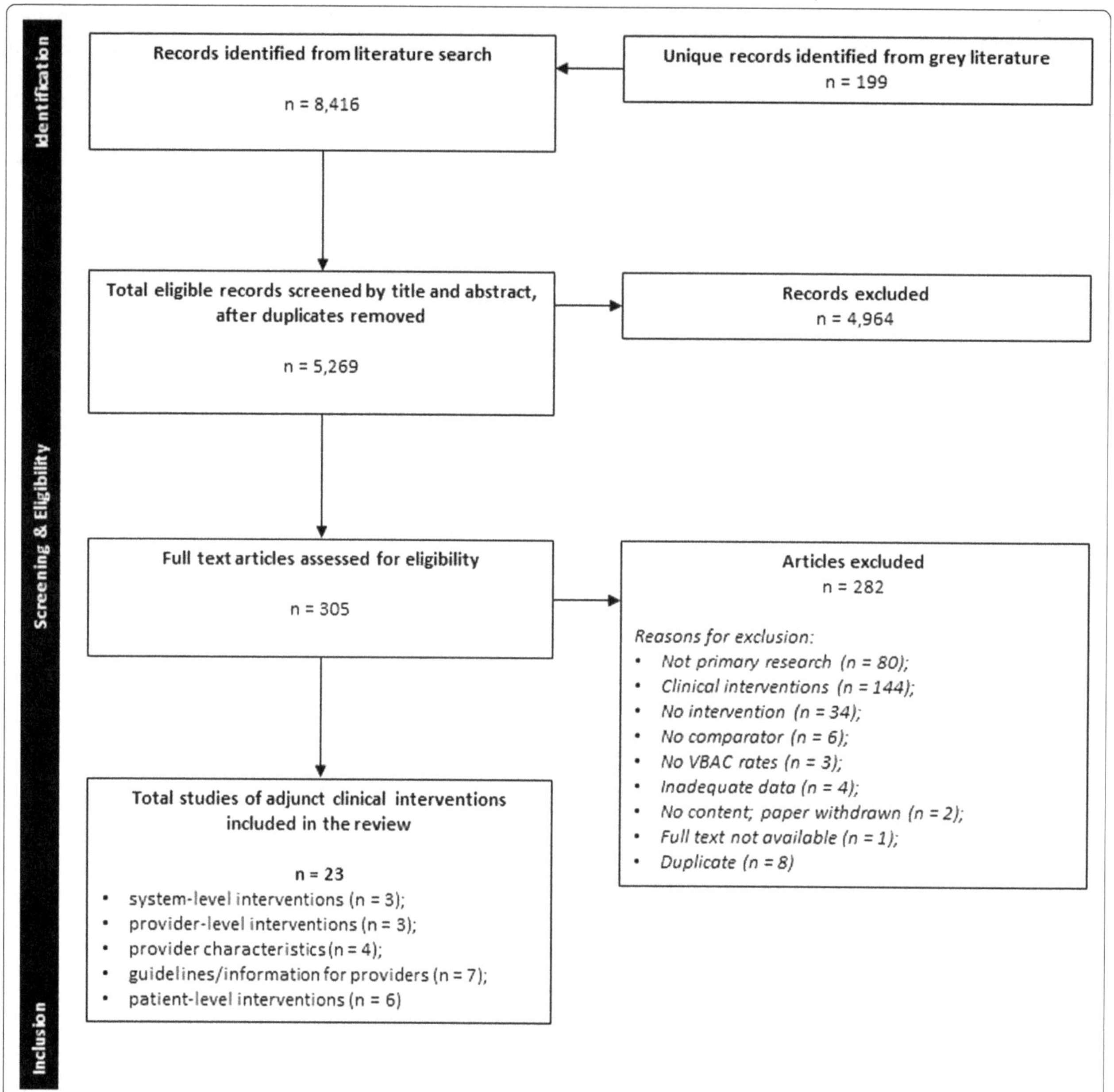

Fig. 1 PRISMA flow of study selection

25, 27, 30, 31, 34–42, 44] studies used appropriate measurements for the interventions/exposures and outcomes, and used interventions that did not present potential contamination between groups. Only seven (39%) studies [23, 24, 27, 39, 40, 42, 44] accounted for important differences between groups, or controlled for such differences in the data analysis. Many studies (n = 16; 89%) [22–25, 27, 29, 31, 34–40, 42, 44] had complete outcome data for at least 80% of the participants, or an acceptable response or follow-up rate (i.e., 60% or above). Overall, seven (39%) [23, 24, 27, 39, 40, 42, 44] studies scored four stars (out of four).

Methodological quality assessments are summarized in Table 7; detailed study assessments are in Additional file 1: Appendix 3.

TOLAC and VBAC rates

System-level interventions

Three studies [22, 24, 31] examined system-level interventions (Table 2). One non-concurrent cohort compared deliveries in continental Portugal before and after a concerted action to reduce cesarean section rates based on transmission and training of healthcare professionals as well as targeted cesarean delivery rates for

Table 1 Summary of adjunct clinical interventions of included studies

Intervention Category	Strategy/Outcome Themes	TOLAC[a]	VBAC[a]	Study (study design)
System-level	Education and training of providers	NA	+	Ayres-de-Campos 2015 (NCC)
	Targeted CD rates with hospital funding	NA	+	Ayres-de-Campos 2015 (NCC)
	Targeted VBAC rates with hospital funding	NA	+	Liu 2013 (NCC)
	Hospital peer-review of CD/VBAC	NA	NS;	Bickell 1996 (BA);
			+, NC	Liu 2013 (NCC)
Provider-level	Opinion leader VBAC	+	+	Lomas 1991 (RCT)
	Hospital with laborists	+	+NS	Feldman 2015 (CS)
	Second opinion requirement for all CDs	+	+	Myers 1993 (NCC)
Provider characteristics	Midwifery vs. non-midwifery provider	+	+	Zhang 2016 (RCT);
				White 2016 (NCC)
	Family physician vs. obstetrician	+	+	Russillo 2008 (CS)
	Night float call vs. traditional call	+	+	Yee 2017 (RC)
Provider guidelines/information	Education and management direction	+	+	Bellows 2016 (NCC);
				Kosecoff 1987 (RC);
				Sanchez-Ramos 1990 (NCC);
				Santerre 1996 (NCC);
		–	–	Pinette 2004 (NCC);
				Zweifler 2006 (NCC);
		NA	NC	Studnicki 1997 (NCC)
Patient-level	Obstetric information vs. no information	+	+	Wong 2014 (PC)
	Verbal vs. written patient information	+NS	+NS	Fraser 1997 (RCT);
	Dedicated VBAC clinic vs. standard care	NA	+	Gardner 2014 (NCC)
	Decision analysis (computerized) vs. brochures	NA	+NS	Eden 2014 (RCT)
	Decision analysis vs. information vs. usual care	NA	+NS	Montgomery 2007 (RCT)
	One-on-one antenatal VBAC counseling vs. standard care	+	–	Cleary-Goldman 2005 (PC)

TOLAC trial of labor after cesarean, *VBAC* vaginal birth after cesarean, *NCC* non-concurrent cohort, *CD(s)* cesarean delivery, *BA* before-after, *RCT* randomized clinical trial, *CS* cross-sectional, vs. versus, *RC* retrospective cohort, *PC* prospective cohort

[a]Rates reported as increased (+), increased but not statistically significant (+NS), decreased (–), no change (NC), or not applicable/not assessed (NA)

contingency-based hospital funding, and found an increase in the VBAC rate from 16.4% (13,399 of 81,750 VBACs) in 2009 to 32.8% (16,859 of 51,478 VBACs) in 2014 ($p < 0.001$) [22]. Another non-concurrent cohort of deliveries at a tertiary hospital in Taiwan found that rates of vaginal deliveries in women with previous cesarean deliveries increased (from 4.8% [38 of 800 deliveries] to 12.2% [231 of 1887 deliveries]) after implementation of direct government funding of hospitals from 2002 to 2005 (rate ratio 0.82, 95% CI 0.74–0.90, $p = 0.0001$), but the rate did not improve further (from 12.2% [231 of 1887 deliveries] to 11.4% [298 of 2621 deliveries]) with the additional employment of a hospital-based post-operative peer review and audit strategy from 2005 to 2010 (rate ratio 0.98, 95% CI 0.96–0.99, $p = 0.0003$) [31]. One study compared peer reviewed with non-reviewed hospitals (45 [mean 1430 deliveries in 1988 and mean 1503 deliveries in 1993] versus 120 hospitals [mean 1720 deliveries in 1988 and 1993]), and found that VBAC rates increased between the years by 14.6 and 12.7% (reviewed and non-reviewed hospitals, respectively), although the difference between reviewed and non-reviewed hospitals was not statistically significant [24].

Provider-level interventions

Three studies examined provider-level interventions [27, 32, 34] (Table 3). One RCT of community hospitals compared opinion leader education (739 women from four hospitals) and audit and feedback (524 women from four hospitals) to mailed guideline recommendations (1233 women from eight hospitals), and found that women were more likely to attempt a TOLAC when delivering in obstetric departments with influential opinion leaders (38.2%) compared to units with audit and feedback (21.4%) or mailed practice guidelines (28.3%) (46% higher in the opinion leaders group versus the other groups, $p = 0.007$) [32]. Women were also more likely to have VBACs in the

Table 2 Summary of studies – system-level interventions

Study; Design; Country, setting; Funding	Population; Study period	Intervention & comparator (no. of participants)			TOLAC rate[a]	VBAC rate[a]	VBAC/ TOLAC rate[a]
Ayres-De-Campos (2015) Non-concurrent cohort Portugal, state-owned hospitals, private hospitals & home births No funding	All deliveries from state-owned hospitals, private hospitals & home births during study period January 1, 2000–September 30, 2014	Grp 1 (2000–2009): no concerted action (n = 913,219)	Grp 2 (2010–2014): concerted action by independent committee (visits to state—owned hospitals with CS rates > 35%; meetings with obstetric & midwifery staff; training courses) (n = 346,157)		NR	2000: 14,993 (14.5%); 2001: 13,298 (13.7%); 2002: 15,360 (15.8%); 2003: 13,890 (14.8%); 2004: 13,710 (15.0%); 2005: 13,147 (14.6%); 2006: 15,700 (17.9%); 2007: 15,431 (18.1%); 2008: 13,837 (16.2%); 2009: 13,399 (16.4%) vs. 2010: 14,834 (17.9%); 2011: 17,624 (22.8%); 2012: 18,076 (25.1%); 2013: 16,365 (25.8%); Jan–Sept 2014: 16,859 (32.8%)	NR
Bickell (1996) Controlled before-after US, hospitals with high/average/low cesarean rate Funding NR	Hospitals from eight designated Health Service Areas of New York State 1988 & 1993	I: reviewed hospitals, external peer reviews by ACOG trained team (audit & feedback) (45 hospitals; mean 1400–1500 deliveries)	C: non-reviewed hospitals, had an obstetric service (120 hospitals; mean 1700 deliveries)		NR	1988: I: mean 10.1 ± 1.4% C: mean 12.1 ± 0.9% NS (p > 0.01) 1993: I: mean 24.8 ± 2.0% C: mean 24.8 ± 1.1% NS (p > 0.01)	NR
Liu (2013) Non-concurrent cohort Taiwan, tertiary hospital Funding NR	All pregnant women delivering by cesarean section June 2001–August 2010	Period 1 (June 2001–July 2002): before implementation of budget systems (n = 800)	Period 2 (July 2002–August 2005): global budget system (n = 1887)	Period 3 (August 2005–2010): hospital-based self-management program (n = 2621)	NR	P1: 38 (4.8%) P2: 231 (12.2%) P3: 298 (11.4%) Period 1 vs. 2, p < 0.001 Period 2 vs. 3, p = 0.3950	NR

no. number, *TOLAC* trial of labor after cesarean, *VBAC* vaginal birth after cesarean, *Grp* group, *n* number, *CS* cesarean section, *NR* not reported, vs. versus, *US* United States, *I* intervention, *ACOG* American College of Obstetricians and Gynecologists, *C* comparator, *NS* not significant
[a]Results of statistical tests or summary statistics were extracted whenever these were reported within studies

opinion leader group (25.3%) compared with the audit and feedback (11.8%) and guideline groups (14.5%) (85% higher in the opinion leaders group versus the other groups, $p = 0.003$) [32]. A cross-sectional study found that a higher proportion of women with prior cesarean delivery had a TOLAC in hospitals employing laborists (356 of 2621 women; 13.6%) compared with hospitals without laborists (201 of 2111 women; 9.5%) [27]. A higher rate of successful VBACs occurred in the same group, however the result was not statistically significant (9.7% versus 6.5%; adjusted odds ratio (aOR) 1.10, 95% CI 0.82–1.47, $p = 0.5417$) [27]. A non-concurrent cohort comparing deliveries in 1985 with deliveries in 1986 to 1991 after the implementation of a hospital initiative utilizing a second opinion by an obstetrician for primary and repeat cesarean deliveries, found increased rates of TOLAC (45.0% versus range 68.4 to 91.3%, pre- versus post--intervention, respectively) and VBAC (23.8% versus range 54.9 to 67.4%, pre- versus post-intervention, respectively) [34].

Provider characteristics

Four studies [36, 40, 42, 43] examined the effect of provider characteristics on VBAC rates (Table 4). A small RCT of women in labor compared midwifery care (n = 48) with standard maternity care (n = 48); the authors reported a higher proportion of VBAC among women receiving continuous midwifery care from the antenatal to postnatal period (87.5% versus 66.7% of women, $p < 0.05$) [43]. Another study examined midwifery care and found that among women with one previous cesarean delivery, there was a higher rate of attempted VBACs in the post-intervention (midwifery-led antenatal care; 153 of 196 women; 78.1%) compared with the pre-intervention group (traditional obstetrician-led antenatal care; 143 of 209 women; 68.4%) [40]. More VBACs occurred in the group who received care from a midwife in 2011 (120 of 196 women; 61.2%) than among women who received obstetrician-led antenatal care in 2008 (98 of 209 women; 46.9%, aOR 1.79; 95% CI 1.17–2.75, $p < 0.05$). One retrospective cohort compared physicians with a traditional call schedule (946 women) with physicians on a night float call schedule (556 women); eligible women were more likely to undergo a TOLAC when delivered by physicians on a night float call system (OR 2.50, 95% CI 1.96–3.20, $p < 0.001$) and the effect persisted when the groups were adjusted for body-mass index (BMI), gestational age (GA) and physician (aOR 2.64, 95% CI 1.65–4.25, $p < 0.001$) [42]. A cross-sectional study of women with at least one previous cesarean delivery with a singleton delivery compared women delivered by an obstetrician ($n = 3493$) with women delivered by a family physician ($n = 201$), and found that more TOLACs occurred in the latter than the former group (81.1% versus 50.6%, $p < 0.001$) as well as VBACs (61.7% versus 32.5%) [36].

Guidelines or information for providers

Seven non-concurrent cohort studies in the US [23, 30, 35, 37–39, 44] examined VBAC rates before and after guidelines or information for providers were implemented (Table 5). Kosecoff et al. compared VBAC rates in 1979 and 1980 (35 and 64 women, respectively) before the National Institutes of Health conference recommendations, with rates in 1981 to 1982 (70 women); a greater proportion of women had a TOLAC (5.7 and 11.0% pre- versus 28.6% post-recommendations) and a VBAC (5.7 and 6.3% pre- versus 15.7% post-recommendations) after the conference recommendations (adjusted positive linear trend of 2.4 [5.8%] for TOLAC and 2.1 [4.5%] for VBAC) [30]. Another study comparing before (1987–1988) and after (1988–1991) the ACOG practice guidelines were implemented reported that VBAC rates increased by 5.6 percentage points as a result of the guideline and its information dissemination [38]. Pinette et al. also compared rates of VBAC before (1998) and after (1999–2001) ACOG guidelines were revised to require the presence of surgical personnel throughout a trial of labour, and found a marked decline in hospital VBAC data (relative risk 3.5, 95% CI 3.1–4.2, $p < 0.01$), citing factors such as patient refusal post-counselling, inability of institutions to meet requirements, and lack of support from the obstetric service [35]. Zweifler et al. examined the effect of the ACOG revision to provide immediate cesarean capability (1996 to 1999 versus 2000 to 2002, before versus after, respectively) and found that there were comparatively fewer TOLACs (24.0% before versus 13.5% after guideline revision, $p < 0.001$) and successful VBACs among women with TOLACs (82.8% [41,961 of 50,670 deliveries] before versus 81.8% [19,273 of 23,573 deliveries] after guideline revision) [44]. In a study focused on the impact of state-legislated practice guidelines, the authors reported that dissemination alone did not significantly increase the VBAC rate (7151 of 23,142 deliveries; 30.9% post-guideline in 1993) compared with the years leading up to the change (4816 of 22,091 deliveries [21.8%] in 1990; 5540 of 21,461 deliveries [25.6%] in 1991; and, 6133 of 22,970 deliveries [26.7%] in 1992) [39]. A study compared intrapartum management of women with prior cesareans before (1986–1987) and after (1988–1989) hospital guideline changes incorporated centralized decision-making, and found that rates of TOLAC increased from 31.7% (139 out of 438 women in 1986) to 84.0% (487 out of 580 women in 1989; $p < 0.0001$), and that the proportion of these women with subsequent VBACs also increased (from 64.7% [90 out of 139 women in 1986] to 82.8% [403 out of 487 women in 1989, $p < 0.0001$) [37]. Bellows et al. examined changes to hospital policies for TOLAC eligibility and labor induction guidelines; the authors reported that while the "overall VBAC rate" (number of women with a prior cesarean who had a VBAC) increased (26.0% pre- versus 33.0% post-guidelines, $p <$ 0.0001), the "VBAC rate" (number of women who underwent a TOLAC and had a successful VBAC) was unchanged (78.9% pre- versus 78.1% post-guidelines, $p =$ 0.75) [23].

Patient-level interventions

Six studies [25, 26, 28, 29, 33, 41] examined patient-level interventions (Table 6). One RCT of women with a single previous low transverse cesarean delivery compared a verbal prenatal education program (641 women) with a written prenatal education program (634 women) and found no evidence of a clinically significant difference for TOLAC rate (72.5% versus 69.4%; relative risk 1.1, 95% CI 1.0–1.1) or VBAC rate (52.9% versus 48.9%; relative risk 1.1, 95% CI 1.0–1.2) [28]. Another RCT compared two interventions (decision analysis aid [235 women] and information program [241 women]) with usual care (239 women), reporting the highest rate of VBAC in the decision analysis group (37.4% versus 29.2% versus 30.3%, decision analysis versus information program versus usual care, respectively; no significant differences between groups) and concluded that women who received any decision aid had greater knowledge and less anxiety than women receiving standard obstetric care [33]. Another trial compared an evidence-based computerized decision aid (66 women) with evidence--based educational ACOG brochures (65 women) and reported that women experienced less decisional conflict in the former group compared with the latter, however, there was no significant difference in VBACs (41.0% versus 37.0%, $p = 0.724$) [26]. A cohort study of patient satisfaction with mode of delivery found that women who received formal one-on-one antenatal counseling ($n =$ 95) had comparatively higher rates of TOLAC (46.3% versus 38.5%) but lower rates of VBAC (27.4% versus 31.7%) than women who didn't participate in VBAC counseling ($n = 221$) [25]. A non-concurrent cohort of

Table 3 Summary of studies – provider-level interventions

Study; Design; Country, setting; Funding	Population; Study period	Intervention & comparator (no. of participants)	TOLAC rate[a]	VBAC rate[a]	VBAC/TOLAC rate[a]	Study; Design; Country, setting; Funding
Feldman (2015) Cross-sectional US, community hospitals Non-industry funded	Women with live-born, singleton, vertex gestations, with prior CS January 2012–January 2014	I: hospitals employing laborists (≥1 physician in hospital, primary focus is to care for patients in labor and delivery) ($n = 2621$)	C: hospitals without laborists ($n = 2111$)	I: 356 (13.6%) C: 201 (9.5%), $p = 0.0318$	I: 253 (9.7%) C: 137 (6.5%), $p = 0.0302$	I: 253 (71.0%) C: 136 (67.9%), $p = 0.2943$
Lomas (1991) RCT, 3-arm Canada, community hospitals Non-industry funded	Study site inclusion needed 100 beds (10+ obstetrical), no status as teaching institution, not in county with teaching institution 1988–1989	I 1: audit and feedback ($n = 524$) I 2: opinion leader education ($n = 739$)	C: eight control hospitals, practice guideline mailed to obstetrical care ($n = 1233$)	I 1: 112 (21.4%) I 2: 282 (38.2%) C: 349 (28.3%), $p = 0.007$	I 1: 62 (11.8%) I 2: 187 (25.3%) C: 179 (14.5%), $p = 0.003$	I 1: 62 (55.4%) I 2: 187 (66.3%) C: 179 (51.3%)
Myers (1993) Follow-up to non-concurrent cohort (1985–1987) US, level 3 prenatal center Funding NR	All patients in obstetric department 1985–1991	Grp 1 (1985): before hospital initiative ($n = 122$)	Grp 2 (1986–1991): after hospital initiative; 2nd opinion required for all CS, VD was preferred, dystocia accepted as indication for CD ($n = 1840$)	1985: 55 (45.0%) vs. 1986: 132 (68.4%) 1987: 233 (86.0%) 1988: 243 (88.3%) 1989: 255 (91.3%) 1990: 312 (85.4%) 1991:374 (81.8%)	1985: 29 (23.8%) vs. 1986: 106 (54.9%) 1987: 162 (59.8%) 1988: 167 (60.1%) 1989: 188 (67.4%) 1990: 242 (66.3%) 1991: 291 (63.7%)	1985: 29 (52.7%) vs. 1986: 106 (80.3%) 1987: 162 (69.5%) 1988: 167 (73.7%) 1989: 188 (73.7%) 1990: 242 (77.5%) 1991: 291 (77.8%)

no. number, *TOLAC* trial of labor after cesarean, *VBAC* vaginal birth after cesarean, *US* United States, *CS* cesarean section, *I* intervention, *C* comparator, *RCT* randomized controlled trial, *NR* not reported, *Grp* group, *VD* vaginal delivery, *CD* cesarean delivery

[a]Results of statistical tests or summary statistics were extracted whenever these were reported within studies

Table 4 Summary of studies – provider characteristics

Study; Design; Country, setting; Funding	Population; Study period	Intervention & comparator (no. of participants)		TOLAC rate[a]	VBAC rate[a]	VBAC/TOLAC rate[a]
Russillo (2008) Cross-sectional Canada, secondary care urban hospital Non-industry funded	Pregnant women with at least one previous CS, singleton delivery, birth weight at least 500 g January 1995–December 2003	Grp 1: deliveries performed by obstetricians ($n = 3493$)	Grp 2: deliveries performed by family physicians ($n = 201$)	Grp 1: 1768 (50.6%) Grp 2: 163 (81.1%), $p < 0.001$	Grp 1: 1136 (32.5%) Grp 2: 124 (61.7%)	Grp 1: 1136 (64.3%) Grp 2: 124 (76.1%), $p = 0.002$
White 2016 Non-concurrent cohort UK, tertiary teaching hospital Non-industry funded	Women with one previous CS who received antenatal and intrapartum care during study period 2008 & 2011	Grp 1 (2008): obstetrician-led antenatal care ($n = 209$)	Grp 2 (≥2011): midwife-led antenatal care ($n = 196$)	Attempted VBAC: Grp 1: 143 (68.4%) Grp 2: 153 (78.1%)	Actual VBAC: Grp 1: 98 (46.9%) Grp 2: 120 (61.2%); aOR 1.79 (95% CI 1.17–2.75), $p < 0.05$ Spontaneous VBAC: Grp 1: 67 (32.1%) Grp 2: 85 (43.4%); OR 1.62 (95% CI 1.08–2.43)	Successful/attempted VBAC: Grp 1: 98 (68.5%) Grp 2: 120 (78.4%); OR 1.67 (95% CI 0.99–2.82), NS ($p > 0.05$)
Yee 2017 Retrospective cohort US, large teaching hospital Funding NR	Women ≥18 years old with one prior low transverse CD, a term, cephalic singleton gestation, and no prior VD January 2008–June 2013	Grp 1: night float schedule ($n = 556$)	Grp 2: traditional call schedule ($n = 946$)	Grp 1: 184 (33.1%) Grp 2: 156 (16.5%), $p < 0.001$	Grp 1: 104 (18.7%) Grp 2: 88 (9.3%), $p < 0.001$	Grp 1: 104 (56.5%) Grp 2: 88 (56.4%), $p = 0.98$
Zhang 2016 RCT China, hospital obstetric department No funding	Women with a history of previous CS in labor willing to undergo a VD May 2013–November 2014	I: continuing midwifery care ($n = 48$)	C: standard maternity care ($n = 48$)	NR	I: 42 (87.5%) C: 32 (66.7%), $p < 0.05$	NR

no. number, *TOLAC* trial of labor after cesarean, *VBAC* vaginal birth after cesarean, *CS* cesarean section, *g* grams, *Grp* group, *UK* United Kingdom, *aOR* adjusted odds ratio, *CI* confidence interval, *OR* odds ratio, *NS* not significant, *US* United States, *CD* cesarean delivery, *VD* vaginal delivery, *RCT* randomized controlled trial, *I* intervention, *C* comparator, *NR* not reported

[a]Results of statistical tests or summary statistics were extracted whenever these were reported within studies

Table 5 Summary of studies – guidelines or information for providers

Study; Design; Country, setting; Funding	Population; Study period	Intervention & comparator (no. of participants)		TOLAC rate[a]	VBAC rate[a]	VBAC/TOLAC rate[a]
Bellows (2016) Non-concurrent cohort US, tertiary care academic hospital Funding NR	All women who underwent TOLAC, at least one prior CD & live, singleton gestation in cephalic presentation, 24 0/7 weeks of gestation July 1, 2009-December 31, 2013	Grp 1 (2009–2011): pre-2011 guideline ($n = 450$)	Grp 2 (2011–2013): post-2011 guideline implementation (offering TOLAC; inducing labor; administering oxytocin) ($n = 781$)	NR	Grp 1: NR (26.0%) Grp 2: NR (33.3%)	Grp 1: 351 (78.1%) Grp 2: 616 (78.9%), $p = 0.75$
Kosecoff (1987) Retrospective cohort US, acute, non-specialty, nonfederal hospitals > 150 beds. Non-industry funded	Women with previous low transverse CS January 1979–December 1979 (time 1) January 1980–September 1980 (time 2) July 1981–June 1982 (time 3)	Period 1 (January–December 1979) & Period 2 (January–September 1980): before NIH Consensus Development conference recommendations ($n = 35$ & $n = 64$)	Period 3 (1981–1982): after conference recommendations; women should be given TOLAC for potential VD ($n = 70$)	Period 1: 2 (5.7%) Period 2: 7 (10.9%) vs. Period 3: 20 (28.6%)	Period 1: 2 (5.7%) Period 2: 4 (6.3%) vs. Period 3: 11 (15.7%)	Period 1: 2 (100%) Period 2: 4 (57.1%) vs. Period 3: 11 (55.0%)
Pinette (2004) Non-concurrent cohort US, birth certificate & hospital reported data Funding NR	All women with previous CS giving birth at 20 weeks of gestation or more 1998–2001	Grp 1 (1998): pre-exposure (birth certificate $n = 1410$; hospital data $n = 1386$)	Grp 2 (1999–2001): ACOG guideline revision (birth certificate data $n = 4463$; hospital data $n = 4015$)	NR	Birth certificate data: 1998: 424 (30.1%) vs. 1999: 327 (22.6%) 2000: 277 (17.9%) 2001: 193 (13.1%) 1988 vs. 2001, RR 2.8 (95% CI 2.5–3.2), $p < 0.01$ Hospital-reported data: 1998: 489 (35.3%) vs. 1999: 411 (28.2%) 2000: 321 (23.1%) 2001: 156 (13.3%) RR 3.5 (95% CI 3.1–4.2), $p < 0.01$	NR
Sanchez –Ramos (1990) Non-concurrent cohort US, regional perinatal center Funding NR	Women with one or two previous CS, with low transverse or vertical scars not extending into uterine corpus 1986–1989	Grp 1 (1986–1987): before July 1, 1987 department-wide guideline change ($n = 899$)	Grp 2 (1988–1989): after July 1, 1987, new guidelines for intrapartum management ($n = 1105$)	1986: 139 (31.7%) 1987: 193 (41.9%) vs. 1988: 402 (76.6%) 1989: 487 (84.0%); Difference: 52.2%, $p < 0.0001$	1986: 90 (20.5%) 1987: 142 (30.8%) vs. 1988: 342 (65.1%) 1989: 403 (69.5%); Difference: 48.9%; $p < 0.0001$	1986: 90 (64.7%) 1987: 142 (73.6%) vs. 1988: 342 (85.1%) 1989: 403 (82.8%); Difference: 18.0%; $p < 0.0001$
Santerre (1996)	Women with a previous CS	Grp 1 (before 1987–1988):	Grp 2 (after Oct. 1988): ACOG	NR	VBAC rate in US	NR

Table 5 Summary of studies – guidelines or information for providers *(Continued)*

Study; Design; Country, setting; Funding	Population; Study period	Intervention & comparator (no. of participants)		TOLAC rate[a]	VBAC rate[a]	VBAC/TOLAC rate[a]
Non-concurrent cohort US, hospitals Funding NR	1987–1991	before practice guideline implementation (n = NR)	practice guideline, prior cesarean section no longer a reason for repeat cesarean (n = NR)		(data for Massachusetts hospitals NR) 1985: 6.6% 1986: 8.5% 1987: 9.8% 1988: 12.6% vs. 1989: 18.5% 1990: 20.4% 1991: 24.2% 1992: 25.1% 1993: 25.4%	
Studnicki (1997) Non-concurrent cohort US, nonfederal acute care provider hospitals Funding NR	Women with prior CS 1990–1993	Grp 1 (1990–1992): before practice guidelines (n = 66,702)	Grp 2 (1993): after legislatively imposed practice guidelines (n = 23,142)	NR	1990: 4816 (21.8%) 1991: 5540 (25.6%) 1992: 6133 (26.7%) vs. 1993: 7151 (30.9%)	NR
Zweifler (2006) Non-concurrent cohort US, California Department of Health Services Birth Statistical Master Files Funding NR	Women who previously gave birth by cesarean delivery & had singleton birth planned in a California hospital 1996–2002	Grp 1 (1996–1999): before ACOG VBAC guideline revision (n = NR[b])	Grp 2 (2000–2002): after ACOG VBAC guideline revision (n = NR[b])	Attempted VBAC: Grp 1: NR (24.0%) Grp 2: NR (13.5%) Difference: 44% decrease, $p < 0.001$	1996–2002: 61,684 (16.0%)	NR

no. number, *TOLAC* trial of labor after cesarean, *VBAC* vaginal birth after cesarean, *US* United States, *NR* not reported, *CD* cesarean delivery, *Grp* group, *CS* cesarean section, *NIH* National Institute of Health, *VD* vaginal delivery, vs. versus, *ACOG* American College of Obstetricians and Gynecologists, *RR* relative risk, *CI* confidence interval

[a]Results of statistical tests or summary statistics were extracted whenever these were reported within studies

[b]Study reported number of live births separately from number of women; table reflects data for number of women whenever this was reported

Table 6 Summary of studies – patient-level interventions

Study; Design; Country, setting; Funding	Population; Study period	Intervention & comparator (no. of participants)	TOLAC rate[a]	VBAC rate[a]	VBAC/TOLAC rate[a]	Population; Study period
Cleary-Goldman (2005) Prospective cohort with controls US, tertiary care center Non-industry funded	Women eligible for a TOLAC 12-month period	I: one-on-one VBAC counselling, in 2nd and 3rd trimesters ($n = 95$)	C: no extra counselling, standard care ($n = 221$)	I: 44 (46.3%) C: 85 (38.5%)	I: 26 (27.4%) C: 70 (31.7%)	I: 26 (59.1%) C: 70 (82.4%)
Eden (2014) RCT US, clinics Non-industry funded	Pregnant women with one prior CS, 18 years or older, pregnant with one fetus, low transverse uterine scar, and providers had given option of TOLAC September 17, 2005-May 4, 2007	I: Evidence-based, interactive decision aid ($n = 66$)	C: two evidence-based educational brochures about cesarean delivery and VBAC ($n = 65$)	NR	I: NR (41.0%) C: NR (37.0%), $p = 0.724$	NR
Fraser (1997) RCT Canada, hospitals Non-industry funded	Women with single previous low transverse CS, gestational age < 28 weeks. April 1992–November 1994	I: Verbal prenatal education program – pamphlet + 2 individualized contacts ($n = 641$)	C: Document prenatal education program – written information ($n = 634$)	I: 465 (72.5%) C: 440 (69.4%); RR 1.1 (95% CI 1.0–1.1)	I: 339 (52.9%) C: 310 (48.9%); RR 1.1 (95% CI 1.0–1.2)	I: 339 (72.9%) C: 310 (70.5%)
Gardner (2014) Non-concurrent cohort Australia, metropolitan teaching hospital Funding NR	Women with a single prior CS, presenting in their next pregnancy 2006 (before) & May 2009–October 2010	Grp 1 (2006): routine care, counselling for mode of birth on ad-hoc basis (n = NR)	Grp 2 (2009–2010): two combined management strategies – Risk Associated Pregnancy consultant & NBAC clinic ($n = 396$)	Grp 1: NR Grp 2: 164 (41.4%)	VBAC rate for NBAC Grp 1: NR (17.2%) Grp 2: 107 (27.0%), $p < 0.001$	Grp 1: NR Grp 2: 107 (65.2%)
Montgomery (2007) RCT UK, maternity units Non-industry funded	Pregnant women with one previous lower segment CS, delivery expected at ≥37 weeks; most recent delivery is cesarean. May 2004–August 2006	I 1: decision analysis aid ($n = 235$) I 2: information program ($n = 241$)	C: usual care ($n = 239$)	NR	I 1: 88 (37.4%) I 2: 70 (29.2%) C: 72 (30.3%) I 1 vs. C: aOR 1.42 (95% CI 0.94–2.14), $p = 0.22$ I 2 vs. C: aOR 0.93 (95% CI 0.61–1.41), $p > 0.9$ I1 vs. I2: aOR 1.53 (95% CI 1.01–2.30), $p = 0.11$	NR
Wong (2014) Prospective cohort UK, district general hospital Funding NR	Women with one previous lower segment CS, no contraindications for VBAC 12-month period commencing January 1, 2012	I: one-stop obstetrician-led cesarean education and antenatal sessions (OCEANS) ($n = 188$)	C: did not attend OCEANS ($n = 78$)	I: 108 (57.4%) C: 33 (42.3%), $p = 0.02$	I: 59 (31.4%) C: 20 (25.6%)	I: 59 (54.6%) C: 20 (60.6%) $p = 0.69$†

no. **number,** ***TOLAC*** **trial of labor after cesarean,** ***VBAC*** **vaginal birth after cesarean,** ***US*** **United States,** ***I*** **intervention,** ***C*** **comparator,** ***RCT*** **randomized controlled trial,** ***CS*** **cesarean section,** ***NR*** **not reported,** ***RR*** **relative risk,** ***CI*** **confidence interval,** ***Grp*** **group,** ***NBAC*** **next birth after cesarean,** ***UK*** **United Kingdom,** ***aOR*** **adjusted odds ratio,** ***OCEANS*** **obstetrician-led cesarean education and antenatal session**

[a]Results of statistical tests or summary statistics were extracted whenever these were reported within studies

†study reports difference as $p = 0.69$ (Table 2) and $p = 0.55$ (abstract)

Table 7 Summary of methodological quality of included studies

MMAT[a] criteria	Screening questions		Quantitative/ control group				Quantitative non-randomized				Total[b]
Study	Clear research questions or objectives?	Do collected data address the research questions/ objective?	2.1 Clear description of randomization?	2.2 Clear description of allocation concealment (or blinding)?	2.3 Complete outcome data (≥80%)?	2.4 Low withdrawal/ drop-out (< 20%)?	3.1 Participants/ organizations recruitment - minimizes selection bias?	3.2 Appropriate measurements used for intervention & outcomes?	3.3 Participants/ organizations comparable, or are differences accounted for?	3.4 Complete outcome data (80% or above) or acceptable follow-up rate?	
Ayres-De-Campos (2015)	☆	☆	NA	NA	NA	NA	☆	☆	–	☆	☆☆☆ (75%)
Bickell (1996)	☆	☆	NA	NA	NA	NA	☆	☆	☆	☆	☆☆☆☆(100%)
Bellows (2016)	☆	☆	NA	NA	NA	NA	☆	☆	☆	☆	☆☆☆☆(100%)
Cleary-Goldman (2005)	☆	☆	NA	NA	NA	NA	–	☆	–	☆	☆☆ (50%)
Eden (2014)	☆	☆	☆	–	–	☆	NA	NA	NA	NA	☆☆ (50%)
Feldman (2015)	☆	☆	NA	NA	NA	NA	☆	☆	☆	☆	☆☆☆☆(100%)
Fraser (RCT)	☆	☆	☆		☆	☆	NA	NA	NA	NA	☆☆☆ (75%)
Gardner (2014)	☆	☆	NA	NA	NA	NA	☆	–	–	☆	☆☆ (50%)
Kosecoff (1987)	☆	☆	NA	NA	NA	NA	☆	☆	–	–	☆☆ (50%)
Liu (2013)	☆	☆	NA	NA	NA	NA	☆	☆	–	☆	☆☆☆ (75%)
Lomas (1991)	☆	☆	☆	–	☆	–	NA	NA	NA	NA	☆☆ (50%)
Montgomery (2007)	☆	☆	☆	☆	☆	☆	NA	NA	NA	NA	☆☆☆☆(100%)
Myers (1993)	☆	☆	NA	NA	NA	NA	–	☆	–	☆	☆☆ (50%)
Pinette (2004)	☆	☆	NA	NA	NA	NA	☆	☆	–	☆	☆☆☆ (75%)
Russillo (2008)	☆	☆	NA	NA	NA	NA	☆	☆	–	☆	☆☆☆ (75%)
Sanchez-Ramos (1990)	☆	☆	NA	NA	NA	NA	☆	☆	–	☆	☆☆☆ (75%)
Santerre (1996)	☆	☆	NA	NA	NA	NA	☆	☆	–	☆	☆☆☆ (75%)
Studnicki (1997)	☆	☆	NA	NA	NA	NA	☆	☆	☆	☆	☆☆☆☆(100%)
White (2016)	☆	☆	NA	NA	NA	NA	☆	☆	☆	☆	☆☆☆☆(100%)
Wong (2014)	☆	☆	NA	NA	NA	NA	☆	☆	–	–	☆☆ (50%)
Yee (2017)	☆	☆	NA	NA	NA	NA	☆	☆	☆	☆	☆☆☆☆(100%)
Zhang (2016)	☆	☆	–	–	☆	–	NA	NA	NA	NA	☆ (25%)
Zweifler (2016)	☆	☆	NA	NA	NA	NA	☆	☆	☆	☆	☆☆☆☆(100%)

[a] Assessed using the Mixed Methods Appraisal Tool; [b] Total score is out of four stars (☆☆☆☆), whereby each assessment criterion met by a study was awarded a star (☆), and a criterion not met by a study was marked with a dash (–); *NA* not applicable

women with a single prior cesarean delivery presenting in their next pregnancy had a higher VBAC rate after the implementation of standardized consultant labor management with a dedicated antenatal clinic (27.0% versus 17.2%, $p < 0.001$) compared with women who received routine antenatal care with mode of birth counseling on an ad-hoc basis [29]. Another cohort study reported higher rates of TOLAC (57.4% versus 42.0%, $p = 0.02$) and VBAC (31.4% versus 25.6%) among women who attended an obstetrician-led cesarean delivery education and antenatal session ($n = 188$) compared with women who chose not to attend the session ($n = 78$), although the authors concluded that the overall rate of successful vaginal deliveries among women who attempted VBAC was not influenced by the education session [41].

Discussion

This systematic review of adjunct clinical interventions aimed at influencing the rate of VBACs identified 23 studies which suggest that some provider-level interventions (e.g. opinion leader education in hospitals, employing laborists as providers, and utilizing obstetrician 'second opinion' for all cesarean deliveries), and provider characteristics (i.e., midwifery-led antenatal care, physicians working a night call float schedule, and birth deliveries by a family physician) are associated with higher TOLAC and VBAC rates, while system-level interventions (i.e., education and training of healthcare providers, contingency-based funding for delivery rates, and peer review/audit), patient-level interventions (i.e., different modes of information delivery, and antenatal counseling for women) and provider guidelines/information report mixed findings. The significant study heterogeneity in research designs, interventions and outcomes did not allow for a meta-analysis to be completed.

Other systematic reviews of adjunct clinical interventions to increase VBAC rates have reported similar findings, although eligibility criteria among these reviews differed slightly from the present study. Catling-Paull et al. [45] examined non-clinical interventions (27 studies) and concluded that local guidelines, opinion leaders and individualized information for women can impact the uptake and/or success of VBAC. While the present study also found that opinion leaders increased VBACs, evidence from guidelines had conflicting findings and information for women did not show significant differences between groups. Lundgren et al. [46] evaluated clinician-centered interventions designed to increase VBAC rates (three studies) and concluded that educational strategies delivered by opinion leaders significantly increased VBAC rates, while external peer review and audit and feedback had no significant effect; the present review also found the impact of opinion leader education on VBACs. A systematic review of women-centered interventions to increase VBACs (three studies) concluded that while decision aids and information programs during pregnancy did not appear to affect the rate of VBAC, they reduced women's decisional conflict and increased their knowledge regarding birth options [47]. The present study echoed the findings that information for women was associated with increased VBAC in one study but without significant difference in two studies.

Strengths and limitations of study

A methodologically rigorous systematic review of the literature was undertaken to capture a broad range of studies of adjunct clinical interventions directed at increasing maternal VBAC rates. However, several factors limit our confidence in effects of interventions, such as inclusion of non-randomized study designs, small number of studies per intervention category, and inconsistent results across heterogeneous studies. Moreover, many studies did not report important maternal baseline characteristics in a consistent manner, including antenatal history (e.g., parity, number of previous cesarean deliveries and vaginal births, medical history/risk factors) or indications (e.g., age, gestational age, fetal risk factors).

Implications for practice

Based on the available evidence, attempts to increase vaginal births among women with prior cesareans need to incorporate different types of provider or provider-level interventions to achieve a greater likelihood of success. Hospitals that utilize the 'influential opinion leader model' to educate colleagues and patients can effect a behavior/clinical change by offering more women the opportunity of a VBAC. Staffing community hospitals with laborists may encourage more support for women to attempt a vaginal delivery. Requiring an expert second opinion prior to a cesarean may decrease the proportion of women who undergo cesarean deliveries (exclusive of those performed for acute emergencies) through counseling, thereby increasing choice and the number of attempted VBACs. Low risk maternity providers (e.g., midwives, family physicians) or the continuity of midwifery care may provide women with support and confidence to undergo a VBAC through a personalized and responsive approach. Overall, these are aligned with the SOGC recommendation that women be given the opportunity to consult with her obstetric care provider on the risks and benefits of TOLAC as well as awareness of availability of hospital resources for an elective cesarean section if indicated [12]. Adoption of any strategy or intervention to increase rates of TOLAC and subsequent VBAC must carefully weigh the potential benefits against the possible risks for mother and baby.

As the scope of the current review was sufficiently broad, the authors did not search for studies that examined barriers to VBAC or factors related to women's motivations, preferences or decision-making. Studies of clinicians' and women's perspectives may provide insight on system, provider-level, and patient-oriented factors that influence rates of attempted and successful VBAC [48, 49]. For example, a qualitative study examined barriers associated with the ACOG VBAC guidelines and found that fear of liability affected the willingness of midwives and obstetricians in offering VBAC [6]. Other factors such as the continual presence of a physician, travel distance to a hospital that offers TOLAC (although 56% of California hospitals permit TOLAC, significantly fewer VBACs were actually carried out), and hospital policy for patient TOLAC eligibility presented as other systemic barriers restricting women's access to a TOLAC [50]. Additionally, there is a paucity of studies on supports intended to facilitate shared decision-making between women and their healthcare providers [51]. Such evidence may provide context for effectiveness, acceptability and feasibility of interventions aimed at individual patients' needs, decisions and satisfaction regarding mode of birth.

Conclusion

This 'up-to-date' systematic review evaluated adjunct clinical interventions directed at increasing the rate of vaginal delivery among women with a prior cesarean delivery and provides evidence that some provider-level interventions and provider characteristics are associated with higher maternal TOLAC and VBAC rates. Further research, using robust study designs with documentation of population characteristics, is needed to provide stronger outcome evidence for the use and effect of adjunct clinical interventions. Enhancing the woman's education and her opportunity to consider and choose VBAC over a repeat cesarean delivery is an important clinical outcome and goal to examine in future research and reviews.

Abbreviations

ACOG: American College of Obstetrics and Gynecology; aOR: adjusted odds ratio; BMI: Body mass index; CI: Confidence interval; GA: Gestational age; GRADE: Grading of Recommendations Assessment, Development and Evaluation; MMAT: Mixed Methods Appraisal Tool; NRCT: Non-randomized clinical trial; OR: Odds ratio; RCT: Randomized clinical trial; RR: Risk ratio; SMFM: The Society for Maternal-Fetal Medicine; SOGC: The Society of Obstetricians and Gynaecologists of Canada; TOLAC: Trial of labor after cesarean; VBAC: Vaginal birth after cesarean

Acknowledgements

We would like to thank: Tara Landry, MLIS, for peer reviewing the search strategy; Ms. MacKinna Hauff for article retrieval; Dr. Allison Gates and Dr. Michelle Gates for assistance with the French translations.

Funding

This study was funded by the Maternal, Newborn, Child and Youth Strategic Clinical Network (MNCY SCN) of Alberta Health Services (AHS) and the Alberta Strategy for Patient-Oriented Research (SPOR) SUPPORT Unit Knowledge Translation Platform. The funders had no role in the design of the study, the collection, analysis or interpretation of data, the writing of the manuscript, or the decision to submit the article for publication.

Authors' contributions

All authors contributed to the conception and design of the project. RF conducted the literature searches. AW and CJ conducted screening, quality assessments, and data extraction and verification. AW drafted the manuscript. AW, CJ, MS, LH and RDW contributed to interpretation of data and revised the manuscript for important intellectual content. All authors contributed to revisions of the manuscript and approved the final version for submission.

Consent for publication

Not applicable.

Competing interests

All authors declare funding from MNCY SCN of AHS and Alberta SPOR SUPPORT Unit KT Platform; LH, MS and RF are employed in part or whole by the Alberta SPOR SUPPORT KT Platform; LH was funded in part by a New Investigator Salary Award from CIHR; there are no other relationships or activities that could appear to have influenced the submitted work.

Author details

[1]Alberta Research Centre for Health Evidence, Department of Pediatrics, University of Alberta, Edmonton, AB, Canada. [2]Alberta Strategy for Patient-Oriented Research (SPOR) SUPPORT Unit Knowledge Translation Platform, University of Alberta, Edmonton, AB, Canada. [3]Department of Obstetrics and Gynecology, Cumming School of Medicine, University of Calgary, 1403 – 29 Street NW, Calgary, AB T2N 2T9, Canada.

References

1. Canadian Institute of Health Information. Inpatient hospitalizations, surgeries and childbirth indicators in 2010–2013. https://secure.cihi.ca/estore/productFamily.htm. Accessed 5 May 2017.
2. Kelly S, Sprague A, Fell DB, Murphy P, Aelicks N, Guo Y, et al. Examining caesarean section rates in Canada using the Robson classification system. J Obstet Gynaecol Can. 2013;35(3):206–14.
3. Canadian Institute for Health Information. Health indicators 2014: caesarean section. 2014. https://yourhealthsystem.cihi.ca/. Accessed 5 May 2017.
4. World Health Organization. WHO statement on caesarean section rates. 2015. http://www.who.int/reproductivehealth/publications/maternal_perinatal_health/cs-statement/en/. Accessed 5 May 2017.
5. Brown HK, Hill J, Natale R. Caesarean section rates in southwestern Ontario: changes over time after adjusting for important medical and social characteristics. J Obstet Gynaecol Can. 2014;36(7):578–89.
6. Cox KJ. Providers' perspectives on the vaginal birth after cesarean guidelines in Florida, United States: a qualitative study. BMC Pregnancy Childbirth. 2011;11(1):72.
7. Johnson J-A, Tough S, SOGC Genetics Committee. Delayed child-bearing. J Obstet Gynaecol Can. 2017;34(1):80–93.
8. Joseph KS, Young DC, Dodds L, O'Connell CM, Allen VM, Chandra S, et al. Changes in maternal characteristics and obstetric practice and recent increases in primary cesarean delivery. Obstet Gynecol. 2003;102(4):791–800.
9. Kawakita T, Reddy UM, Landy HJ, Iqbal SN, Huang CC, Grantz KL. Indications for primary cesarean delivery relative to body mass index. Am J Obstet Gynecol. 2016;215(4):e1–9.
10. Born K, Konkin J, Tepper J, Okan N. Pulling back the curtain on Canada's rising c-section rate. 2014. http://healthydebate.ca/2014/05/topic/quality/c-section-variation. Accessed 5 May 2017.

11. Degani N, Sikich N. Caesarean delivery rate review: an evidence-based analysis. Ont Health Technol Assess Ser. 2015;15(9):1–58.
12. Martel MJ, MacKinnon CJ. Clinical practice obstetrics committee. Guidelines for vaginal birth after previous caesarean. J Obstet Gynaecol. 2018;40(3): e195–207.
13. Sabol B, Denman MA, Fuise JM. Vaginal birth after cesarean: an effective method to reduce cesarean. Clin Obstet Gynecol. 2015;58(2):309–19.
14. Grobman WA, et al. The change in the rate of vaginal birth after caesarean section. Paediatr Perinat Epidemiol. 2011;25(1):37–43.
15. American Congress of Obstetricians and Gynecologists. ACOG practice bulletin: vaginal birth after cesarean delivery. Practice bulletin; 2017. p. 130.
16. American Congress of Obstetricians and Gynecologists. New VBAC guidelines. What they mean to you and your patients. ACOG Today. 2010; 54(4):6–7.
17. American Congress of Obstetricians and Gynecologists. ACOG practice bulletin no. 115: vaginal birth after previous cesarean delivery. Obstet Gynecol. 2010;116:450–463.
18. Higgins J, Green S (editors). The Cochrane Handbook for Systematic Reviews of Interventions 5.1.0 [updated: March 2011]. The Cochrane Collaboration; 2011. www.cochrane-handbook.org. Accessed: 14 Nov 2017.
19. Moher D, Liberati A, Tetzlaff J, Altman DG. Preferred reporting items for systematic reviews and meta-analyses: the PRISMA statement. J Clin Epidemiol. 2009;62(10):1006–12.
20. Pace R, Pluye P, Bartlett G, Macaulay AC, Salsberg J, Jagosh J, et al. Testing the reliability and efficiency of the pilot mixed methods appraisal tool (MMAT) for systematic mixed studies review. Int J Nurs Stud. 2012;49(1):47–53.
21. Guyatt GH, Oxman AD, Schunemann HJ, Tugwell P, Knottnerus A. GRADE guidelines: a new series of articles in the journal of clinical epidemiology. J Clin Epidemiol. 2011;64(4):380–2.
22. Ayres-De-Campos D, Cruz J, Medeiros-Borges C, Costa-Santos C, Vicente L. Lowered national cesarean section rates after a concerted action. Acta Obstet Gynecol Scand. 2015;94(4):391–8.
23. Bellows P, Shah U, Hawley L, Drexler K, Gandhi M, Sangi-Haghpeykar H, et al. Evaluation of outcomes associated with trial of labor after cesarean delivery after a change in clinical practice guidelines in an academic hospital. J Matern Fetal Neonatal Med. 2016:1–5.
24. Bickell NA, Zdeb MS, Applegate MS, Roohan PJ, Sui AL. Effect of external peer review on cesarean delivery rates: a statewide program. Obstet Gynecol. 1996;87(5 Pt 1):664–7.
25. Cleary-Goldman J, Cornelisse K, Simpson LL, Robinson JN. Previous cesarean delivery: understanding and satisfaction with mode of delivery in a subsequent pregnancy in patients participating in a formal vaginal birth after cesarean counseling program. Am J Perinatol. 2005;22(4):217–21.
26. Eden KB, Perrin NA, Vesco KK, Guise JM. A randomized comparative trial of two decision tools for pregnant women with prior cesareans. J Obstet Gynecol Neonatal Nurs. 2014;43(5):568–79.
27. Feldman DS, Bollman DL, Fridman M, Korst LM, El Haj IS, Fink A, et al. Do laborists improve delivery outcomes for laboring women in California community hospitals? Am J Obstet Gynecol. 2015;213(4):587 e1-13.
28. Fraser W, Maunsell E, Hodnett E, Moutquin JM. Randomized controlled trial of a prenatal vaginal birth after cesarean section education and support program. Childbirth alternatives post-cesarean study group. Am J Obstet Gynecol. 1997;176(2):419–25.
29. Gardner K, Henry A, Thou S, Davis G, Miller T. Improving VBAC rates: the combined impact of two management strategies. Aust N Z J Obstet Gynaecol. 2014;54(4):327–32.
30. Kosecoff J, Kanouse DE, Rogers WH, McCloskey L, Winslow CM, Brooks RH. Effects of the National Institutes of Health consensus development program on physician practice. JAMA. 1987;258(19):2708–13.
31. Liu CM, Lin YJ, Su YY, Chang SD, Cheng PJ. Impact of health policy based on the self-management program on cesarean section rate at a tertiary hospital in Taiwan. J Formos Med Assoc. 2013;112(2):93–8.
32. Lomas J, Enkin M, Anderson GM, Hannah WJ, Vayda E, Singer J. Opinion leaders vs audit and feedback to implement practice guidelines. Delivery after previous cesarean section. JAMA. 1991;265(17):2202–7.
33. Montgomery AA, Emmett CL, Fahey T, Jones C, Ricketts I, Patel RR, et al. the DiAMOND Study Group. Two decision aids for mode of delivery among women with previous caesarean section: randomised controlled trial. BMJ. 2007;334(7607):1305.
34. Myers SA, Gleicher N. The Mount Sinai cesarean section reduction program: an update after 6 years. Soc Sci Med. 1993;37(10):1219–22.
35. Pinette MG, Kahn J, Gross KL, Wax JR, Blackstone J, Cartin A. Vaginal birth after cesarean rates are declining rapidly in the rural state of Maine. J Matern Fetal Neonatal Med. 2004;16(1):37–43.
36. Russillo B, Sewitch MJ, Cardinal L, Brassard N. Comparing rates of trial of labour attempts, VBAC success, and fetal and maternal complications among family physicians and obstetricians. J Obstet Gynaecol Can. 2008; 30(2):123–8.
37. Sanchez-Ramos L, Kaunitz AM, Peterson HB, Martinez-Schnell B, Thompson RJ. Reducing cesarean sections at a teaching hospital. Am J Obstet Gynecol. 1990;163(3):1081–7.
38. Santerre RE. The effect of the ACOG guideline on vaginal births after cesarean. Med Care Res Rev. 1996;53(3):315–29.
39. Studnicki J, Remmel R, Campbell R, Werner DC. The impact of legislatively imposed practice guidelines on cesarean section rates: the Florida experience. Am J Med Qual. 1997;12(1):62–8.
40. White H, Le May A, Cluett E. Evaluating a midwife-led model of antenatal care for women with a previous caesarean section: a retrospective, comparative cohort study. Br J Obstet Gynaecol. 2016;123:200–8.
41. Wong KW, Thomas JM, Andrews V. Are women's and obstetricians, views on mode of delivery following a previous cesarean section really OCEANS apart? J Obstet Gynaecol India. 2014;64(6):400–2.
42. Yee LM, Liu LY, Grobman WA. Obstetrician call schedule and obstetric outcomes among women eligible for a trial of labor after cesarean. Am J Obstet Gynecol. 2017;216(1):75 e1-6.
43. Zhang T, Liu C. Comparison between continuing midwifery care and standard maternity care in vaginal birth after cesarean. Pak J Med Sci. 2016; 32(3):711–4.
44. Zweifler J, Garza A, Hughes S, Stanich MA, Hierholzer A, Lau M. Vaginal birth after cesarean in California: before and after a change in guidelines. Ann Fam Med. 2006;4(3):228–34.
45. Catling-Paull C, Johnston R, Ryan C, Foureur MJ, Homer CS. Non-clinical interventions that increase the uptake and success of vaginal birth after caesarean section: a systematic review. J Adv Nurs. 2011;67(8):1662–76.
46. Lundgren I, Smith V, Nilsson C, Vehvilainen-Julkunen K, Nicoletti J, Devane D, et al. Clinician-centred interventions to increase vaginal birth after caesarean section (VBAC): a systematic review. BMC Pregnancy Childbirth. 2015;15(16):1–9.
47. Nilsson C, Lundgren I, Smith V, Vehnilainen-Julkunen K, Nicoletti J, Devane D, et al. Women-centred interventions to increase vaginal birth after caesarean section (VBAC): a systematic review. Midwifery. 2015;31(7):657–63.
48. Lundgren I, van Limbeek E, Vehvilainen-Julkunen K, Nilsson C. Clinicians' views of factors of importance for improving the rate of VBAC (vaginal birth after caesarean section): a qualitative study from countries with high VBAC rates. BMC Pregnancy Childbirth. 2015;15(196):1–12.
49. Nilsson C, van Limbeek E, Vehvilainen-Julkunen K, Lundgren I. Vaginal birth after cesarean: views of women from countries with high VBAC rates. Qual Health Res. 2017;27(3):325–40.
50. Barger MK, Dunn JT, Bearman S, DeLain M, Gates E. A survey of access to trial of labor in California hospitals in 2012. BMC Pregnancy Childbirth. 2013;13:83.
51. Horey D, Kealy M, Davey MA, Small R, Crowther CA. Interventions for supporting pregnant women's decision-making about mode of birth after a caesarean. Cochrane Database Syst Rev. 2013;7:CD010041.

13

Do provider birth attitudes influence cesarean delivery rate

Emily White VanGompel[1,2*], Elliott K. Main[3], Daniel Tancredi[4] and Joy Melnikow[5]

Abstract

Background: When used judiciously, cesarean sections can save lives; but in the United States, prior research indicates that cesarean birth rates have risen beyond the threshold to help women and infants and become a contributor to increased maternal mortality and rising healthcare costs. Healthy People 2020 has set the goal for nulliparous, term, singleton, vertex (NTSV) cesarean birth rate at no more than 23.9% of births. Currently, cesarean rates vary from 6% to 69% in US hospitals, unexplained by clinical or demographic factors. This wide variation in cesarean use is also seen among individual providers of intrapartum care. Previous research of birth attitudes found providers of intrapartum care hold widely differing views, which may be a key underlying factor influencing practice variation; however, further study is needed to determine if differences in attitudes are associated with differences in clinical outcomes. The purpose of this study was to estimate the association between individual provider attitudes towards birth and their low-risk primary cesarean rate.

Methods: Four hundred providers were drawn from a stratified random sample of all California providers of intrapartum care in 2013 and surveyed for their attitudes towards various aspects of labor and birth. Providers' NTSV cesarean birth rates were obtained for 2013 and 2014. Covariates included gender, years of experience, practice location, and primary hospital's NTSV cesarean rate. We used adjusted multivariate Poisson regression to compare cesarean rates and linear regression to compare attitude scores of providers meeting versus not meeting the Healthy People 2020 (HP2020) goal.

Results: Two hundred nine total participants (obstetricians, family physicians, and midwives) completed surveys, of which 109 perform cesareans. Providers' NTSV cesarean rate was significantly associated with their composite attitudes score [IRR for each one-point increase 1.21 (95% CI 1.002–1.45)]. Physicians meeting the HP2020 goal held attitudes which were significantly more favorable towards vaginal birth: mean 2.70 (95% CI 2.58–2.83) versus 2.91 (95% CI 2.82–3.00), $p < 0.01$.

Conclusions: Provider attitudinal differences are associated with NTSV cesarean rates. Those meeting the HP2020 goal hold attitudes more favorable towards vaginal birth. These findings may present a modifiable target for quality improvement initiatives to decrease low risk primary cesareans.

Keywords: Cesarean section, Provider attitudes, Quality improvement, Primary cesarean, Culture

* Correspondence: EWhiteVanGompel@northshore.org
[1]Department of Family Medicine, The University of Chicago, Pritzker School of Medicine, NorthShore University HealthSystem Research Institute, 1001 University Place, Evanston, IL 60201, USA
[2]Department of Obstetrics and Gynecology, The University of Chicago, Pritzker School of Medicine, NorthShore University HealthSystem Research Institute, 1001 University Place, Evanston, IL 60201, USA
Full list of author information is available at the end of the article

Background

Cesarean sections, when used judiciously, save lives; however, research indicates that the use of cesareans in the United States has risen well above the level of necessity and has become a contributor to maternal morbidity and mortality [1–5]. Women who are nulliparous, at full term, with a singleton pregnancy in vertex presentation (NTSV) have been established as a standard population and used as a target group for reducing the cesarean birth rate [6–8]. Healthy People 2020 has set the goal for NTSV cesarean rate at no more than 23.9% of births [6]. Currently, cesarean rates vary from 6% to 69% in US hospitals [9]. Substantial variation persists after adjustment for hospital demographics, referral categories, or teaching status, and after adjustment for patient clinical or sociodemographic factors [9, 10].

Wide variation is also seen between providers, even those practicing within the same hospital and utilizing a laborist model [11]. Over 90% of the variation in the NTSV cesarean rate is due to two indications: "fetal intolerance of labor" and "failure to progress"; indications requiring subjective decision-making by the intrapartum provider [12]. The American Congress of Obstetricians and Gynecologists' Committee Opinion on limiting intervention during labor highlights the labor management techniques that, despite prevailing evidence, vary significantly among providers [13]. Evidence is filtered through the lens of a provider's experiences and attitudes [14]; yet how these attitudes affect clinical outcomes has not been evaluated.

Previous research found differences in birth attitudes between providers of different disciplines (obstetrics, family medicine, midwifery) [15, 16]; yet did not examine clinical outcomes. The objective of this study was to examine the association of individual provider NTSV cesarean rates with their attitudes towards birth. In contrast to earlier studies examining physician demographic factors [17–19], this study sought to evaluate a potentially *modifiable* personal attribute that may contribute to cesarean overuse.

Aim

Our primary aim was to assess the association between providers' birth attitudes and their NTSV cesarean rates.

Methods

Design

A stratified random sample of providers listed as delivering clinicians on California birth certificates in 2013 were surveyed with a previously validated survey instrument of provider birth attitudes [16]. We linked providers' scores on this survey with their individual NTSV cesarean rates for the years of 2013 and 2014, as calculated by the California Maternal Data Center (CMDC), a service of the California Maternal Quality Care Collaborative. Baseline demographics and survey scores were analyzed using SAS Version 9.4. Poisson regressions were performed using Stata 12.1. This study was approved under expedited review by University of California Davis Internal Review Board. Participants received the consent document, but signed consent was waived by the IRB.

Setting

California has approximately 3500 providers that are listed as delivering clinicians in a given year; these include obstetricians (OB), Maternal-Fetal Medicine specialists, family medicine physicians, Certified Nurse Midwives (CNM), and California Licensed Midwives (LM). Practice settings are diverse, and include rural, urban, and frontier geographic locations, teaching hospitals, community hospitals, and tertiary care centers. Provider mix at each hospital may include only obstetricians or family physicians, or may include Maternal-Fetal Medicine specialists or midwives. The CMDC combines existing datasets, including monthly discharge and clinical data, birth certificate data, and semi-annual patient discharge data from the California Office of Statewide Health Planning and Development, to create hospital and physician-level quality improvement metrics. We obtained a stratified random sample from 2013 - the latest available year of complete data. At the time of final data collection, 2014 complete data became available, thus we included provider and hospital metrics from both 2013 and 2014 combined. Our primary sample size consideration was based on the six domain scores' ability to account for variation in NTSV cesarean delivery rate. Using pilot data, we determined that a sample size of 116 patients would provide 80% power to detect an 11.1% partial R-square. To account for intermittent missing variables, we targeted a sample of 130 survey participants.

Inclusion criteria for providers were: having been listed on a birth certificate as the delivering clinician in the year 2013, belonging to one of the key study disciplines (maternal-fetal medicine, OB, family medicine, CNM, LM), and having performed at least 10 deliveries per year. Providers with a license address outside the state of California and those without an identifiable discipline based either on license number prefix or NPI taxonomy code were excluded from sampling.

Based on prior research pointing to important influences on provider practice [17–19], stratification was performed based on three variables: provider discipline (maternal-fetal medicine, OB, family medicine, CNM, LM), geographic location as defined by the federally designated Medical Service Study Areas (rural = population density < 250 persons/square mile; frontier = population density < 11 persons/square mile; urban = anything not rural or frontier) [20], and years in practice (< 5 years,

5–15 years, 16–25 years, > 25 years). The stratified random sample was drawn in two rounds of 200, for a total of 400 sampled providers. To ensure adequate power for analysis, oversampling was performed on provider groups other than obstetricians (who perform the vast majority of all births in California). Researchers were blinded to individual providers' cesarean rates during sample selection.

Attitudes survey

The birth attitudes survey, previously validated by Klein and colleagues, included 9 different domains assessing provider attitudes towards different aspects of labor and birth [16]. Six of these domains, comprising 31 Likert-style items, were chosen as those most likely to have an effect on the targeted outcome – low-risk primary cesareans. They included (renumbered for this study): Domain 1: attitudes regarding use of electronic fetal monitoring (Cronbach alpha [α] = 0.704), Domain 2: factors that increase cesarean rates ($\alpha = 0.810$), Domain 3: fears of birth mode by respondents or their partners/spouses ($\alpha = 0.929$), Domain 4: factors that decrease cesarean rates ($\alpha = 0.819$), Domain 5: maternal choice and mothers' roles in birth ($\alpha = 0.646$), and Domain 6: safety by mode or place of birth ($\alpha = 0.748$). The composite scale combined the individual domain scores. Coding of domains 4 and 5 was reversed for directional consistency to create a total mean score. Lower scores on the composite scale indicate attitudes more favorable toward vaginal birth, while higher scores indicate attitudes that favor cesarean birth. Providers were also asked to give their discipline and years of experience. Each provider was assigned a random identifier, so that survey responses were not associated with provider name.

We used best practices for achieving maximal survey response as detailed by Dillman et al. [21] Survey data collection began in October 2015 and ended in April 2016. We sent the attitudes survey via postal mail and included a web address for optional completion online. The initial mailing included the 4-page survey, a cover letter, informed consent document, a self-addressed stamped envelope, and an incentive of a $10 Starbucks gift card. Providers could opt to provide their email addresses to be entered into a drawing at the conclusion of the study for an iPad of approximately $400 value at the conclusion of the study. One to two weeks after the initial mailing, we sent a postcard reminder to complete the survey. Between one and 2 months after the initial mailing, all non-responders were sent a second complete packet including cover letter, consent, survey document, and self-addressed stamped envelope.

Provider-level cesarean rate

The CMDC database uses the standard NQF-endorsed algorithm [4] to calculate the total number of births attended by a provider that qualify as primary low-risk cesareans. This criteria includes all nulliparous, term (> 37 weeks gestation), singleton gestations in vertex presentation at delivery. These are termed NTSV births for nulliparous, term, singleton, and vertex, and remain the primary target for quality improvement initiatives to decrease cesarean section overuse in the United States [6–8]. We obtained both the total number of NTSV births providers attended in 2013–2014, and the total number of those births that were delivered via cesarean from the CMDC database.

Not all providers included in the survey sample had privileges to perform cesareans. In order to provide a complete picture of the spectrum of attitudes held by all providers practicing as independent clinicians in California, we chose to include all those listed as delivering clinicians on at least 10 deliveries per study year. As it would not be appropriate to assess provider-level cesarean rates in providers who cannot perform cesareans, we excluded these providers from the NTSV predictive model. Both CNMs and LMs do not perform cesareans under any circumstances. A majority of family medicine physicians who do prenatal and intrapartum care do not perform cesareans; however, there are family medicine physicians who have done additional training to qualify to perform cesareans. There is no central database that tracks these privileges, thus this was ascertained by anonymously calling individual family medicine physicians' offices.

Covariates

Provider demographic data, including discipline (maternal-fetal medicine, Average Risk OB, family medicine, CNM, LM), gender, years since graduation from medical school (< 5 years, 5–15 years, 16–25 years, > 25 years), practice geographic location (rural/urban), and hospital-level demographics including hospital-level NTSV rate, neonatal intensive care unit level, and percent Medicaid were obtained from the CMDC database. Some providers practiced at multiple hospitals; however, the hospital where they had their greatest number of NTSV births was assigned as their primary hospital of delivery.

Statistical methods

Due to the large range of providers' total NTSV birth volume, we used multivariate Poisson regression to maximize precision of our estimation model, using counts of NTSV cesarean deliveries per provider as the dependent variable and total deliveries per provider as an "exposure" variable whose log-transformed value is included as an offset term, to account for between-provider variation. We used robust standard error estimators to protect against model misspecification. Simple regression with predicted margins was used to compare attitudinal scores between discipline groups. Attitude domain and composite means were calculated from all non-missing items. For the dichotomous

Healthy People 2020 provider comparison, we compared providers' attitudes based on whether or not their NTSV cesarean rates met the Healthy People 2020 (HP2020) goal of less than 23.9% [6]. We used multiple linear regression, adjusting for provider gender, practice geography, and experience level to compare predicted means for each group. In order to adjust for the provider's hospital cultural environment, we adjusted each regression model for the primary hospital's NTSV rate *exclusive* of provider's contribution to this rate.

Results

We received 209 completed surveys, a total response rate of 52.3%, including 22 maternal-fetal medicine, 101 OB, 53 family medicine, 16 CNM, and 17 LM responding. There was a higher response rate for midwives, 97% of who were female, but no difference in disciplinary distribution or gender of physician respondents versus non-respondents. Experience level, practice geographic location, and primary hospital nursery level did not vary between respondents versus non-respondents. Respondents' primary hospitals had higher annual birth volumes than non-respondents' hospitals (mean = 5,203.9 versus 2,666.8, $p < 0.001$). Hospital NTSV rates were slightly lower for respondents compared with non-respondents (25.3% versus 26.8%, $p < 0.01$). (Table 1).

Attitudes varied significantly according to provider discipline (Fig. 1). Each domain displayed a spectrum of provider attitudes towards birth, with midwives on one end of the spectrum and OBs on the other (Fig. 2). Family medicine physicians either fell between the two or held attitudes more similar to midwives. Maternal-fetal medicine physicians held attitudes most consistent with average risk OBs, but tended to express attitudes that fell between average risk OBs and family medicine physicians. The OB group had widest variation in composite attitude scores (range = 1.37 to 4.33).

Of the 53 responding family medicine physicians, only 8 had privileges to perform cesareans, though 22 had "first assist" privileges. Family medicine physicians with cesarean privileges (family medicine-CS) were identical to family medicine physicians without privileges on the

Table 1 Demographic and Practice Characteristics of Responders and Non-responders

	Responders (n)	Percent	Non-Responders (n)	Percent	*p*-value
N	209		191		
Discipline					*0.35*[a]
MFM	22	10.5	19	9.9	
OB	101	48.3	120	62.8	
Family Medicine	53	25.4	46	24.1	
CNM	16	7.7	3	2.1	
LM	17	8.1	3	1.6	
Gender					*0.29*[a]
Female	132	63.2	102	53.4	
Male	77	36.8	89	46.6	
Experience					*0.49*
< 5 years	35	18.3	28	13.9	
5–15 years	58	30.4	70	34.7	
16–25 years	46	24.1	43	21.3	
> 25 years	52	27.2	61	30.2	
Hospital NICU Level					*0.64*
Basic Nursery	50	23.9	57	29.8	
Community Nursery	82	39.2	73	38.2	
Intermediate Nursery	36	17.2	33	17.3	
Regional Nursery	20	9.6	25	13.1	
Continuous Variables	Mean	SD	Mean	SD	p-value
Hospital Birth Volume[b]	5203.9	3835.9	2666.8	2012.8	< 0.0001
Hospital NTSV CS Rate[b]	25.30	4.80	26.80	6.10	< 0.01

Abbreviations: *MFM* maternal fetal medicine, *OB* obstetricians, *Family Medicine* family medicine physicians, *CNM* certified nurse midwives, *LM* licensed midwives, *NICU* neonatal intensive care unit, *NTSV CS* nulliparous, term, singleton, vertex cesarean section

[a]P-value includes physicians only. Midwives were all female except for one participant and had exceptionally high response rate

[b]Calculated for provider's primary delivering hospital site

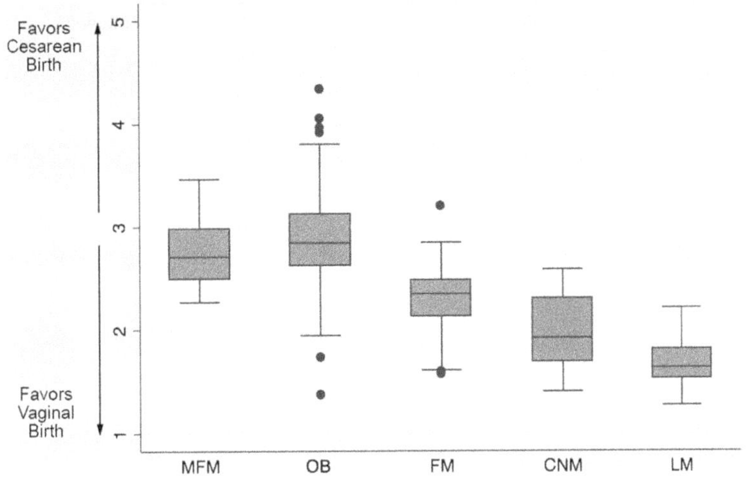

Fig. 1 Mean Provider Attitudes Scores on the Composite Scale by Provider Discipline. Figure 1 is a boxplot of providers' mean attitude scores on the composite attitudes scale categorized by provider membership in a training discipline. Abbreviations: MFM: maternal fetal medicine; OB: obstetricians; family medicine: family medicine physicians; CNM: certified nurse midwives; LM: licensed midwives

composite scale (mean 2.31 with SD 0.16, and 2.31 with SD 0.35, respectively, $p = 0.98$). For the most part, family medicine-CS physicians expressed attitudes on the individual domains that were slightly less favorable towards vaginal delivery than family medicine physicians; however, family medicine-CS tended to endorse *less* fear of vaginal delivery than their family medicine counterparts, though this was not statistically significant (mean 1.19 ± 0.30 versus 1.40 ± 0.74, respectively, $p = 0.43$). The database attributed cesarean deliveries to 14 family medicine physicians without any cesarean privileges and 10 family medicine physicians with first assist privileges.

The analyses of association of provider attitudes with NTSV cesarean rates included only providers with cesarean privileges and at least 20 NTSV deliveries within the 2 year study period: 11 maternal-fetal medicine, 91 OB, and 7 family medicine physicians. The composite attitudes scale scores for these providers ranged from 1.73 to 4.33 (mean 2. 83, standard deviation 0.48). Adjusted incidence rate ratios for domain and composite scale from the Poisson multiple regression are shown in Table 2; this model adjusted for provider gender, practice geography, experience level, and primary hospital's NTSV rate (exclusive of provider's contribution to this rate). The composite attitudes scale had an incident rate ratio of 1.21 (95% CI 1.002–1.45, $p = 0.048$), indicating that, for every 1 point increase in a provider's score on the composite scale, their NTSV cesarean rate *decreased* relatively by 21%. For individual domains, attitudes towards the perceived benefits of cesarean and fear of vaginal birth approached significance [respectively, 1.07 (95% CI 0.99–1.17) and 1.08 (95% CI 0.99–1.17)]. (Table 2).

When dichotomizing providers by the Healthy People 2020 NTSV cesarean goal cut-off of 23.9%, our sample reflected the overall California distribution, with 35% of providers meeting this goal and 65% of providers whose rate exceeded the goal. Providers meeting the HP2020 goal held attitudes more favorable toward vaginal birth compared with those over the HP2020 goal [adjusted mean 2.70 (95% CI 2.58–2.83) versus 2.91 (95% CI 2.82–3.00), $p < 0.01$].

Discussion

We found a significant association between providers' attitudes and beliefs about birth to their own NTSV cesarean rate. This study was consistent with the findings of the original Canadian survey validation study [16], finding that California providers' attitudes towards birth were primarily divided along disciplinary lines. One of the most surprising findings in the disciplinary analysis was the wide range of obstetricians' attitudes, spanning views more pro-cesarean than maternal-fetal medicine providers all the way to those consistent with midwives. This large variation within a single discipline suggests that there may be key acculturation differences in obstetric training and practice environment, where a provider's attitudes and beliefs are influenced.

We took prior work an important step further by connecting provider attitudes to their own measured clinical outcomes. For providers with cesarean privileges, those meeting the Healthy People 2020 goal held attitudes that were more favorable toward vaginal birth than those not meeting this goal. In our regression analysis, as attitudes became more favorable toward cesarean and less favorable toward vaginal birth, a provider's NTSV cesarean rate increased proportionately. Additionally, we used a novel adjustor to account for local hospital culture – the primary hospital's NTSV cesarean rate less the provider's contribution to that rate. This adjustment highlights the

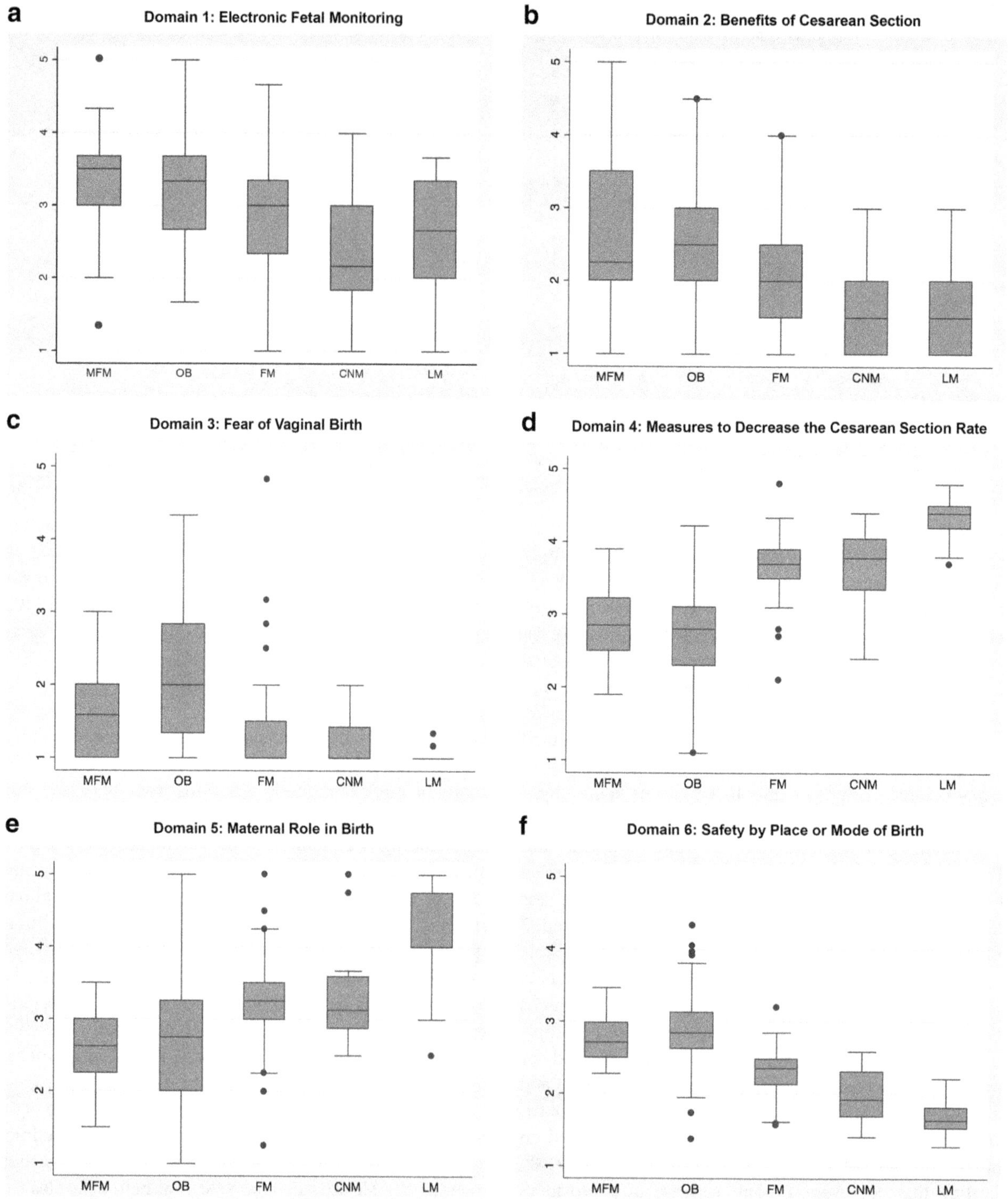

Fig. 2 a-f Boxplots of Provider Attitudes Scores on the Individual Domain Scales by Provider Discipline. Figure 2 **a-f** includes individual boxplots of providers' mean attitude scores for each individual attitudinal domain categorized by provider membership in a training discipline. Abbreviations: MFM: maternal fetal medicine; OB: obstetricians; family medicine: family medicine physicians; CNM: certified nurse midwives; LM: licensed midwives

Table 2 Adjusted[a] Associations between Attitude Scores and Provider NTSV CS Rate[b]

Domain	Incidence Rate Ratio[c]	95% CI	*p*-value
Fetal Monitoring	1.01	0.94–1.10	0.71
Benefits of CS	1.07	0.99–1.17	0.10
Fear of Vaginal Birth	1.08	0.99–1.17	0.09
Measures to Decrease CS[d]	0.91	0.77–1.08	0.28
Maternal Role in Birth[d]	0.93	0.85–1.02	0.14
Safety by Place or Mode of Birth	1.12	0.97–1.30	0.14
Composite Scale	1.21	1.002–1.45	0.048

Abbreviations: *NTSV CS* nulliparous, term, singleton, vertex cesarean section, *CS* cesarean section, *CI* confidence interval
[a]Results are from individual Poisson regression models of the NTSV cesarean outcome, with one model for each row, with that variable the focal predictor and with additional covariates used to adjust for gender, experience level, geographic location of practice, primary hospital's NTSV cesarean rate calculated without the individual provider's contribution
[b]Only includes providers with confirmed privileges to perform cesarean sections who had at least 20 NTSV births over the two-year study period of 2013–2014
[c]Higher scores indicate attitudes more favorable toward cesarean section except for the two reverse-coded scales (as below)
[d]Higher scores indicate attitudes more favorable toward vaginal birth on these scales

impact of individual provider attitudes on top of that of local hospital norms and practices. These findings suggest that a provider's underlying attitudes, values, and beliefs play an important role in intrapartum decisions that ultimately affect birth outcomes.

Our results are consistent with, and provide a possible underlying mechanism for, other studies that have found provider differences such as demographics, litigation history, and practice environment are associated with provider self-report personal thresholds to perform cesareans [22, 23]. By independently measuring attitudes while protecting the confidentiality of providers and using administrative data to associate attitudes with an unbiased measure of the individual provider-level cesarean rate, our study minimized social desirability bias, which can confound self-report data.

Of note, the actual magnitude of the point estimate of the association between composite attitudinal score and NTSV cesarean rate is quite large. For every 1 point increase in agreement with attitudes favoring cesarean, NTSV cesarean rates increased by a relative 21%. For a provider with a baseline rate of 25%, this would translate into an absolute change of 5.25%. In comparison, the QUARISMA trial found changes to the absolute cesarean rate of 0.7–2.3% resulting from an audit and feedback mechanism in conjunction with hospital-based best practices implementation [24]. Targeting attitudinal change, which is a "bottom-up" method, in conjunction with quality improvement, or "top-down", efforts may enhance the impact of interventions. Research is needed to identify effective interventions to enhance evidence-based attitudes towards vaginal birth.

Training may offer a promising target for influencing attitudes that favor vaginal birth. One study found that providers who trained in hospitals with lower obstetric complication rates continued to have lower complication rates once in practice [25]. Most recently, one hospital program significantly decreased their primary cesarean rate by providing senior obstetric supervision of residents on labor and delivery, highlighting the impact of preceptor experience level on trainees [26]. The impact of integrating midwives into traditional obstetric training has been posited but not yet rigorously tested against clinical outcomes [27]. Finally, ongoing training and support after experiencing a traumatic delivery event may mitigate some of the fear attitudes associated with increased cesarean rate, which appear to impact entire hospital units and not just the providers involved. This was described recently in a study of unplanned hospital cesarean rates, which increased and stayed elevated for 4 weeks after any catastrophic neonatal outcome within that hospital [28].

Limitations

This cross-sectional study cannot draw conclusions regarding causality or time course between independent and dependent variables. Additionally, our a priori sample size justification assumed a linear regression analysis, but we found that a Poisson regression analysis was better suited to the outcome distribution. Thus, in order to assess the adequacy of the realized sample size for the reported effect sizes, one should consider the range of values included within the 95% CI [29]. Where the null value was included along with values that would be clinically meaningful, one could conclude that the effect is ambiguous and would require a more precise estimate in future work. For example, we would assert that a 15% relative increase in the NTSV cesarean rate would be particularly clinically meaningful. When examining the 95% CI for the effect size of the individual attitude items, we find that all of them included the null value (i.e. were not statistically significant) but three of them extended beyond an IRR of 1.15, suggesting that the results for those items are ambiguous and could warrant a study with a larger sample size. For the composite attitude measure, we found statistically significant and clinically significant effects.

Finally, the administrative data used to assess provider-level cesarean rate was restricted to the provider listed on the birth certificate and subject to errors of attribution. For example, the provider listed as "Delivering Clinician" on the Birth Certificate is usually but not always the person that managed the majority of a patient's labor or made the decision to go to cesarean. Unfortunately, this method discounts information about providers who do not carry cesarean privileges but may play a major role in intrapartum care, and may be key decision-makers along the route that ends in either cesarean or vaginal delivery. For example, a provider may decide to admit a patient prior to the onset of active labor or use continuous electronic fetal monitoring despite a patient's low-risk status, both of which increase the likelihood of that patient requiring a cesarean, yet the cesarean birth would be attributed to the clinician who performed the surgery itself and not the provider managing the labor. Further studies are needed to assess the interplay of personnel on labor and delivery wards, how key decisions are made and birth outcomes attributed.

Conclusions

This is the first study we are aware of linking provider attitudinal differences to differences in measured birth outcomes. We found that the more providers' birth attitudes favored cesarean, the higher their NTSV cesarean rate. In contrast to earlier studies that have focused on physician demographics or litigation history, which are rarely modifiable without major policy changes, we sought to evaluate the influence of a modifiable attribute – a provider's personal attitudes and beliefs. These findings suggest further scrutiny is needed of how future providers are acculturated during training and while in practice, and how practice groups, hospital units, and inter-professional interactions may modify these attitudes to ultimately improve quality of care and health outcomes.

Abbreviations

CMDC: California Maternal Data Center; CNM: Certified nurse midwives; family Medicine: Family medicine; family medicine-CS: Family medicine physicians with privileges to perform cesarean; HP2020: Healthy People 2020; LM: California licensed midwives; MFM: Maternal-fetal medicine; NICU: Neonatal intensive care unit; NTSV: Nulliparous, term, singleton, vertex; OB: Obstetrician

Acknowledgements

Jairo Chavez, supported by the Ambulatory Primary Care Innovations Group of the NorthShore University HealthSystem Research Institute assisted in the preparation of this manuscript. Suzanne Eidson-Ton, MD, supported by the University of California Davis Department of Family and Community Medicine, contributed content expertise and assisted with pilot work for this study.

Funding

This work was supported by grant number T32HS022236 from the Agency for Healthcare Research and Quality and grant number S-D936808-MCPAB from the University of California Davis Department of Family and Community Medicine Jump Start Fund. Neither funding body had any role in the design, collection, analysis, interpretation of data, or in writing the manuscript.

Authors' contributions

EWV and JM designed the study with statistical consultation from DT and content area expertise from EM. EM created the provider data file for sampling and supplied outcomes data for participants. EWV and DT analyzed and interpreted the attitudinal and outcomes data. EWV wrote the majority of the manuscript with major contributions from all authors. All authors read and approved the final manuscript.

Competing interests

The authors declare that they have no competing interests.

Author details

[1]Department of Family Medicine, The University of Chicago, Pritzker School of Medicine, NorthShore University HealthSystem Research Institute, 1001 University Place, Evanston, IL 60201, USA. [2]Department of Obstetrics and Gynecology, The University of Chicago, Pritzker School of Medicine, NorthShore University HealthSystem Research Institute, 1001 University Place, Evanston, IL 60201, USA. [3]California Maternal Quality Care Collaborative, Stanford University, Stanford Medical School Office Building, 1265 Welch Road, MS 5415, Stanford, CA 94305, USA. [4]Center for Healthcare Policy and Research and Department of Pediatrics, University of California Davis School of Medicine, 2103 Stockton Blvd, Sacramento, CA 95817, USA. [5]Center for Healthcare Policy and Research and Department of Family and Community Medicine, University of California Davis School of Medicine, 2103 Stockton Blvd, Sacramento, CA 95817, USA.

References

1. Caughey AB, Cahill AG, Guise JM, Rouse DJ. Safe prevention of the primary cesarean delivery. Am J Obstet Gynecol. 2014;210:179–93.
2. Childbirth Connection. Vaginal or cesarean Birth. What is at stake for women and babies. New York: Childbirth Connection; 2012. p. 52.
3. Berg CJ, Atrash HK, Koonin LM, Tucker M. Pregnancy-related mortality in the United States, 1987-1990. Obstet Gynecol. 1996;88:161–7.
4. Berg CJ, Callaghan WM, Syverson C, Henderson Z. Pregnancy-related mortality in the United States, 1998 to 2005. Obstet Gynecol. 2010;116: 1302–9.
5. Berg CJ, Chang J, Callaghan WM, Whitehead SJ. Pregnancy-related mortality in the United States, 1991-1997. Obstet Gynecol. 2003;101:289–96.
6. Office of Disease Prevention and Health Promotion. Healthy people 2020: maternal, infant, and child health. Washington (DC), 2016. Retrieved from https://www.healthypeople.gov/2020/topics-objectives/topic/maternal-infant-and-child-health/objectives. Accessed 22 Nov 2016.
7. National Quality Forum (NQF). National Voluntary Consensus Standards for perinatal care 2008: a consensus report. Washington, DC: NQF; 2009. Retrieved from https://www.qualityforum.org/Publications/2009/05/National_Voluntary_Consensus_Standards_for_Perinatal_Care_2008.aspx. Accessed 22 Nov 2016.
8. Main EK, Moore D, Farrell B, Schimmel LD, Altman RJ, Abrahams C, et al. Is there a useful cesarean birth measure? Assessment of the nulliparous term singleton vertex cesarean birth rate as a tool for obstetric quality improvement, Am J Obstet Gynecol. 2006;194:1644-51. discussion 51-2
9. Kozhimannil KB, Law MR, Virnig BA. Cesarean delivery rates vary tenfold among US hospitals; reducing variation may address quality and cost issues. Health Aff (Millwood). 2013;32:527–35.
10. Caceres IA, Arcaya M, Declercq E, Belanoff CM, Janakiraman V, Cohen B, et al. Hospital differences in cesarean deliveries in Massachusetts (US) 2004-2006: the case against case-mix artifact. PLoS One. 2013;8:e57817.
11. Metz TD, Allshouse AA, Gilbert SA, Doyle R, Tong A, Carey JC. Variation in primary cesarean delivery rates by individual physician within a single-hospital laborist model. Am J Obstet Gynecol. 2016;214:531 e1-6.
12. Main EK, Morton CH, Melsop K, Hopkins D, Giuliani G, Gould JB. Creating a

public agenda for maternity safety and quality in cesarean delivery. Obstet Gynecol. 2012;120:1194–8.
13. Committee Opinion No. 687: approaches to limit intervention during labor and birth. Obstet Gynecol. 2017;129:e20–e8.
14. Olatunbosun OA, Edouard L, Pierson RA. Physicians' attitudes toward evidence based obstetric practice: a questionnaire survey. BMJ. 1998;316:365–6.
15. Reime B, Klein MC, Kelly A, Duxbury N, Saxell L, Liston R, et al. Do maternity care provider groups have different attitudes towards birth? BJOG. 2004;111:1388–93.
16. Klein MC, Kaczorowski J, Hall WA, Fraser W, Liston RM, Eftekhary S, et al. The attitudes of Canadian maternity care practitioners towards labour and birth: many differences but important similarities. J Obstet Gynaecol Can. 2009;31:827–40.
17. Burns LR, Geller SE, Wholey DR. The effect of physician factors on the cesarean section decision. Med Care. 1995;33:365–82.
18. Mitler LK, Rizzo JA, Horwitz SM. Physician gender and cesarean sections. J Clin Epidemiol. 2000;53:1030–5.
19. Tussing AD, Wojtowycz MA. The effect of physician characteristics on clinical behavior: cesarean section in New York state. Soc Sci Med. 1993;37:1251–60.
20. State of California, Office of Statewide Health Planning and Development, Healthcare Workforce Development Division. Medical service study areas. Sacramento: Office of Statewide Health Planning and Development; 2013. Retrieved from https://www.oshpd.ca.gov/HWDD/CalPCO.html#Maps-GIS. Accessed 21 Mar 2017.
21. Dillman DA, Smyth JD, Christian LM, Dillman DA. Internet, mail, and mixed-mode surveys : the tailored design method. 3rd ed. Hoboken: Wiley & Sons; 2009.
22. Cheng YW, Snowden JM, Handler S, Tager IB, Hubbard A, Caughey AB. Clinicians' practice environment is associated with a higher likelihood of recommending cesarean deliveries. J Matern Fetal Neonatal Med. 2014;27:1220–7.
23. Cheng YW, Snowden JM, Handler SJ, Tager IB, Hubbard AE, Caughey AB. Litigation in obstetrics: does defensive medicine contribute to increases in cesarean delivery? J Matern Fetal Neonatal Med. 2014;27:1668–75.
24. Chaillet N, Dumont A, Abrahamowicz M, Pasquier JC, Audibert F, Monnier P, et al. A cluster-randomized trial to reduce cesarean delivery rates in Quebec. N Engl J Med. 2015;372:1710–21.
25. Asch DA, Nicholson S, Srinivas S, Herrin J, Epstein AJ. Evaluating obstetrical residency programs using patient outcomes. JAMA. 2009;302:1277–83.
26. Bardos J, Loudon H, Rekawek P, Friedman F, Brodman M, Fox NS. Association between senior obstetrician supervision of resident deliveries and mode of delivery. Obstet Gynecol. 2017;129:486–90.
27. King TL, Laros RK, Parer JT. Interprofessional collaborative practice in obstetrics and midwifery. Obstet Gynecol Clin N Am. 2012;39:411–22.
28. Dan O, Hochner-Celnikier D, Solnica A, Loewenstein Y. Association of Catastrophic Neonatal Outcomes with Increased Rate of subsequent cesarean deliveries. Obstet Gynecol. 2017;129:671–5.
29. Colegrave N, Ruxton G. Confidence intervals are a more useful complement to nonsignificant tests than are power calculations. Behav Ecol. 2003;14:446–7.

14

Birth by caesarean section and school performance in Swedish adolescents

Eileen A. Curran[1], Louise C. Kenny[1], Christina Dalman[2], Patricia M. Kearney[3], John F. Cryan[4], Timothy G. Dinan[5] and Ali S Khashan[1,3*]

Abstract

Background: Our objective was to assess the impact of obstetric mode of delivery, and in particular birth by Caesarean section (CS), on school performance in adolescents using a large, population-based cohort.

Methods: We extracted data from the Swedish Medical Birth Register and National School Register. We included all live singleton births in Sweden from 1982–1995 (n = 1,489,925). School grades were reported on a scale from 0 to 320, scores less than 160 (i.e. "pass") were considered to be "poor school performance." Mode of delivery was categorised as: unassisted vaginal delivery (VD), assisted VD, elective CS and emergency CS. We measured the association between mode of delivery and "poor school performance" using logistic regression. We then used quantile regression to assess the association between mode of delivery and school performance across the distribution of scores. We adjusted for maternal age, parity, small and large for gestational age, gestational age, maternal country of birth, maternal depression, non-affective disorder or bipolar disorder, parental income at time of birth, and parental social welfare at time of birth. We also conducted sensitivity analyses to investigate the association further.

Results: With logistic regression analysis, the adjusted odds ratio (aOR) of assisted VD and poor school performance, compared to unassisted VD, was 1.06 (95% CI: 1.03–1.08). For elective CS it was 1.06 (95% CI:1.03-1.09) and for emergency CS it was 1.12 (95% CI: 1.09–1.15). With quantile regression, assisted VD showed little difference in scores, when compared to unassisted VD, at any point across the distribution. Elective CS was associated with a 1–3 point decrease in scores, and emergency CS was associated with a 2–5 point decrease in scores.

Conclusion: A slight association was found between birth by CS and school performance. However, the effect was quite small and given the complex nature of the relationship, should be interpreted with caution.

Keywords: Caesarean section: School performance, Cohort study, Quantile regression

Background

Rates of Caesarean section (CS) are rising globally. A recent study including data from thirty one European countries, reported the median rate of CS in those countries to be 25%, [1] though this trend is by no means limited to Europe or other high-income countries. Another recent study reported that in 2010–2011, among the 21 countries included, the rate of CS in countries with a high Human Development Index (HDI) was 40.0%, in countries with moderate HDI it was 32.4% and in countries with low HDI it was 20.3% [2]. Given such a large and growing rate of CS, it is becoming of increasing interest to understand potential long-term effects of birth by CS, [3] as even a small increase in risk could potentially have a large impact globally.

It has been hypothesised that birth by CS leads to changes in psychological development, due to "early term" birth [4, 5] or alterations in microbiota or stress response [6]. In animal models, birth by CS and changes in microbiota have been associated with changes in

* Correspondence: a.khashan@ucc.ie
[1]Department of Obstetrics and Gynaecology, The Irish Centre for Fetal and Neonatal Translational Research (INFANT), University College Cork, Cork, Ireland
[3]Department of Epidemiology and Public Health, University College Cork, Cork, Ireland
Full list of author information is available at the end of the article

behaviour, stress response, and anxiety [7]. Notably, these theories apply more to pre-labour or "elective" CS. Previous evidence suggests the association between CS and neurodevelopmental disorders in human populations may be primarily driven by confounding [8]. However, it is also possible that birth by CS may lead to sub-clinical changes in behavioural development, for example increased anxiety, that are not included in official diagnoses. One way to potentially assess the overall impact on psychological well-being is through school performance. School performance has been associated with several psychological outcomes including behavioural problems, [9] attention problems, [10] substance abuse, [10] and insomnia [11]. In addition, school performance as a teenager has been linked to psychological well-being as an adult, including depression and self-harm [12, 13]. Therefore, if CS has an impact on behavioural development, it may lead to changes in overall school performance.

Elective CS has been associated with delays in personal social skills and gross motor function at age 9 months, [14] and early term birth has been associated with increased special education requirements [4]. However, to our knowledge, no one has examined the potential association between obstetric mode of delivery, more specifically birth by CS, and school performance. To that end, the objective of the current study was to investigate the possible impact of birth by CS on school performance in a large, population-based Swedish cohort.

Methods

Data

Study Population

We included data from 4 Swedish Registers: Medical Birth Register, National School Register, Multi-Generation Register, and National Patient Register. Each resident of Sweden is given a personal identification number (PIN) which is the same in each of these registers, and can be used to link data across registers. The Medical Birth Register was established in 1973 and includes data on over 98% of all births in Sweden [15]. For our cohort, we included all live singleton births in the Swedish Medical Birth Register that occurred between 1982 and 1995. As both mode of delivery and school performance are likely to be highly correlated in multiple births, these were excluded. Variables detailing the timing of onset of labour and CS are available from 1982, thus marking the beginning of our cohort births. Ethical approval was obtained from the regional ethical research committee of Stockholm at Karolinska Institutet. Informed consent was waived by the ethics committee.

Exposure-obstetric mode of delivery

Obstetric mode of delivery, extracted from the Medical Birth Register, consisted of "unassisted vaginal delivery VD," "assisted VD," "elective CS" and "emergency CS". Unassisted VD was defined as VD without the use of forceps or vacuum extraction, and assisted VD was VD with the use of forceps or vacuum extraction. Unassisted and assisted VD included both spontaneous and induced VD. Elective CS was defined as CS which started before onset of labour (as indicated on medical charts by water departure, bleeding or regular and sustained pain) and emergency CS was defined as CS which started after onset of labour.

Outcome-school performance

Data on school performance were extracted from the National School Register, which are available beginning in 1988. In Sweden, upon finishing the compulsory years of school (age 16), grades in 16 subjects are recorded. Starting in 1998, these grades were categorised into 4 levels for each subject: not pass (score of 0), pass (score of 10), pass with distinction (score of 15), and pass with great distinction (score of 20). This allowed for a maximum total score of 320 (i.e. a score of 20 in each of the 16 subjects). Prior to 1998 there was a different grading system, but as the oldest children in our cohort turned 16 in 1998 only the current method was included. Children that "drop out" of school before compulsory grading still technically graduate but are recorded as having received a total of 0 for their final grade, and are not able to continue on to high school. These children were included in our population and were recorded as having a total score of 0. Scores were assessed in both categorical and continuous (from 0 to 320 in jumps of 5) form [16, 17].

Co-variates

Based on previous literature and the use of a directed acyclic graph (DAG) [18] (Additional file 1: Figure S1), the following a priori co-variates were included in the analysis: maternal age at time of birth (<25 years, 25–34 years, 35–44 years, 45+ years), [16] birth order (first born), [16] small for gestational age (SGA), [16] large for gestational age (LGA) (defined as birth weight less or greater than 2 standard deviations from the mean for gestational age, respectively), gestational age (<37 weeks, 37, 38, 39, or 40 weeks, >40 weeks), [16] maternal country of birth (Swedish, other Nordic, other), [19] maternal depression, non-affective disorder, or bipolar disorder (never diagnosed, diagnosed before birth, diagnosed after birth), parental income at time of birth (in quintiles), and parental social welfare at time of birth (yes/no, note: available from 1983), [19] and parental highest education (pre-high school, high school, post-high school) [16, 19, 20].

Though not identified as confounders in the DAG, further co-variates that were identified based on previous literature were also assessed, including: year of birth,

[20] year of school completion, smoking at time of first antenatal visit (none, 1–9 cigarettes/day, 10+ cigarettes/day), [16, 20] infant gender, [16, 19] Apgar score at 5 min ("low" [0–3], "intermediate" [4–6], "high" [7–10]), [16, 21] paternal country of birth (Swedish, other Nordic, other), [19] paternal depression, non-affective disorder, and bipolar disorder (never diagnosed, diagnosed before birth, diagnosed after birth), parental co-habitation at time of birth [19, 20].

All co-variates were tested individually in the logistic regression analysis to assess the potential impact on the association between mode of delivery and school performance. As no variable changed the estimate by more than 10% (only maternal age changed the estimate by more than 5%), only the variables decided on a priori were included in final analysis. Notably, parental education was considered an a priori variable, but was only available from 1990, and thus though it was tested individually, and as it had no impact on the estimate, was not included in the model. Distribution of each variable by mode of delivery is outlined in Table 1.

Statistical analysis

Logistic regression

For the logistic regression, we considered "poor school performance" to be a total score of less than160, [16, 17, 22] meaning the individual did not have an average of at least 10 (i.e. "pass") for the 16 subjects. In Sweden, scores are assigned by teachers rather than a standardised test, and thus standards for a particular grade could vary school-to-school. To account for this, we used mixed effects modelling with a random intercept for school ID.

Quantile regression

The data on school performance have been previously reported to be highly skewed [16, 20]. We used quantile regression to analyse school performance in its continuous form. Quantile regression is similar to an ordinary least squares (OLS) model, except the model regresses on the quantile of interest (such as the median), instead of the mean. Quantile regression also does not require an assumption of normality or equal variance, and allows for assessment across the distribution (i.e. at every quantile). In this way we were able to determine if there was an effect of mode of delivery across the distribution of scores (for example, a possible effect only on the high or low scores), rather than an effect only on passing scores as seen with logistic regression. We plotted quantile regression coefficients for every fifth quantile from the 5th to the 95th using the kernel-based method for estimating standard errors [23]. We also looked at coefficient estimates for specifically the 5th, 25th, 50th, 75th, and 95th quantiles. In adjusted analysis we included the same co-variates as the fully adjusted logistic regression model.

Additional analyses

We conducted several sub-group analyses. In the logistic regression, we restricted to births from 1990 onwards (the year data on parental education became available), and assessed the association with and without adjustment for parental education. We assessed the association only among male babies. We also excluded children born through a secondary CS (children born by CS whose mothers' had previously given birth through CS), and children with a low Apgar score at 5 min. Though the vast majority of the population finishes compulsory years of school at age 16 (95%), there are some students who finish younger or older. To that end, we also restricted the population to those who were 16 at the time they finished compulsory school to determine what effect age may have had on school performance. To account for potential clustering of academic performance within families, we restricted the population to one-child families and first born children. We then repeated overall analysis with a random intercept for maternal ID instead of school ID. For both logistic and quantile regression we conducted sensitivity analyses by excluding children who received a "0" as a grade (i.e. children who did not complete the compulsory years of schooling).

Additionally, we conducted logistic regression to assess the association between birth by CS and school performance in five subject categories: [12] natural sciences (biology, chemistry and physics), social sciences (geography, religion, history and society knowledge), arts (art and handicraft), sports, and Swedish. An average below "pass" (10 points per subject) was considered poor performance in each category. Similar to overall school performance analysis, sub-group analyses were conducted where children who were recorded as a "0" in any subject were excluded from that category.

The logistic regression analysis was conducted in SAS v9.3 (Cary, N.C) using PROC GLIMMIX [24] and quantile regression analysis was conducted in R v3.2.2 using the QUANTREG package [23]. Missing data were addressed using the missing indicator method, with a category for each variable used to indicate "missing" status [25].

Results

Descriptive statistics

There were 1,489,925 live births in Sweden from 1982–1995. We excluded 34,199 (2.3%) multiple births, and 52,562 (3.5%) births missing mode of delivery, leaving a total of 1,403,164 births. Of these, 176,836 (12.6%) did not have grades recorded in the National School Register. Possible reasons for not being recorded in the National School Register include death, emigration, and attendance

Table 1 Distribution of descriptive variables by mode of delivery

	Unassisted VD	Assisted VD	Elective CS	Emergency CS
Total Population	1036424 (84.51)	78441 (6.40)	52107 (4.25)	59357 (4.84)
Poor grade	138202 (13.33)	8880 (11.32)	7064 (13.56)	8203 (13.82)
Gender (Male)	522988 (50.46)	45361 (57.83)	26165 (50.21)	32357 (54.51)
Maternal age				
<20	30367 (2.93)	2679 (3.42)	698 (1.34)	1551 (2.61)
21–29	633991 (61.17)	50482 (64.36)	24004 (46.07)	33689 (56.76)
31–39	356370 (34.38)	24176 (30.82)	2486 (47.71)	22406 (37.75)
40+	15696 (1.51)	1104 (1.41)	2545 (4.88)	1711 (2.88)
First born child	599463 (57.84)	69919 (89.14)	31350 (60.16)	44922 (75.68)
Smoking at time of first antenatal visit				
None	704557 (67.98)	52772 (67.28)	35328 (67.80)	39483 (66.52)
1–9 Cigarettes/day	148178 (14.30)	11924 (15.20)	7746 (14.87)	9586 (16.15)
10+ Cigarettes/day	91075 (8.79)	6401 (8.16)	4979 (9.56)	5864 (9.88)
Missing	92614 (8.94)	7344 (9.36)	4054 (7.78)	4424 (7.45)
SGA	20383 (1.97)	2178 (2.78)	2969 (5.70)	5017 (8.45)
LGA	31455 (3.03)	2279 (2.91)	2996 (5.75)	2605 (4.39)
Parental education				
Pre-Highschool	34151 (3.30)	209 (2.67)	1878 (3.60)	2342 (3.95)
Highschool	232551 (22.44)	17107 (21.81)	11862 (22.76)	15568 (26.23)
Post-Highschool	151078 (14.58)	12916 (16.47)	8555 (16.42)	10506 (17.70)
Missing	9145 (0.88)	680 (0.87)	344 (0.66)	703 (1.18)
Born Prior to 1990	609499 (58.81)	45647 (58.19)	29468 (56.55)	30238 (50.94)
Parental income				
First	201292 (19.42)	8839 (11.27)	8943 (17.16)	9095 (15.32)
Second	210046 (20.27)	9836 (12.54)	10020 (19.23)	9407 (15.85)
Third	209679 (20.23)	13499 (17.21)	10215 (19.60)	10713 (18.05)
Fourth	204240 (19.71)	19267 (24.56)	10316 (19.80)	13159 (22.17)
Fifth	191366 (18.46)	25526 (32.54)	11730 (22.51)	15816 (26.65)
Missing	1981 (1.91)	1474 (1.88)	883 (1.69)	1167 (1.97)
Parental social welfare status				
Yes	84609 (8.16)	5597 (7.14)	4173 (8.10)	5490 (9.25)
No	864190 (83.38)	65913 (83.03)	44174 (84.78)	50000 (84.24)
Missing	19132 (1.85)	1416 (1.81)	858 (1.65)	1133 (1.91)
Born Prior to 1983	68493 (6.61)	515 (7.03)	2902 (5.57)	2734 (4.61)
Apgar Score (5 min)				
Low (0–3)	1484 (0.14)	241 (0.31)	141 (0.27)	417 (0.70)
Intermediate (4–6)	3375 (0.33)	1501 (1.91)	479 (0.92)	1836 (3.09)
High (7–10)	1004980 (96.97)	75464 (96.20)	50105 (96.16)	55775 (93.97)
Missing	26585 (2.57)	1235 (1.57)	1382 (2.65)	1329 (2.24)
Gestational age				
<37 Weeks	39384 (3.80)	1971 (2.51)	5941 (11.40)	10820 (18.23)
37 Weeks	48430 (4.67)	2546 (3.25)	5923 (11.37)	4508 (7.59)
38 Weeks	122702 (11.84)	6707 (8.55)	25006 (47.99)	7487 (12.61)
39 Weeks	255027 (24.61)	15235 (19.42)	9990 (19.17)	8416 (14.18)
40 Weeks	311130 (30.02)	23094 (29.44)	2714 (5.21)	11056 (18.63)
>40 Weeks	257116 (24.81)	28678 (36.56)	2400 (4.61)	16892 (28.46)

Table 1 Distribution of descriptive variables by mode of delivery *(Continued)*

Missing	2635 (0.25)	210 (0.27)	133 (0.26)	178 (0.30)
Maternal Depression				
Never Diagnosed	952661 (91.92)	71714 (91.42)	46936 (90.08)	53615 (90.33)
Diagnosed before birth	6051 (0.58)	457 (0.58)	584 (1.12)	540 (0.91)
Diagnosed after birth	77712 (7.50)	6270 (7.99)	4587 (8.80)	5202 (8.76)
Maternal Non-affective Disorder				
Never Diagnosed	1026908 (99.08)	77638 (99.98)	51460 (98.76)	58644 (98.82)
Diagnosed before birth	2392 (0.23)	227 (0.29)	209 (0.40)	201 (0.34)
Diagnosed after birth	7124 (0.69)	576 (0.73)	438 (0.84)	501 (0.84)
Maternal Bipolar Disorder				
Never Diagnosed	1026027 (99.00)	77649 (98.99)	51507 (98.85)	58702 (98.90)
Diagnosed before birth	818 (0.08)	82 (0.10)	80 (0.15)	61 (0.10)
Diagnosed after birth	9579 (0.92)	710 (0.91)	520 (1.00)	594 (1.00)
Paternal Depression				
Never Diagnosed	983156 (94.86)	74367 (94.81)	49255 (94.53)	56114 (94.54)
Diagnosed before birth	4697 (0.45)	309 (0.39)	309 (0.59)	325 (0.55)
Diagnosed after birth	48571 (4.69)	3765 (4.80)	2543 (4.88)	2918 (4.92)
Paternal Non-affective Disorder				
Never Diagnosed	1028187 (99.21)	77816 (99.20)	51705 (99.23)	58823 (99.10)
Diagnosed before birth	2360 (0.23)	171 (0.22)	134 (0.26)	167 (0.28)
Diagnosed after birth	5877 (0.57)	454 (0.58)	268 (0.51)	367 (0.62)
Paternal Bipolar Disorder				
Never Diagnosed	1029320 (99.31)	77915 (99.33)	51703 (99.22)	58919 (99.26)
Diagnosed before birth	805 (0.08)	65 (0.08)	68 (0.13)	43 (0.07)
Diagnosed after birth	6299 (0.61)	461 (0.59)	336 (0.63)	395 (0.67)
Co-habitating with child's father				
Yes	894777 (86.33)	66362 (84.60)	45489 (87.30)	50855 (85.68)
No	47235 (4.56)	4655 (5.93)	2389 (4.58)	3464 (5.84)
Missing	94412 (9.11)	7424 (9.46)	4229 (8.12)	5038 (8.49)
Maternal Country of Birth				
Sweden	917862 (88.56)	69758 (88.93)	45638 (87.59)	51349 (86.51)
Other Nordic	41385 (3.99)	2935 (3.74)	2327 (4.47)	2526 (4.26)
Other	77170 (7.45)	5747 (7.33)	4141 (7.95)	5482 (9.24)
Missing	7 (0.00)	1 (0.00)	1 (0.00)	0 (0.00)
Paternal Country of Birth				
Sweden	905824 (87.40)	68936 (87.88)	45771 (87.84)	51084 (86.06)
Other Nordic	34953 (3.37)	2445 (3.12)	1910 (3.67)	2153 (3.63)
Other	90567 (8.74)	6485 (8.27)	4155 (7.97)	5713 (9.62)
Missing	5080 (0.49)	575 (0.70)	271 (0.52)	407 (0.69)
Natural science poor performance	298903 (28.43)	21026 (26.51)	15266 (28.86)	17513 (29.09)
Civics poor performance	408082 (38.81)	49818 (37.18)	32022 (39.47)	36182 (39.91)
Sports poor performance	70358 (6.79)	4365 (5.56)	3611 (6.93)	4048(6.82)
Arts poor performance	62182 (5.91)	3937 (4.96)	3223 (6.09)	3644 (6.05)
Swedish poor performance	68154 (6.48)	4196 (5.29)	3467 (6.55)	4297 (7.14)

Abbreviations: *VD* vaginal delivery, *CS* Caesarean section, *SGA* small for gestational age, *LGA* large for gestational age

at a specialised school (for example if the child had a disability) [21]. There were 143,740 missing that were born through unassisted VD (12.2%), 11,538 from assisted VD (12.8%), 9,615 from elective CS (15.6%) and 11,943 from emergency CS (16.8%). Our final cohort consisted of 1,243,876 children. Of these, 1,036,424 were born by unassisted VD (84.5%), 78,441 by assisted VD (6.4%), 42,107 by elective CS (4.3%) and 59,357 by emergency CS (4.8%) (Table 1). 162,349 (13.2%) children had poor school performance. Ages at time of grading ranged from 14–21, with 95% of children receiving grades at 16 years of age. The median score was 210 (Interquartile range: 175–250) (Fig. 1).

Logistic regression

In unadjusted analysis, the OR for assisted VD compared to unassisted VD was 0.84 [95% CI:0.82–0.86] (Table 2). After adjustment it was 1.06 [95% CI:1.03–1.08]. For elective CS the unadjusted OR was 1.05 [95% CI: 1.03–1.08] and the adjusted OR was 1.06 [95% CI:1.03–1.09]. For emergency CS the unadjusted OR was 1.05 [95% CI:1.02–1.07] and increased to 1.12 [95% CI:1.09–1.15] after adjustment. Adjusting for birth year, year of receiving grades, and parental education (for those born after 1990) had no effect on results (Additional file 2: Table S1 and Additional file 3: Table S2). Results were consistent among male babies, children born in Stockholm County, children who were 16 years old when they received grades, children without a low Apgar score, and children with a score above 0 (Additional file 4: Table S3). Similarly, there seemed to be no family effect seen by creating a random intercept for maternal ID, or restricting the population based on family size and birth order (Data not shown, available on request).

When school performance was divided into subjects, the association was similar to the overall association between birth by CS and poor school performance (Additional file 5: Table S4).

Quantile regression

There was little difference in the distribution of grades by mode of delivery (Fig. 1). The plots of estimates across the distribution, as well an explanation for how to interpret them, is shown in Fig. 2. Scores for children born through assisted VD were slightly higher than unassisted VD, especially at lower quantiles. There was no association with elective or emergency CS. After adjustment, there was no association between assisted VD and school performance (Fig. 3 and Additional file 6: Figure S2). Elective and emergency CS were associated with a slight decrease (2–5 points) in scores across the distribution.

In unadjusted analysis, the 5th, 25th, 50th, 75th and 95th percentiles for unassisted VD were 70, 175, 210, 250 and 300, respectively. Assisted VD was 20 points

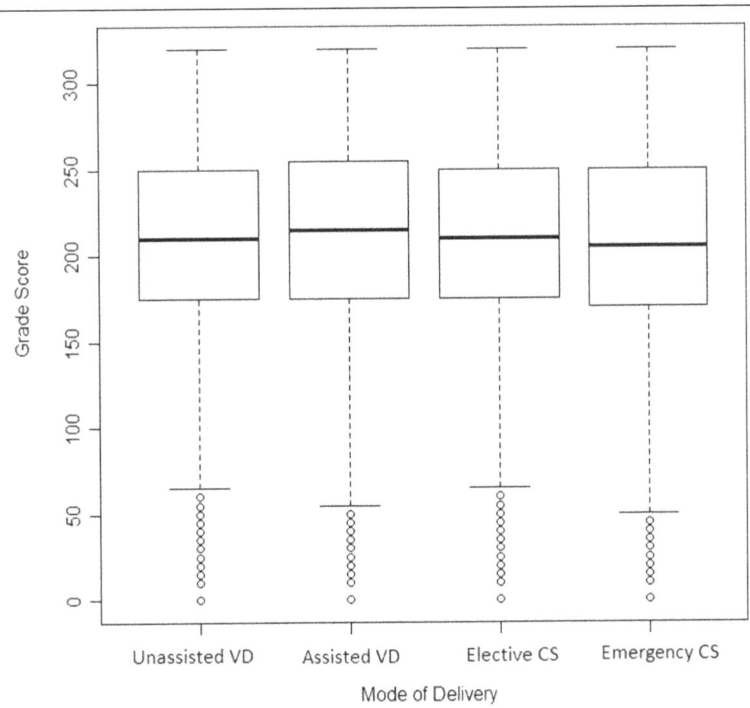

Fig. 1 Distribution of school grades by mode of delivery. *Abbreviations*: OR: odds ratio, VD: vaginal delivery, CS: Caesarean section. *Interpretation: the *bold lines* represent the median (50th percentile), *lines* at the top and bottom of each box represent the 25th and 75th percentiles, respectively. Dotted lines extend to the most extreme data point that is within 1.5 times the inter-quartile range of the box. Circles represent outliers, or data points outside this range

Table 2 Association between mode of delivery and poor school performance

	Exposed Cases	Unadjusted OR (95% CI)	Adjusted OR (95% CI)
Unassisted VD	138202	Ref	Ref
Assisted VD	8880	0.84 (0.82-0.86)	1.06 (1.03-1.08)
Elective CS	7064	1.05 (1.03-1.08)	1.06 (1.03-1.09)
Emergency CS	8203	1.05 (1.02-1.07)	1.12 (1.09-1.15)

Abbreviations: *OR* odds ratio, *VD* vaginal delivery, *CS* Caesarean section

higher for the 5th percentile, and 5 points higher for the 50th and 75th percentiles. Elective CS was the same as unassisted VD at all five percentiles. Emergency CS was 5 points lower than unassisted VD at the 25th and 50th percentiles. In adjusted analysis, the 5th, 25th, 50th, 75th, and 95th percentiles for unassisted VD were 17.2, 132.8, 180, 215, and 274.7, respectively. Assisted VD was largely equal to unassisted VD. Elective CS showed a slight decrease (ranging from −1.4 to −2.78) in scores across the distribution, with the exception of the 75th percentile where it was equal. Similarly, emergency CS also showed a slight decrease in scores (ranging from −2 to −5) with the exception of the 75th percentile, which showed no change. Excluding scores of 0 did not change results (Data not shown, available on request).

Discussion

Main findings

We assessed the impact of obstetric mode of delivery, and in particular birth by CS, on school performance at age 16 using a large, population-based cohort. Two separate analyses were conducted, logistic and quantile regression, assessing school performance in both dichotomous and continuous form. There was a slight association between birth by CS and a reduction in school performance in both analyses. In logistic regression, elective CS was significantly associated with increased likelihood of poor school performance. However, children born by CS were only 6% more likely to receive a poor grade when compared to children born through unassisted VD. The association between emergency CS and poor school performance was somewhat stronger but still small (OR = 1.12, [95% CI:1.09–1.15]). With quantile regression analysis, there again appeared to be a slight association between birth by CS and school performance, primarily in adjusted results. Children born by elective or emergency CS had a 1–5 point decrease in score across the distribution, translating to a 0.31–1.56% decrease.

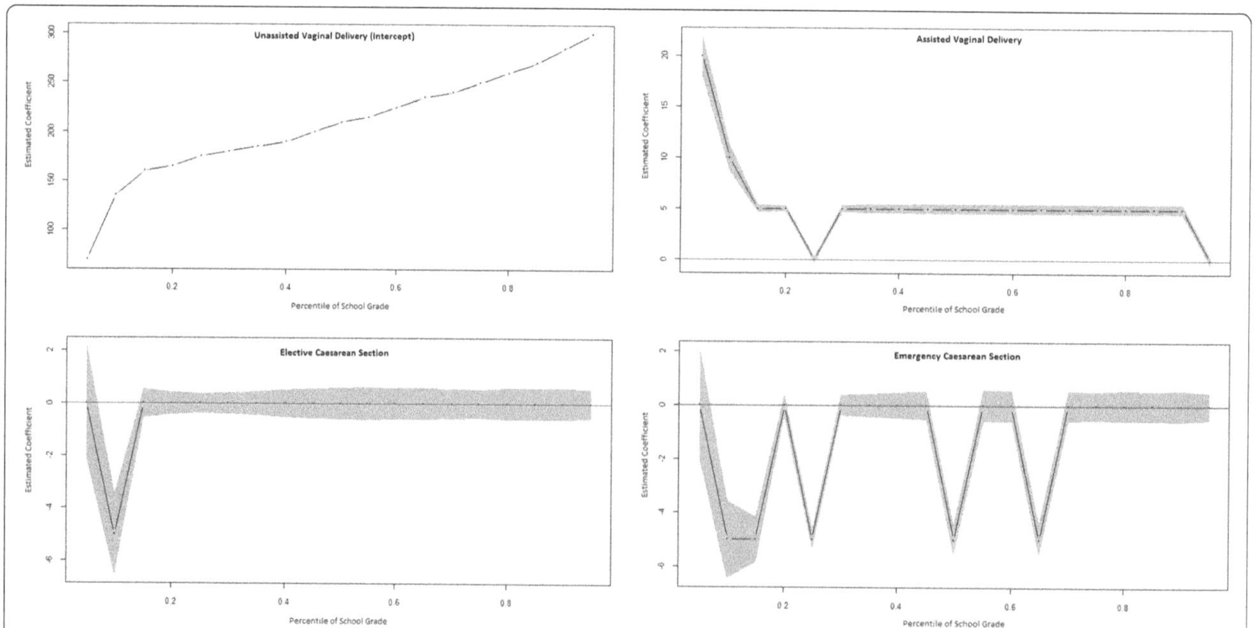

Fig. 2 Unadjusted quantile regression modelling the association between mode of delivery and school performance. *Interpretation: the coefficient values for unassisted vaginal delivery correspond to the school grade at that percentile. Estimated coefficients for other modes of delivery correspond to the estimated difference in score at each percentile. Grey area indicates 95% confidence intervals. *Note*: Percentiles are recorded as proportions. For example, 0.2 corresponds to the 20th percentile etc

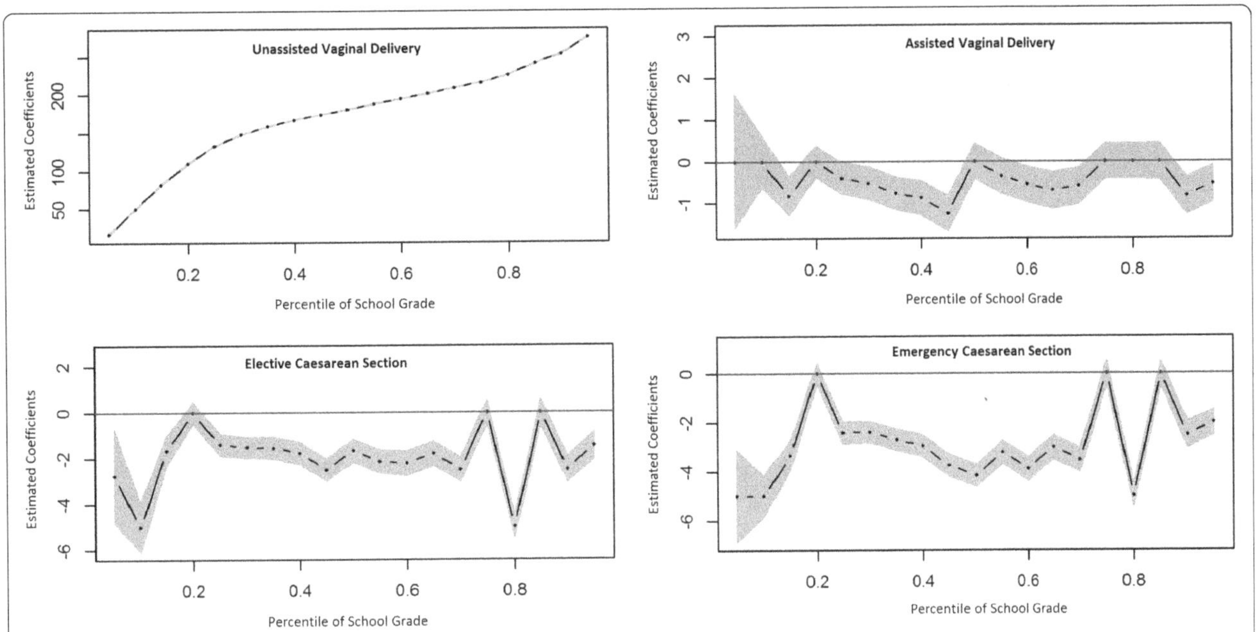

Fig. 3 Adjusted quantile regression modelling the association between mode of delivery and school performance. *Interpretation: the coefficient values for unassisted vaginal delivery correspond to the predicted school grade at that percentile, given reference value for all co-variates. Estimated coefficients for other modes of delivery correspond to the estimated difference in score at each percentile. Grey area indicates 95% confidence intervals

Interpretation

There are several possible explanations for an observed association between birth by CS and a small reduction in school performance. A range of characteristics influence school performance including not only behaviour [9] and personality, [26] but also cognitive ability, [26] and external factors such as ethnic diversity in the district [19]. It is possible that rather than having an effect across this wide range of factors and behaviours, birth by CS is having an effect on only one aspect, such as anxiety. Another potential explanation is that this result is being driven by confounding, such as confounding by indication or residual confounding. Confounding by indication occurs when an outcome is causally associated with an indication for the exposure of interest [27]. For example, foetal distress and maternal anxiety may be indications for emergency or elective CS, [28] and may also have an impact on school performance [29, 30], leading to a non-causal association between CS and poor school performance. Additionally, the association could be driven by residual confounding [27]. The relationship between pre and perinatal risk factors and psychological development is complex, and it can be difficult to rule out the effect of difficult to measure confounders, such as social adversity [31]. Regardless of what is driving the association, the decrease in score is very slight. A previous study on this population reported comparable effect sizes for the association between current asthma, rhinitis, eczema and school performance (change in mean score ranging from −3.1 to 4.1) and similarly concluded that though there were statistically significant associations they were likely not clinically meaningful or causally associated [32]. For comparison, the same study reported that severe nasal symptoms is associated with a 12.1 point decrease in mean grade, [32] and another study reported consumption of fish at least once a week is associated with a 14.5–19.9 point increase in mean grade [33].

Strengths and limitations

The strengths of the present study include the use of population-based registries, limiting selection, information bias and measurement error, as we were able to include the entire population and received data from official records. Also, due to the extensive nature of these registries, we were able to assess the effect of a wide variety of co-variates and potential confounders including not only obstetric information, but also demographic and socio-economic factors. Additionally, due to the grading system in Sweden and the use of quantile regression, we were able to assess the impact of mode of delivery across a range of school grades, rather than merely assessing the likelihood of a "passing" grade.

The present study also has several limitations. First, we had no data on breast feeding, which has been linked to both mode of delivery [34] and school performance [35]. However, Sweden has a very high rate of breast feeding and close to 100% of Swedish-born children have ever been breast fed [36]. Additionally, as breast feeding may be affected by mode of delivery it is more likely to be a mediator rather than a confounder in this situation. Second, a range of factors affect school performance, and we cannot rule out a potential effect on more specific outcomes, such as anxiety, disruptive behaviour, or cognition. Previous results would indicate that mode of delivery does not have an impact on childhood neurodevelopment, [8] but results on behavioural difficulties are conflicting [14, 37]. Finally, it is worth noting that birth by CS in Sweden may not be representative. Access to medical care in Sweden is egalitarian, and the associations between social class and CS seen in other countries are not as prevalent [38]. Additionally, Sweden has a very low rate of birth by CS compared to other European countries, [1] and it is probable that we had a low incidence of non-medically indicated CS. Though we did not have access to information on indications for CS, we were able to separate pre- and post-labour CS, which had no impact on results.

Conclusions

The present study used two analysis methods, adjusted for a wide variety of potential confounders, and conducted several sensitivity analyses to further investigate a potential association. With these robust analysis methods, we have concluded there is a slight association between birth by CS and poor school performance. Given the complex nature of the relationship between perinatal risk factors, such as birth by CS, and development, this small association should be interpreted with caution.

Additional files

Additional file 1: Figure S1. Proposed directed acyclic graph (DAG) describing the association between birth by Caesarean section and poor school performance. Dark grey corresponds to variables which were measured, light grey corresponds to variables which were not measured or are difficult to fully quantify.

Additional file 2: Table S1. Effect of birth year and year of grading on the association between mode of delivery and poor school performance.

Additional file 3: Table S2. Effect of parental education on the association between mode of delivery and poor school performance among children born in 1990 or later.

Additional file 4: Table S3. Sensitivity analyses examining the effect of gender, county of birth, age at grading and Apgar score on the association between mode of delivery and poor school performance. (DOCX 15 kb)

Additional file 5: Table S4. The association between mode of delivery and poor school performance by subject.

Additional file 6: Figure S2. Complete model of the adjusted association between mode of delivery and school performance.

Abbreviations

aOR: Adjusted odds ratio; CS: Cesarean section; DAG: Directed acyclic graph; HDI: Human development index; LGA: Large for gestational age; PIN: Personal identification number; SGA: Small for gestational age; VD: Vaginal delivery

Acknowledgements

We thank Mr. Henrik Dal and Dr. Beata Jablonska, Department of Public Health Sciences, Karolinska Institutet, Stockholm, Sweden, for providing data management support and advice.

Funding

This work was supported by The Irish Centre for Fetal and Neonatal Translational Research (INFANT) (Science Foundation Ireland (SFI) funded centre, Grant number 12|RC|2272). The Alimentary Pharmabiotic Centre (APC) is a research centre also funded by SFI (grant number SFI/12/RC/2273). GC, TGD and JFC are supported by the Health Research Board (HRB) through Health Research Awards (grants no HRA_POR/2011/23; TGD, JFC and GC, and HRA_POR/2012/32; JFC, TGD). GC is supported by a NARSAD Young Investigator Grant from the Brain and Behavior Research Foundation (Grant Number 20771). TD and JFC are also funded by the European Community's Seventh Framework Programme (MyNewGut, FFP7-KBBE/2013–2018, grant agreement no 613979). The APC has conducted studies in collaboration with several companies including GSK, Pfizer, Wyeth and Mead Johnson. Funding bodies had no role in the design of the study and collection, analysis, and interpretation of data and in writing the manuscript.

Authors' contributions

EAC contributed to study design, analysis and interpretation, and drafted the initial manuscript. LCK contributed to study design and interpretation, and critical revision of the manuscript. CD contributed to study design and interpretation, and critical revision of the manuscript. PMK contributed to study design and interpretation, and critical revision of the manuscript. JFC contributed to interpretation of the results and critical revision of the manuscript. TGD contributed to interpretation of the results and critical revision of the manuscript. ASK contributed to study conception, design and interpretation, and critical revision of the manuscript. All authors approved the final manuscript as submitted and agree to be accountable for all aspects of the work in ensuring that questions related to the accuracy or integrity of any part of the work are appropriately investigated and resolved.

Competing interests

The authors declare that they have no competing interests.

Consent for publication

Consent for publication was not required, as data were anonymised and informed consent was waived by the ethics committee.

Author details

[1]Department of Obstetrics and Gynaecology, The Irish Centre for Fetal and Neonatal Translational Research (INFANT), University College Cork, Cork, Ireland. [2]Department of Public Health Sciences, Division of Public Health Epidemiology, Karolinska Institutet, Stockholm, Sweden. [3]Department of Epidemiology and Public Health, University College Cork, Cork, Ireland. [4]Department of Anatomy and Neuroscience, APC Microbiome Institute, University College Cork, Cork, Ireland. [5]Department of Psychiatry, APC Microbiome Institute, University College Cork, Cork, Ireland.

References

1. Macfarlane AJ, Blondel B, Mohangoo AD, Cuttini M, Nijhuis J, Novak Z, et al. Wide differences in mode of delivery within Europe: risk stratified analyses of aggregated routine data from the Euro-Peristat study. BJOG. 2016;123(4):559–68.
2. Vogel JP, Betrán AP, Vindevoghel N, Souza JP, Torloni MR, Zhang J, et al. Use of the Robson classification to assess caesarean section trends in 21 countries: a secondary analysis of two WHO multicountry surveys. Lancet Glob Health. 2015;3(5):e260–e70.
3. Blustein J, Liu J. Time to consider the risks of caesarean delivery for long term child health. BMJ. 2015;350:h2410.

4. MacKay DF, Smith GC, Dobbie R, Pell JP. Gestational age at delivery and special educational need: retrospective cohort study of 407,503 schoolchildren. PLoS Med. 2010;7(6):e1000289.
5. Quigley MA, Poulsen G, Boyle E, Wolke D, Field D, Alfirevic Z, et al. Early term and late preterm birth are associated with poorer school performance at age 5 years: a cohort study. Arch Dis Child Fetal Neonatal Ed. 2012;97(3): F167–73.
6. Cho CE, Norman M. Cesarean section and development of the immune system in the offspring. Am J Obstet Gynecol. 2013;208(4):249–54.
7. Cryan JF, Dinan TG. Mind-altering microorganisms: the impact of the gut microbiota on brain and behaviour. Nat Rev Neruosci. 2012;13(10):701–12.
8. Curran E, Dalman C, Kearney P, Kenny LC, Cryan JF, Dinan T, et al. The association between obstetric mode of delivery and autism spectrum disorder: A population-based sibling design study. JAMA Psychiatry. 2015; 72(9):935–42.
9. Poropat AE. A meta-analysis of adult-rated child personality and academic performance in primary education. Brit J Educ Psychol. 2014;84(2):239–52.
10. McLeod JD, Uemura R, Rohrman S. Adolescent mental health, behavior problems, and academic achievement. J Health Soc Behav. 2012;53(4):482–97.
11. Kronholm E, Puusniekka R, Jokela J, Villberg J, Urrila AS, Paunio T, et al. Trends in self-reported sleep problems, tiredness and related school performance among Finnish adolescents from 1984 to 2011. J Sleep Res. 2015;24(1):3–10.
12. Jablonska B, Lindberg L, Lindblad F, Rasmussen F, Ostberg V, Hjern A. School performance and hospital admissions due to self-inflicted injury: a Swedish national cohort study. Int J Epidemiol. 2009;38(5):1334–41.
13. McCarty CA, Mason WA, Kosterman R, Hawkins JD, Lengua LJ, McCauley E. Adolescent school failure predicts later depression among girls. J Adolesc Health. 2008;43(2):180–7.
14. Khalaf SY, O'Neill SM, O'Keeffe LM, Henriksen TB, Kenny LC, Cryan JF, et al. The impact of obstetric mode of delivery on childhood behavior. Soc Psychiatry Psyciatr Epidmiol. 2015;50(10):1557–67.
15. The Swedish Centre for Epidemiology. The Swedish medical birth register- a summary of content and quality. 2003 [cited 2016 May 18] Available from: https://www.socialstyrelsen.se/Lists/Artikelkatalog/Attachments/10655/2003-112-3_20031123.pdf.
16. Lambe M, Hultman C, Torrång A, MacCabe J, Cnattingius S. Maternal smoking during pregnancy and school performance at age 15. Epidemiology. 2006; 17(5):524–30.
17. Gardner RM, Lee BK, Magnusson C, Rai D, Frisell T, Karlsson H, et al. Maternal body mass index during early pregnancy, gestational weight gain, and risk of autism spectrum disorders: Results from a Swedish total population and discordant sibling study. Int J Epidemiol. 2015;44(3):870–83.
18. Textor J, Hardt J, Knuppel S. DAGitty: a graphical tool for analyzing causal diagrams. Epidemiology. 2011;22(2):745.
19. Szulkin R, Jonsson JO. Ethnic segregation and educational outcomes in Swedish comprehensive schools. Stockholm: The Stockholm University Linnaeus Center for Integration Studies (SULCIS); 2007.
20. D'Onofrio BM, Singh AL, Iliadou A, Lambe M, Hultman CM, Neiderhiser JM, et al. A quasi experimental study of maternal smoking during pregnancy and offspring academic achievement. Child Dev. 2010;81(1):80–100.
21. Stuart A, Otterblad Olausson P, Källen K. Apgar scores at 5 minutes after birth in relation to school performance at 16 years of Age. Obstet Gynecol. 2011;118(2, Part 1):201–8.
22. D'Onofrio BM, Rickert ME, Frans E, Kuja-Halkola R, Almqvist C, Sjolander A, et al. Paternal age at childbearing and offspring psychiatric and academic morbidity. JAMA Psychiatry. 2014;71(4):432–8.
23. Koenker R. Quantile regression in R: a vignette. 2015 [cited; Available from: https://cran.r-project.org/web/packages/quantreg/vignettes/rq.pdf
24. Li J, Alterman T, Deddins JA. Analysis of large hierarchical data with multilevel logistic modeling using PROC GLIMMIX. [cited 2016 May 18] Available from: http://www2.sas.com/proceedings/sugi31/151-31.pdf.
25. Rosander P, Bäckström M, Stenberg G. Personality traits and general intelligence as predictors of academic performance: A structural equation modelling approach. Learn Individ Differ. 2011;21(5):590–6.
26. Bosco JL, Silliman RA, Thwin SS, Geiger AM, Buist DS, Prout MN, et al. A most stubborn bias: no adjustment method fully resolves confounding by indication in observational studies. J Clin Epidemiol. 2010;63(1):64–74.
27. Stjernholm YV, Petersson K, Eneroth E. Changed indications for cesarean sections. Acta Obstet Gynecol Scand. 2010;89(1):49–53.
28. Galler JR, Ramsey FC, Harrison RH, Taylor J, Cumberbatch G, Forde V. Postpartum maternal moods and infant size predict performance on a national high school entrance examination. J Child Psychol Psyciatr. 2004;45(6):1064–75.
29. van Handel M, Swaab H, de Vries LS, Jongmans MJ. Long-term cognitive and behavioral consequences of neonatal encephalopathy following perinatal asphyxia: a review. Eur J Pediatr. 2007;166(7):645–54.
30. Thapar A, Rutter M. Do prenatal risk factors cause psychiatric disorder? Be wary of causal claims. Br J Psychiatry. 2009;195(2):100–1.
31. Sundberg R, Toren K, Hoglund D, Aberg N, Brisman J. Nasal symptoms are associated with school performance in adolescents. J Adolesc Health. 2007; 40(6):581–3.
32. Kim JL, Winkvist A, Aberg MA, Aberg N, Sundberg R, Toren K, et al. Fish consumption and school grades in Swedish adolescents: a study of the large general population. Acta Paediatr. 2010;99(1):72–7.
33. Prior E, Santhakumaran S, Gale C, Philipps LH, Modi N, Hyde MJ. Breastfeeding after cesarean delivery: a systematic review and meta-analysis of world literature. Am J Clin Nutr. 2012;95(5):1113–35.
34. Heikkila K, Kelly Y, Renfrew MJ, Sacker A, Quigley MA. Breastfeeding and educational achievement at age 5. Matern Child Nutr. 2014;10(1):92–101.
35. OECD Family Database. CO1.5: Breastfeeding rates. 2009. [cited 2016 May 18] Available from: http://www.oecd.org/els/family/43136964.pdf.
36. Curran EA, Cryan JF, Kenny LC, Dinan TG, Kearney PM, Khashan AS. Obstetrical mode of delivery and childhood behavior and psychological development in a British Cohort. J Autis Dev Disord. 2015;46(2):603–14.
37. Thomas J, Hildingsson I. Sweden. In: Kennedy P, Kodate N, editors. Maternity Services and Policy in an International Context: Risk, Citizenship and Welfare Regimes: Routledge; 2009.

15

Management of persistent caesarean scar pregnancy after curettage treatment failure

Zhi-Da Qian[1*], Yue Weng[1], Yong-Jiang Du[1], Chun-Fen Wang[2] and Li-Li Huang[1]

Abstract

Background: Caesarean scar pregnancy (CSP) is a late serious complication of caesarean section. The incidence of CSP has increased worldwide in recent years. Early diagnosis and prompt therapy are crucial to avoid catastrophic complications. There are various strategies for CSP treatment, but there is no consensus on the best management for CSP. Dilation and curettage (D&C) and hysteroscopy are common and effective treatments with their advantages and disadvantages. No in-depth study of the clinical effects of hysteroscopic management of CSP after D&C treatment failure has been conducted. The purpose of this study is to evaluate the effectiveness and safety of hysteroscopic removal of residual CSP tissue (persistent CSP) as a rescue after failed D&C management.

Methods: This is a retrospective clinical research study. Forty-five patients underwent operative hysteroscopy to remove the residual gestational tissue in the caesarean scar after failed D&C treatment. The clinical characteristics and outcomes of hysteroscopic surgeries of 45 CSP cases were investigated. All data analyses were conducted with SPSS 17.0.

Results: Forty-three CSP cases after unsuccessful curettage treatment were successfully treated by operative hysteroscopy. The estimated intraoperative blood loss was 20.00 (10.00–500.00) mL, the hysteroscopic operating time was 20.00 (15.00–45.00) min, the decline of serum β-hCG the day after surgery was 71.91 ± 14.05%, the total hospitalisation time was 7.87 ± 2.26 days, the medical cost was 13,682.71 ± 3553.77 China Yuan (CNY), the time of bleeding after surgery was 7.42 ± 2.48 days, and the time of serum β-hCG resolution after surgery was 13.84 ± 9.83 days. Follow-up after discharge demonstrated that there were no severe complications for any patients.

Conclusions: Hysteroscopy therapy could treat persistent CSP effectively and safely after curettage treatment failure. Therapy should be individualised, and the risks and cost of the hysteroscopy procedure and anaesthesia must be considered and fully discussed with the patients before surgery.

Keywords: Caesarean scar pregnancy, Dilatation and curettage, Hysteroscopy, Uterine artery embolisation, Treatment

Background

A caesarean scar pregnancy (CSP) is a late serious complication of caesarean section (CS). CSP is defined as a gestational sac located in the scar of an earlier caesarean delivery. As a special form of ectopic pregnancy, CSP was first reported by Larsen and Solomon in 1978 [1]. The incidence of CSP is one in 1800–2216 pregnancies [2]. Prior CS represents the most common predisposing factor for CSP [3]. There has been a rapid increase in the incidence of CSP worldwide, especially in China in recent years. This increased incidence may have contributed to the in-depth understanding of CSP, the high CS rate, and the more wide-spread use of colour Doppler sonography [4, 5]. The phasing out of the one child policy in China has also contributed to the increasing incidence of CSP. If such a pregnancy is allowed to continue, the patient is at risk for uterine scar rupture with haemorrhage (even in the first trimester), hysterectomy, and loss of sequent fertility.

Accurate diagnosis and prompt therapy are important to avoid catastrophic complications. There are various strategies for CSP therapy, and the uterine conserving termination of CSP (medical or surgical) in the first

* Correspondence: qianada@163.com
[1]Women's Hospital, School of Medicine, Zhejiang University, 1 Xueshi Road, Hangzhou, Zhejiang Province 310006, People's Republic of China
Full list of author information is available at the end of the article

trimester has been strongly preferred [2]. As less-invasive management options, a variety of medications (methotrexate (MTX), etoposide, and potassium chloride) have been adopted in the treatment of CSP [2, 4, 6]. Surgical managements include dilation and curettage (D&C) [7–9], uterine artery embolisation (UAE) [10] coupled with MTX arterial injection [11], hysteroscopy [12–15], and laparoscopy [16]. Hysterectomy is usually performed in emergencies such as heavy bleeding or uterine rupture. It is hard to decide on the optimal management for individual CSP cases.

As a traditional and primary treatment of CSP [7–9], D&C under transabdominal sonography (TAS) guidance after preventive UAE is simple and effective in most cases [5, 10]. D&C carries low cost and good curative effect, but it is accompanied by risks, including sever haemorrhage, low success rate, and even uterine perforation due to lack of direct visualisation. It often takes a longer time for the normalisation of the serum beta-human chorionic gonadotropin (β-hCG) level and resolution of the CSP mass. Some patients require further treatments and even hysterectomy [17, 18]. As reported, for CSP patients who had continuous vaginal bleeding and abnormal serum levels of β-HCG after medication and D&C, the remaining ectopic gestational tissue could be successfully hysteroscopically removed [15, 19, 20]. According to recent small case series, hysteroscopic removal of CSP is an alternative minimally invasive operation that offers direct visualisation, definitive confirmation of the diagnosis, removal of the gestational tissue entirely, short operative time and postoperative stay, and rapid normalisation of β-hCG. Although it is effective and safe, it requires experienced surgeons who are familiar with the anatomy of the uterine cavity and who are skilful at manipulating hysteroscopic instruments to prevent heavy bleeding and to keep the operative field clear. Facilities for immediate laparotomy or laparoscopy must be available. As a minimally invasive treatment, UAE is alternatively used to prevent and control severe haemorrhage and to preserve the patient's uterus and future fertility. Women with CSP who experienced preventive UAE before surgery have a high success rate and a low complication rate [21].

Although they have been reported with success, both D&C and hysteroscopy treatments have their advantages and disadvantages. Furthermore, most of literature reports were small case series or case reports. There are no in-depth studies of the clinical effects of hysteroscopic treatment of persistent CSP after D&C management failure. We conducted this retrospective clinical research to evaluate the clinical outcomes of hysteroscopic removal of residual gestational tissue as a rescue in the treatment of CSP patients with failed D&C. We found that the operative hysteroscopy was safe and effective.

Methods

This retrospective clinical investigation was conducted in the Department of Obstetrics and Gynaecology, Women's Hospital, School of Medicine, Zhejiang University, People's Republic of China, between March 2011 and September 2014. This hospital is the largest tertiary obstetrics and gynaecology medical treatment centre in Zhejiang province. Informed consent for the surgery and participation was obtained from each patient in the study, and the protocol was approved by the Institutional Review Board in the Women's Hospital, School of Medicine, Zhejiang University.

Subjects' criteria

Women with CSP who underwent hysteroscopic management after D&C were enrolled in the study if they were ≤12 weeks of gestation (at the time of D&C), haemodynamically stable without internal bleeding, and had an unruptured type of CSP. The actual gestational age was calculated based on last menstrual period and adjusted according to the date of the positive early pregnancy test, the ultrasound examination, the appearance of morning sickness, and whether the patient's menstruation was regular or not. Exclusion criteria included cervical pregnancy, inevitable abortion, incomplete abortion, missed abortion, caesarean scar choriocarcinoma, and significant maternal hepatic, renal, cardiac or blood system disease.

Diagnosis standard of CSP

The CSP was diagnosed using the following criteria: a history of low-transverse caesarean delivery in the lower uterine segment, positive urine pregnancy test or serum β-HCG level, and fulfilment of the following ultrasonography criteria [22] (Fig. 1): (a) Development of the gestational sac in the anterior portion of the lower uterine segment; (b) Empty uterine cavity and cervical canal; and (c) Absence of healthy myometrium between the gestational sac and the bladder. Magnetic resonance imaging (MRI) and three-dimensional (3-D) power Doppler ultrasound might be useful in the cases in which the diagnosis remains unclear after transvaginal sonography (TVS) examination.

Management

Patients were readmitted due to intermittent vaginal bleeding, severe bleeding, a prolonged return of β-hCG to normal, or the persistence of a caesarean scar mass after D&C. All patients were initially treated with a D&C regimen only or D&C combined with preventive UAE. They were counselled extensively regarding the abnormal vaginal bleeding, the abnormal β-hCG levels, the residual gestational tissue, and the further treatment indications. With the diagnosis of persistent CSP, medical and surgical

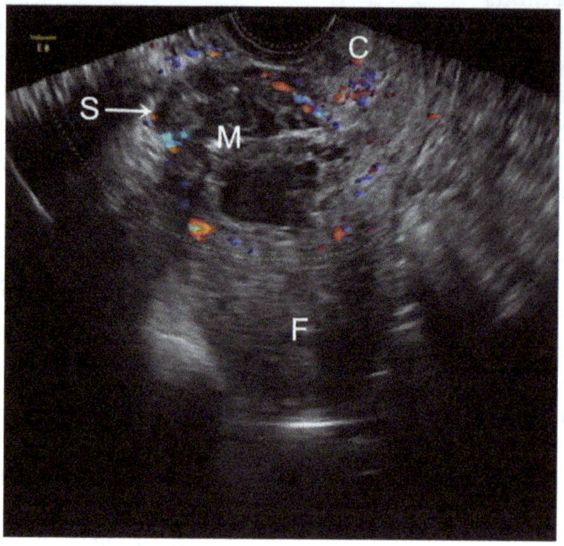

Fig. 1 Transvaginal ultrasonography of the patient with caesarean scar pregnancy after curettage treatment failure. The uterine cavity and cervical canal were empty. A 5.4 × 3.7 × 3.7 cm mass implanted in the anterior wall of the uterine caesarean scar (*arrow*) embedded and surrounded by thin myometrium and separated from the endometrial cavity was visible on the retroverted uterus. Ultrasonography revealed that the mass was heterogeneous with a mixture of cystic and solid echogenicity. C = cervix; F = fundal endometrial cavity; M = mass; S = scar of caesarean section

options (including administration of MTX, hysteroscopic resection, and laparoscopy or laparotomy resection) were discussed with them before they were treated with operative hysteroscopy combined with or without UAE.

Super selective embolisation of both uterine arteries was performed using gelatine sponge powder by two experienced radiologists. Under local anaesthesia, the Seldinger technique was applied to puncture and catheterize via the right femoral artery, into the bilateral internal iliac arteries to perform pelvic artery digital subtraction angiography. Post UAE angiography was performed to confirm that the vessel occlusion was complete.

All patients underwent careful hysteroscopic surgeries (Fig. 2) by experienced gynaecologists to remove the products of conception under TAS (LOGIQ P6, GE, USA) guidance. The cervical dilatation was carefully and successively accomplished by Hegar dilators from 5 mm to 10.5 mm. Under epidural anaesthesia, an operative hysteroscope (CA95138, Stryker, USA) with a 10-mm external diameter was placed inside the uterus. A continuous flow 26F hysteroscopic resectoscope with a 90-degree wire loop electrode was used under the guidance of TAS. Propelled by a uterine expansion instrument, 5% glucose solution was used to obtain uterine distension. An electrosurgical generator (VIO300S, ERBE, Germany) was used on a setting of 70 W of coagulation current and 70 W of cutting current, respectively.

Hysteroscopy recognised the implantation of the persistent ectopic gestational tissue under direct visualisation. The vessel bed of the implantation site was exposed and coagulated for haemostasis first. If the diameter of residual gestational tissue was more than 2 cm, an oval pair of forceps was used to remove it under TAS guidance. Then, the electric loop was used carefully without electricity to curettage the residual gestational tissue on the wall of the diverticulum (disruption of the caesarean scar) to decrease the risk of uterine scar rupture and to remove the residual villous. When the residual gestational tissue was closely attached to the uterus wall, the electric cutting was used to ensure the remaining tissue was removed completely. Finally, the uterine scar diverticulum was checked thoroughly to confirm that there were no obvious residual tissue and active bleeding.

The amount of bleeding during surgery was observed in all patients. Iodoform gauze packing was left in situ for 24–48 h when there was heavy bleeding (800–1500 mL). Hysterectomy was performed immediately if the blood loss was more than 1500 mL. The serum β-hCG level, liver and kidney function tests, and routine blood tests were examined

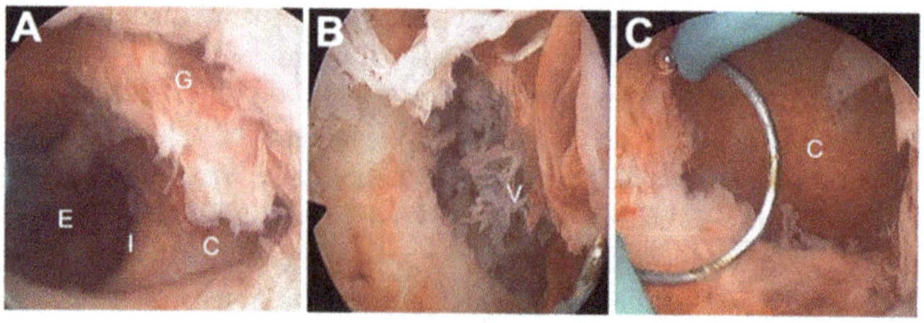

Fig. 2 Hysteroscopic view of the caesarean scar pregnancy. C = caesarean scar diverticulum; E = endometrial cavity; G = gestational tissue; I = internal os; V = villous. **a** Before operation: the endometrial cavity was empty, and the gestational tissue was implanted in a diverticulum located in the left anterior endocervical wall, compatible with prior caesarean section scar. **b** During operation: the residual villous in a niche located in the left endocervical wall (disruption of the caesarean scar). **c** After operation: the residual gestational tissue was removed completely, and there was no obvious bleeding point

before surgery, the day after surgery, and 7 days after surgery. The size of the residual mass was measured by TVS at the same time.

Investigation content

All patients were observed during the hospitalisation. The clinical characteristics of 45 CSP patients were investigated, and the variables included maternal age, gravidity, number of prior CSs, number of abortions, interval between CSP and CS, gestational age, interval between hysteroscopic surgery and D&C, mean size of the residual gestational tissue before hysteroscopic surgery, thickness of the lower uterine segment, estimated intraoperative blood loss, hysteroscopic operating time, serum β-hCG levels before and after hysteroscopic surgery, side effects (such as haemorrhagic shock and infection), number of hysterectomy, medical cost, hospitalisation time after surgery, and total hospitalisation time.

All patients were retrospectively investigated more than 1 year after hysteroscopic surgeries. Their serum β-hCG levels were followed-up weekly until the normalisation. At half a month, 1 month (2 months or 3 months, if needed) postoperation, TVS was performed to evaluate the recovery of the uterus. Other information about the 45 patients were investigated, including their clinical status (lower abdominal pain, bleeding pattern, or any other symptoms), days for β-hCG to return to normal (<5.3 IU/L), and the time of vaginal bleeding after surgery.

Statistical analysis

All the data were analysed by SPSS 17.0 software (SPSS, Inc., USA) for homogeneity of variance with the Levene test and for normal distribution with the Kolmogorov–Smirnov test. If variables met assumptions of homogeneity of variance and normality, the independent samples *t* test was used (mean ± SD), If not, the nonparametric test (the Mann–Whitney *U* test) was used [median (range)].

Results

A total of 1348 women were diagnosed as CSP in our hospital during the study period, and 154 (11.42%) of them were readmitted due to retained products of conception or other symptoms. Forty-five (3.34%) CSP patients underwent operative hysteroscopy after the initial treatment of D&C (41 patients underwent D&C regimen only, and 4 patients underwent D&C combined with preventive UAE) during the study period. They were readmitted due to the persistence of caesarean scar mass (45/45) accompanied by intermittent vaginal bleeding (21/45), severe bleeding (7/45), and a prolonged return time of β-hCG to normal (9/45). With the diagnosis of persistent CSP, they were treated with operative hysteroscopy only (10/45) or in combination with UAE (35/45). In all patients, histopathologic examination performed on residual tissue obtained at hysteroscopic surgery confirmed the diagnosis of persistent CSP.

The patients' characteristics and demographics (Table 1): the maternal age was 32.84 ± 4.37 years old, the gravidity was 4.49 ± 1.41 times, the number of prior abortions was 2.00 (0.00–6.00) times, the number of prior CSs was 1.00 (1.00–2.00) times, the interval between CS and CSP was 71.44 ± 46.17 months, the gestational age was 83.18 ± 28.14 days, the interval between D&C and hysteroscopic surgery was 22.33 ± 13.08 days, the serum β-hCG level before hysteroscopic surgery was 2623.00 (0.55–39,992.00) IU/L, the size of the residual gestational tissue before hysteroscopic surgery was 3.44 ± 1.12 cm, and the thickness of the lower uterine segment was 1.20 (0.50–8.00) mm.

The outcomes of hysteroscopic surgeries (Table 2): the estimated intraoperative blood loss was 20.00 (10.00–500.00) mL, the hysteroscopic operating time was 20.00 (15.00–45.00) min, the serum β-hCG level the day after hysteroscopic surgery was 675.80 (0.20–16,336.00) IU/L, the decline of serum β-hCG the day after surgery was 71.91 ± 14.05%, the medical cost was 13,682.71 ± 3553.77 China Yuan (CNY), the hospitalisation time after hysteroscopic surgery was 4.47 ± 1.83 days, the total hospitalisation time was 7.87 ± 2.26 days, the time of bleeding after surgery was 7.42 ± 2.48 days, and the time of serum β-hCG resolution after surgery was 13.84 ± 9.83 days. Follow-up after discharge showed that there were no severe complications for any women.

The success rate was 95.56% (43/45) (definition of success: patient needs no more operations or medication therapy during or after hysteroscopic surgery, and her fertility is preserved), and no patient underwent hysterectomy. A

Table 1 The patients' characteristics and demographics

Characteristic	Value
Maternal age (years)	32.84 ± 4.37
Gravidity (times)	4.49 ± 1.41
Prior abortion (times)	2.00 (0.00–6.00)[a]
Prior CS (times)	1.00 (1.00–2.00)[a]
Interval between CS and CSP (months)	71.44 ± 46.17
Gestational age (days)	83.18 ± 28.14
Interval between D&C and hysteroscopic surgery (days)	22.33 ± 13.08
Serum β-hCG level before hysteroscopic surgery (IU/L)	2623.00 (0.55–39,992.00)[a]
Size of the residual gestational tissue before hysteroscopic surgery (cm)	3.44 ± 1.12
Thickness of the lower uterine segment (mm)	1.20 (0.50–8.00)[a]

Normal distribution (mean ± SD), Non-normal distribution (median [range]).
Unless noted [a]otherwise, values are presented as mean ± SD
CS cesarean section, *CSP* cesarean scar pregnancy, *D&C* dilatation and curettage

Table 2 Outcomes of hysteroscopic surgeries

Characteristic	Value
Success rate (%)	95.56
Side effect (%)	8.89
Estimated intraoperative blood loss (mL)	20.00 (10.00–500.00)[a]
Hysteroscopic operating time (min)	20.00 (15.00–45.00)[a]
Serum β-hCG level the day after hysteroscopic surgery (IU/L)	675.80 (0.20–16,336.00)[a]
Decline of serum β-hCG the day after surgery (%)	71.91 ± 14.05
Total hospitalization time (days)	7.87 ± 2.26
Hospitalization time after hysteroscopic surgery (days)	4.47 ± 1.83
Medical cost (CNY)	13,682.71 ± 3553.77
Time of bleeding after surgery (days)	7.42 ± 2.48
Time of serum β-hCG resolution after surgery (days)	13.84 ± 9.83

Normal distribution (mean ± SD), Non-normal distribution (median [range]).
Unless noted [a]otherwise, values are presented as mean ± SD
CS cesarean section, *CSP* cesarean scar pregnancy, *CNY* China Yuan

30-year-old woman was treated with a single dose of intramuscular MTX (50 mg/m^2 body surface area) and mifepristone (50 mg twice a day for 3 days) 4 days after hysteroscopic operation combined with UAE owing to a serum β-hCG level that was decreased less than 50% from the preoperative level, and it decreased to normal 21 days after surgery. Another 35-year-old woman was offered operative hysteroscopy without preventive UAE. Emergency UAE was performed successfully after unsuccessful iodoform gauze tamponade in this patient owing to haemorrhage (500 mL) during hysteroscopic surgery. There were no other severe complications for this patient.

The side effect rate was 8.89% (4/45), and there were no severe side effects in the research. One patient had a pelvic infection after hysteroscopy. She was a 36-year-old woman, and she had a history of irregular vaginal bleeding for 131 days at the hysteroscopic operation. On the first day after surgery, she started to have fever (38.7 °C) accompany with a mild lower abdominal pain. Bimanual examination revealed uterine tenderness, and motion of the cervix and uterus caused increased pain. Intravenous antibiotics were continued until the patient had been afebrile for 48 h. The patient was discharged 9 days after operation. There were 2 patients who suffered mild abnormalities of liver function after hysteroscopy combined with UAE. Their liver functions were normal a few days after the liver-protecting treatment. Another patient had experienced chest congestion at the end of hysteroscopy, and her vital signs were stable at that time. The symptom disappeared soon after the procedure was stopped immediately. The other 41 patients were discharged without any side effects and complications.

The hysteroscopy revealed a large caesarean scar defect (diverticulum) embedded with residual gestational tissues and an empty uterine cavity (Fig. 2). Thirteen patients with intrauterine adhesions were diagnosed during the hysteroscopy procedure and were simultaneously treated with hysteroscopic adhesiolysis.

Discussion

As a rare type of ectopic pregnancy, it is crucial to make an accurate diagnosis and to provide prompt therapy to avoid catastrophic complications. According to earlier reports, expectant management is not recommended owing to a low success rate and poor prognosis [3, 23]. It is generally recommended to terminate CSP in the first trimester as soon as possible after diagnosis. Haemodynamically stable cases have more conservative management options.

Although D&C is used as a traditional and simple treatment of CSP, it often coupled with a high rate of haemorrhage even when sonographically guided [6] and is accompanied by prolonged resolution time of β-hCG levels and of the CSP mass. Other problems might not be acceptable for doctors and patients, such as extended surveillance time and intermittent vaginal bleeding, and some patients require further management. Sadeghi et al. [18] reported that 8.33% of CSP patients initially treated with D&C ultimately required hysterectomy.

It is controversial whether intervention is clinically justified based on a slow decline in β-hCG level or ultrasound evidence of retained tissue. Jurkovic et al. [24] reported that 15% of CSP patients attending for follow-up had ultrasound evidence of retained products of conception, but only 6% required repeat intervention based on their clinical symptoms. They did not use β-hCG for follow up. In this study, 11.42% (154/1348) CSP patients were readmitted due to a persistent caesarean scar mass, abnormal β-hCG level, and other symptoms. Only 45 (3.34%) underwent operative hysteroscopy to remove the residual gestational tissue due to the persistence of caesarean scar mass (45/45) accompanied by intermittent vaginal bleeding (21/45), severe bleeding (7/45), and a prolonged return time of β-hCG to normal (9/45). The other 8 patients only had ultrasound evidence of retained tissue. These 17 asymptomatic patients were so worried about their retained tissue and the slow decline in β-hCG level that they underwent hysteroscopy surgeries after full discussion and informed consent. It is important to follow-up with patients after D&C management to identify evidence of persistent CSP. The surgical indication for persistent CSP is contentious, and it is valuable to carry out further research to reach a more definitive conclusion.

Further management of persistent CSP after D&C treatment failure includes expectant management, systemic or local MTX, repeat curettage, hysteroscopy, laparoscopy, laparotomy, and hysterectomy. MTX treatment is a less-invasive and appropriate management option when the woman is clinically stable and has an unruptured CSP [6]. However, it might also be associated with nausea, stomatitis, impairment of liver and renal function, abnormal vaginal spotting or even severe bleeding, and a prolonged return time of β-hCG. Due to the lack of direct visualisation, repeat curettage under ultrasound guidance carries the possibility of residue, haemorrhage, uterine perforation, and low success rate. Laparotomy and laparoscopy could remove the residual gestational tissue and repair the uterine defect (or 'niche') simultaneously. Ben et al. [25] reported a CSP case that underwent successful repair of the uterine defect, resulting in subsequent normal intrauterine pregnancy. However, abdominal surgery and uterine repair might be complicated by postoperative intra-abdominal adhesions and poor scar healing, both of which might have adverse effects on women's future fertility. Hysterectomy is usually performed in emergency situations (heavy bleeding or uterus rupture) in the treatment of persistent CSP.

Hysteroscopic removal of CSP might be used as an effective rescue after D&C or medical management failure [15, 19, 20]. It offers an accurate diagnosis by observing the gestational tissue at the implantation site. Operative hysteroscopy also offers appropriate management by separating the gestational tissue from the uterine wall and coagulating the blood vessels directly. Deans et al. [15] and Chao et al [19] reported that hysteroscopy is an important alternative method for CSP with less blood loss, shorter operating time, and rapid normalisation of the β-hCG level. We retrospectively investigated the use of TAS guided operative hysteroscopy to manage persistent CSP after unsuccessful D&C treatment. Our findings were similar with their studies. Laparoscopically assisted operative hysteroscopy has the additional advantages of minimally invasive caesarean scar resection, rapid and effective management of haemorrhage, and immediate detection and address uterine and/or bladder perforation [26, 27].

We found that the readmission reasons included the persistence of caesarean scar mass, abnormal vaginal bleeding, and prolonged decrease of β-hCG. It suggests that whatever treatment is selected, follow-up of symptoms, caesarean scar mass, and β-hCG level are necessary to ensure complete resolution of CSP. When surgical removal is performed in ectopic pregnancy without residual chorionic villi, the serum β-hCG level should be no more than 1/2 of its pre-surgical level at 24 h after operation and should continually decrease 1/2 for each subsequent 24 h [28]. If the serum β-hCG level falls less than that, it suggests the possibility of trophoblastic tissue remaining (persistent CSP) [26]. In this study, the curve of the serum β-hCG level decline after D&C in some patients is less dramatic due to the residual gestational tissue. It seems that simple suction evacuation and curettage would frequently leave chorionic villi imbedded within the caesarean scar defect.

Preventive UAE followed by curettage or hysteroscopy is an alternative, effective, safe, and minimally invasive treatment for CSP [10, 21]. The purpose of UAE before surgery includes blocking the blood flow in uterine arteries, decreasing local vascularisation, and inducing trophoblastic degeneration. Patients treated with UAE before D&C have less intraoperative blood loss, shorter hospitalisation time, lower rate of hysterectomy, quicker normalisation of serum β-hCG level, and shorter recovery time than those without UAE. However, there were only 4 cases who underwent preventive UAE before D&C in this study, and this low rate might be related to persistent CSP. From our experience, preventive UAE before D&C should be recommended in cases with ≥8 weeks of gestation, a CSP mass diameter ≥ 6 cm, a lesion bulging into the uterovesical fold, and abundant blood flow signals around the lesion under pulsed Doppler ultrasonography. In this report, 35 patients were treated with operative hysteroscopy combined with UAE. The performance of hysteroscopy therapy treating the persistent CSP effectively and safely might be partly owed to the fact that most patients underwent preventive UAE before operative hysteroscopy to prevent massive bleeding.

There were two patients who failed in this study. One case was treated with mifepristone and MTX a few days after hysteroscopy owing to a slow decrease in serum β-hCG level. The hysteroscopy revealed a large caesarean scar defect in the left endocervical wall deeply embedded with gestational tissue by direct visualisation. However, it was hard to completely remove the residual tissue in the niche due to the special position and villous implantation. She was diagnosed as persistent CSP after hysteroscopy and was offered medication therapy. Another patient underwent emergency UAE owing to massive bleeding during hysteroscopic surgery. This complication might be due to her big residual gestational mass with abundant blood flow and a thinner myometrium at the implantation site. The presence of a large CS scar defect might lead to haemorrhage because of weakened myometrial contractility. It is hard to prevent severe haemorrhage under hysteroscopy in this situation because active bleeding could impair vision and block the operative field. In the case of heavy bleeding after the residual gestational tissue is removed, Foley tamponade or intrauterine gauze compression might be tried initially. When other management techniques have failed to stop the bleeding, hysterectomy is performed as the last step to save the patient's life. We recommend that the selection of specific surgical procedures should be according to the size of the CSP mass and its implantation site.

Laparoscopy or laparoscopically assisted operative hysteroscopy might be more suitable for a patient with a large CSP mass deeply implanted into a CS defect, especially for a patient with the residual tissue bulge into the uterovesical fold under the caesarean scar.

One patient suffered chest congestion during hysteroscopic surgery, suggesting that cases treated by operative hysteroscopy might have additional risks from anaesthesia and from the hysteroscopy procedure. Although hysteroscopy is considered a safe procedure and is used widely, complications such as cervical laceration, uterine perforation, haemorrhage, absorption of irrigation solutions (water intoxication), and air embolism might occur. Although epidural anaesthesia is safe and effective, some complications might occur, including internal bleeding, epidural haematoma, nerve injury, mucosa or skin oedema, anaesthetic toxicity reaction, and coma. To detect mismanagement and limit the extent of injury, careful monitoring during the hysteroscopy procedure and epidural blocking should be taken. The hysteroscopy hospitalisation cost might be significantly higher than D&C management only. The additional financial burden and risks owing to hysteroscopy and anaesthesia must be considered and carefully discussed with the patients before operation.

Conclusions

A persistent CSP after unsuccessful D&C treatment could be effectively treated by operative hysteroscopy with or without UAE. However, hysteroscopic surgery has additional risks and costs owing to the anaesthesia and hysteroscopy procedures. For an inexperienced surgeon, operative hysteroscopic management of CSP might be very difficult. There is no agreement on the optimum management of CSP; treatment should be individualised, and some conditions must be carefully considered and discussed before making a therapy plan with the patient, including the patient's age, history of gestation, haemodynamic stability, size of gestational tissue, serum β-hCG level, and desire for future fertility. Whatever treatment is selected, follow-up with symptoms, serum β-hCG level, and uterus ultrasound are necessary to ensure complete resolution of the pregnancy. It is important to carry out high-quality, large-sample, longer follow-up trials to reach more definitive conclusions.

Abbreviations

CNY: China Yuan; CS: Caesarean section; CSP: Caesarean scar pregnancy; D&C: Dilation and curettage; MRI: Magnetic resonance imaging; MTX: Methotrexate; TAS: Transabdominal sonography; TVS: transvaginal sonography; UAE: Uterine artery embolisation; β-HCG: Beta-human chorionic gonadotropin

Acknowledgements

None.

Funding

None.

Authors' contributions

ZDQ designed the study, collected the patients' information, performed statistical analysis, and drafted the manuscript. YW collected the patients' information and drafted the manuscript. YJD and CFW collected the patients' information and performed statistical analysis. LLH designed the study and drafted the manuscript. All authors read and approved the final manuscript.

Competing interests

The authors declare that they have no competing interests.

Author details

[1]Women's Hospital, School of Medicine, Zhejiang University, 1 Xueshi Road, Hangzhou, Zhejiang Province 310006, People's Republic of China. [2]Maternal and Child Health Institute of Lin'an City, 25 Jiangnan Road, Lin'an, Zhejiang Province 311300, People's Republic of China.

References

1. Larsen JV, Solomon MH. Pregnancy in a uterine scar sacculus: an unusual case of postabortal hemorrhage. South Afr Med J. 1978;53:142–3.
2. Rotas MA, Haberman S, Levgur M. Cesarean scar ectopic pregnancies: etiology, diagnosis, and management. Obstet Gynecol. 2006;107:1373–81.
3. Ash A, Smith A, Maxwell D. Caesarean scar pregnancy. BJOG. 2007;114:253–63.
4. Timor-Trisch IE, Monteagudo A. Unforeseen consequences of the increasing rate of cesarean deliveries: early placenta accreta and cesarean scar pregnancy: a review. Am J Obstet Gynecol. 2012;297:14–29.
5. Wang JH, Qian ZD, Zhuang YL, Du YJ, Zhu LH, Huang LL. Risk factors for intraoperative hemorrhage at evacuation of a cesarean scar pregnancy following uterine artery embolization. Int J Gynaecol Obstet. 2013;123:240–3.
6. Maymon R, Halperin R, Mendlovic S, Schneider D, Herman A. Ectopic pregnancies in a caesarean scar: review of the medical approach to an iatrogenic complication. Hum Reprod Update. 2004;10:515–23.
7. Arslan M, Pata O, Dilek TU, Aktas A, Aban M, Dilek S. Treatment of viable cesarean scar ectopic pregnancy with suction curettage. Int J Gynaecol Obstet. 2005;89:163–6.
8. Huang L, Du Y, Zhao C. High-intensity focused ultrasound combined with dilatation and curettage for cesarean scar pregnancy. Ultrasound Obstet Gynecol. 2014;43:98–101.
9. Tekin YB, Ural UM, Balık G, Ustuner I, Şahin FK, Güven ESG. Management of cesarean scar pregnancy with suction curettage: a report of four cases and review of the literature. Arch Gynecol Obstet. 2014;289:1171–5.
10. Zhuang YL, Huang LL. Uterine artery embolization compared with methotrexate for the management of pregnancy implanted within a cesarean scar. Am J Obstet Gynecol. 2009;201:152.e1–3.
11. Yin X, Su S, Dong B, Ban Y, Li C, Sun B. Angiographic uterine artery chemoembolization followed by vacuum aspiration: an efficient and safe treatment for managing complicated cesarean scar pregnancy. Arch Gynecol Obstet. 2012;285:1313–8.
12. Wang CJ, Yuen LT, Chao AS, Lee CL, Yen CF, Soong YK. Caesarean scar pregnancy successfully treated by operative hysteroscopy and suction curettage. BJOG. 2005;112:839–40.
13. Wang CJ, Chao AS, Yuen LT, Wang CW, Soong YK, Lee CL. Endoscopic management of cesarean scar pregnancy. Fertil Steril. 2006;85:494. e1–4
14. Wang CJ, Tsai F, Chen C, Chao A. Hysteroscopic management of heterotopic cesarean scar pregnancy. Fertil Steril. 2010;94:1529. e15–18
15. Deans R, Abbott J. Hysteroscopic management of cesarean scar ectopic pregnancy. Fertil Steril. 2010;93:1735–40.
16. Wang G, Liu X, Bi F, Yin L, Sa R, Wang D, et al. Evaluation of the efficacy of laparoscopic resection for the management of exogenous cesarean scar pregnancy. Fertil Steril. 2014;101:1501–7.

17. Kim K, Pietrzak A, Gonzalez S, Podgony K. Severe hemorrhage in a first-trimester cesarean scar pregnancy during dilation and curettage. Int J Obstet Anesth. 2010;19:348–9.
18. Sadeghi H, Rutherford T, Rackow BW, Campbell KH, Duzyj CM, Guess MK, et al. Cesarean scar ectopic pregnancy: case series and review of the literature. Am J Perinatol. 2010;27:111–20.
19. Chao A, Wang TH, Wang CJ, Lee CL, Chao AS. Hysteroscopic management of cesarean scar pregnancy after unsuccessful methotrexate treatment. J Minim Invasive Gynecol. 2005;12:374–6.
20. Chou YM, Wu D, Wu KY, Lee CL. Hysteroscopic removal of cesarean scar pregnancy after methotrexate treatment failure. Gynecol Minim Invasive Ther. 2013;2:70–2.
21. Zhang B, Jiang ZB, Huang MS, Guan SH, Zhu KS, Qian JS, et al. Uterine artery embolization combined with methotrexate in the treatment of cesarean scar pregnancy: results of a case series and review of the literature. J Vasc Interv Radiol. 2012;23:1582–8.
22. Fylstra DL. Ectopic pregnancy within a cesarean scar: a review. Obstet Gynecol Surv. 2002;57:537–43.
23. Herman A, Weinraub Z, Avrech O, Maymon R, Ron-Ei R, Bukovsky Y. Follow up and outcome of isthmic pregnancy located in a previous caesarean section scar. Br J Obstet Gynaecol. 1995;102:839–41.
24. Jurkovic D, Knez J, Appiah A, Farahani L, Mavrelos D, Ross JA. Surgical treatment of cesarean scar ectopic pregnancy: efficacy and safety of ultrasound-guided suction curettage. Ultrasound Obstet Gynecol. 2016;47:511–7.
25. Ben Nagi J, Ofili-Yebovi D, Sawyer E, Aplin J, Jurkovic D. Successful treatment of a recurrent cesarean scar ectopic pregnancy by surgical repair of the uterine defect. Ultrasound Obstet Gynecol. 2006;28:855–6.
26. Robinson JK, Dayal MB, Gindoff P, Frankfurter D. A novel surgical treatment for cesarean scar pregnancy: laparoscopically assisted operative hysteroscopy. Fertil Steril. 2009;92:1497. e13–6
27. Fylstra DL. Hysteroscopy and suction evacuation of cesarean scar pregnancies: a case report and review. J Obstet Gynaecol Res. 2014;40:853–7.
28. Billieux MH, Petignat P, Anguenot JL, Campama A, Bischof P. Early and late half-life of human chorionic gonadotropin as a predictor of persistent trophoblast after laparoscopic conservative surgery for tubal pregnancy. Acta Obstet Gynecol Scand. 2008;82:550–5.

16

Trial of labour or elective repeat caesarean delivery: are women making an informed decision at Kenyatta national hospital?

Phocas Biraboneye S[1*], Omondi Ogutu[2], Jos van Roosmalen[3], Samson Wanjala[4], Kizito Lubano[5] and John Kinuthia[6]

Abstract

Background: Trial of labour is a safe option for most women after one previous caesarean delivery. However, the proportion of women attempting trial of labour after previous caesarean delivery (TOLAC) has been declining in many countries. In addition, women with prior caesarean delivery appear to know little regarding their mode of delivery and healthcare providers' recommendations. The doctors' preferences exert a strong influence on patient's decision whether or not to pursue TOLAC. In Kenya, it is unclear whether women who opt for trial of labour after caesarean delivery (TOLAC) or elective repeat caesarean delivery (ERCD) do that based on clear understanding of risks and benefits of both modes of delivery. This study aimed at determining whether patients with one previous caesarean delivery make an informed decision on preferred mode of delivery following their interactions with doctors.

Methods: A cross-sectional descriptive study was carried out on 202 pregnant women with one previous caesarean delivery at Kenyatta National Hospital (KNH) antenatal clinic. Data was collected from both the patients' records and women were interviewed using a structured questionnaire.

Results: Out of 202 women with mean age of 30.2 years 136 (67.2%) chose Elective Repeat Caesarean Delivery (ERCD), while 66 (32.8%) opted for TOLAC. Only 61/202 (30.6%; 95% C.I: 24.4 to 37.6%) made informed decisions. Few women (65: 32.2%) knew that the chance of successful TOLAC was high (60-80%) and 97 (48%) were not aware of the chances for a successful TOLAC. More than half of the women (109: 53.9%) were unaware of the risk of uterine rupture after one previous delivery and only few patients (64: 31.7%) knew that the risk of uterine rupture in TOLAC is low (< 1%). The majority of the women (112: 55.4%) did not know that the indications for previous caesarean delivery are an important factor in determining the chance of a successful Vaginal Birth after Caesarean Delivery (VBAC). For 47(23.3%) of the women, there was no documented indication for the previous caesarean delivery. The women's mode of delivery was significantly associated with the preference of the counseling doctor ($p < 0.001$) and their qualification ($p = 0.020$). Only 23 (11.4%) women signed the consent form for ERCD while none of the women for TOLAC signed any consent form.

Conclusions: There was an overall lack of information on both modes of delivery while doctor's preferences affected women's decisions. Only just under one third of the women made an informed decision. There is a need to develop clear standard protocols and checklists for information to be disseminated to doctors and all patients with previous caesarean deliveries in subsequent pregnancies in Kenya.

* Correspondence: biraboneye@gmail.com

[1]Department of Obstetrics and Gynaecology, Jeanne de Navarre Hospital Center, Château-Thierry, France

Full list of author information is available at the end of the article

Background

A successful trial of labour culminating in vaginal birth, a failed trial resulting in an emergency repeat caesarean delivery, or an elective repeat caesarean delivery are the three possible outcomes for the woman who has had a prior caesarean section. Planning the mode of delivery should be addressed early during prenatal care, and can begin even pre-conceptionally. With either approach, women who have undergone a prior caesarean delivery are at risk for serious maternal and perinatal complications and should be counselled about these risks [1].

In the USA, Federal Acts and regulations as well as professional guidelines clearly demonstrate that every pregnant woman has the right to base her maternity care decisions on accurate, up-to-date, comprehensible information [2]. Informed consent is "the willing acceptance of a medical intervention by a patient after adequate disclosure by the physician of the nature of the intervention and its alternatives with its risks and benefits " [3, 4]. It is thus more than just signing a consent form.

The decision for elective repeat caesarean delivery or trial of labour should be made by the woman in consultation with her provider. Both clinicians and patients desire individualized information about the chance of successful TOLAC and the balance between the risk of maternal or foetal morbidity if TOLAC is unsuccessful and the risk of maternal and foetal morbidity with ERCD [5]. Women in the USA report that their healthcare providers' recommendations and preferences exert a strong influence on their decision whether or not to pursue TOLAC [6].

This information is also important on a population level, especially in the setting of rising caesarean delivery rates, as selection of candidates who are most likely to deliver vaginally after a previous operation can minimize the costs of ERCD and failed TOLAC [5]. In fact, improving patient education may not affect the increasing section rate; it would, however, empower women to make a well informed, educated decision [7].

The aim of this study was to determine whether patients with one previous caesarean delivery were making an informed decision about their preferred mode of delivery at "Kenyatta National Hospital".

Methods

Study sites

The study was conducted in the Antenatal Clinic at KNH, which is the national referral hospital located in Nairobi. It is also the main teaching hospital for the College of Health Sciences, University of Nairobi. The hospital caters for patients from Nairobi and its neighbourhoods as well as referrals from other hospitals in the country.

Study design

This was a cross-sectional descriptive study that targeted pregnant women with one previous caesarean delivery attending ANC at KNH for delivery from September 2013 to January 2014. On average approximately 50 women with one previous caesarean delivery attend ANC per month.

Data collection

Consenting women completed structured questionnaires to assess their demographic characteristics, awareness about risks and benefits of both modes of delivery, doctors' preferences, knowledge about complications following prior caesarean delivery as well as indications of previous caesarean delivery, and knowledge about the mode of delivery in the current pregnancy. Data abstraction was also done from patients' records through a structured questionnaire to assess parity, level of provider, family planning goals, and relevant clinical examination including estimated foetal weight, obstetrical ultrasound data, timing on decision of mode of delivery and any other medical or obstetric complication (Additional file 1).

Statistical analysis

Data was entered into a micro-computer through Epidata designed database and exported to STATA 11.0 and Statistical Package for Social Science (SPSS-20) for analysis. Comparative analysis focused on patient knowledge, baseline characteristics, obstetric characteristics and antenatal care provided, and chosen mode of delivery. $P < 0.05$ was considered statistically significant.

Ethics

Approval was obtained from the KNH/UoN Ethics and Research committee before carrying out the study. Informed consent of women was obtained before participating in the study. Antenatal care was provided to all women regardless of whether they consented or declined to participate in the study. The records were coded and anonymised. The information collected remained confidential and was only used for the purpose of the study. No incentives were given to the study subjects.

Results

Socio-demographic characteristics

A total of 202 women participated in the study with a mean age of 30.2 years. The highest proportion of women (77; 38.1%) was in the group between 30 and 34 years (Table 1). Most women were married (94%). Many women (n = 92; 45.6%) had secondary level of education and 46% of the participants were self-employed. The majority of women with one previous caesarean delivery were para one (75.7%). The outcome

Table 1 Socio-demographic characteristics of the study participants

Parameters	N (%)
Woman's age (years)	
20-24	25 (12.4%)
25-29	64 (31.7%)
30-34	77 (38.1%)
> 35	36 (17.8%)
Educational level	
Primary	38 (18.8%)
Secondary	92 (45.6%)
University	72 (35.6%)
Marital Status	
Married	190 (94.0%)
Single	10 (5.0%)
Separated	2 (1.0%)
Occupation	
Employed	49 (24.3%)
Business /self employed	92 (45.5%)
Student	2 (1%)
Housewive	59 (29.2%)

Table 2 Obstetric characteristics of the study participants

Parameters	N (%)
Woman's parity	
1	153 (75.7%)
2-3	45 (22.3%)
> 3	4 (2%)
Outcome of previous caesarean delivery	
live infant	166 (82.1%)
Live infant in distress	4 (2%)
Premature baby	1 (0.5%)
Still birth	11 (5.4%)
Neonatal death	10 (5%)
Infant death	6 (3%)
Not documented	4 (2%)
Medical or obstetrical complications after the previous c/s according to the participant's interview (n = 32)	
Bleeding (PPH)	3 (7.9%)
Eclampsia	8 (21.1%)
Maternal infections	8 (21.1%)
Death of the baby(neonatal death)	15 (39.5%)
Burst abdomen	3 (7.9%)
Post partum psychosis	1 (2.6%)
Women's family planning method choice following the current delivery	
Bilateral Tubal Ligation	12 (5.9%)
Natural	1 (0.5%)
Pills	6 (3%)
Injections	2 (1%)
Not yet decided	181 (89.6%)
Women's preferred mode of delivery before attending KNH	
Trial of labour	86 (42.6%)
Elective repeat c/s	95 (47.0%)
Not sure	17 (8.4%)
Any	4 (2.0%)

of the previous caesarean delivery was a live birth for 82.1%. About 15.8% (n = 32) reported medical or obstetric complications following the previous caesarean delivery, with 39.5% among them reporting early neonatal death. The majority of the women (89.6%) opted for no contraceptive choice following the current delivery, with only 5.9% of the women preferring bilateral tubal ligation. Before attending ANC –KNH, 47% of the patients preferred ERCD as mode of delivery while 42.6% of the patients preferred TOLAC (Table 2).

Antenatal clinical assessment

Non reassuring foetal heart rate (NRFS) was the most common indication for the previous caesarean delivery documented at 27.2% (Table 3). However, for 23.3% of the women there was no documented indication. The medical or obstetric complications postpartum were not documented for the majority (98%). During the time of decision of mode of delivery, the estimated foetal birth weight was not documented in 90.6% and only 11.4% of the consent forms for ERCD was signed and documented in the file, while patients for TOLAC did not sign any consent form.

Participants' knowledge on risks and benefits of both modes of delivery.

On complications of surgery, most women knew little about complications of anaesthesia (8.3%), injury to organs, severe haemorrhage, hysterectomy and even maternal death (1.1%) as associated risks of repeat caesarean delivery.

Only 32.2% of the women knew that the overall chances of success of TOLAC is >50%. Regarding the risks of uterine scar rupture, more than half of the women (53.9%) did not know about this risk, while only 31.7% knew that the risk is very low (< 1%), but increasing with the number of repeat caesarean deliveries (Table 4). More than half of the women (55.4%) did not know that the reasons for previous caesarean delivery are an important factor in determining the chance of successful TOLAC.

The majority of the participants (70.3%) had attended ANC at KNH more than three times and in 62.4% of the

Table 3 Antenatal clinical assessment of women with one previous caesarean delivery attending KNH ANC

Parameters	*N* (%)
Medical or obstetrical complication documented during ANC	
Preeclampsia	8 (4%)
Diabetes	2 (1%)
Anemia	1 (0.5%)
HIV-positive	7 (3.4%)
Placenta praevia	2 (1%)
Malpresentation	5 (2.5%)
Fibroids	5 (2.5%)
No complication documented/indicated	172 (85.1%)
Documented reasons for the previous caesarean delivery	
CPD/big baby	31 (15.3%)
Malpresentation	15 (7.4%)
APH	4 (2%)
Failed induction	18 (8.9%)
Prolonged labour	32 (15.8%)
Non reassuring foetal distress	55 (27.2%)
Not documented	47 (23.3%)
Medical or obstetrical complication postpartum documented after the previous caesarean delivery	
Infections	2 (1%)
Preeclampsia	2 (1%)
Not documented	198 (98%)
Estimated foetal birth weight (Kg) clinically or by U/S documented at the time of the decision of mode of delivery	
< 3.5	15 (7.4%)
≥ 3.5	4 (2%)
Not documented	183 (90.6%)
Consent form signed and documented in the file at the time of decision for mode of delivery	
Yes (Women admitted for ERCD from ANC)	23 (11.4%)
Booked in elective diary	92 (45.8%)
Not documented	86 (42.8%)

cases women were informed on ERCD as the only mode of delivery.

Few women knew that a classical scar (7 out of 116) and unavailability of 24 h theatre and skilled providers (1/116) are reasons to consider recommending ERCD (Table 5). The majority of doctors at ANC- KNH were senior house officers (174: 86.1%), while consultants were represented at 28 (13.9%).

The decision made on mode of delivery during ANC was ERCD in 136 (67.2%) women and trial of labour in 66 (32.8%). After counselling during ANC a significant reduction in the choice of TOLAC was observed from 42.6% to 32.8% with an increase from 47% to 67.2% of ERCD (Table 6).

Table 4 Knowledge on risks and benefits of both modes of delivery amongst one previous caesarean delivery women attending KNH ANC

Parameters	*N* (%)
Women's knowledge on risks associated with repeat C/S than TOLAC (*n* = 163)	
Increased blood loss	124 (28.4%)
High risk of infection	106 (24.3%)
Complication of anaesthesia	36 (8.3%)
Uterine scar rupture in case of big baby	10 (2.3%)
Injury to organs	5 (1.1%)
Recovery is longer	140 (32.2%)
Limb numbness	15 (3.4%)
Women's knowledge on risks associated with TOLAC than ERCD (*n* = 155)	
Uterine scar rupture resulting in emergency C/S	54 (20.8%)
Failed trial of labour	114 (44%)
Uterine rupture is > with VBAC than repeat C/S	81 (31.3%)
Increased blood loss	5 (1.9%)
Increased risk of infection	2 (0.8%)
Foetal death	3 (1.2%)
Women's knowledge regarding overall chances of success of TOLAC	
Very high (>50%)	65 (32.2%)
Very low (<25%)	40 (19.8%)
Don't know	97 (48%)
Women's knowledge regarding the risks of uterine scar rupture	
Very low (<1%) but increased with number of c/s	64 (31.7%)
Very high (>50%)	29 (14.4%)
Don't know	109 (53.9%)
Women's knowledge on recovery from vaginal delivery against repeat C/S	
Same	1 (0.5%)
Longer for repeat C/S	166 (82.2%)
Longer for vaginal delivery	2 (1%)
I don't know	33 (16.3%)
Reasons for previous C/S as important factor in determining the chance of successful TOLAC according to the participants	
Yes	60 (29.7%)
No	30 (14.9%)
Don't know	112 (55.4%)

In Table 7, the minimum proposed criteria for informed decision on mode of delivery at KNH are given. On average, it was reported that 61 (30.2%; 95% CI: 24 to 37%) of the women were making informed decisions.

There was no association with preferred mode of delivery in terms of women's age (p = 0.654), level of education (p = 0.224), marital status (p = 0.419) number of ANC visits (p = 0.574), patient's parity (p = 0.286, and

Table 5 Number of antenatal visits and information provided to women with one previous caesarean delivery attending KNH ANC

Parameters	*N* (%)
Number of ANC visits at the time of recruitment	
< 3	60 (29.7%)
≥ 3	142 (70.3%)
Women informed on available options of mode of delivery	
Elective repeat c/s	126 (62.4%)
Trial of labour	61 (30.2%)
None	15 (7.4%)
Women counselled on reasons for ERCD against TOLAC (*n* = 116)	
Big baby (>3.5 kg)	21 (18.1%)
Classical scar	7 (6%)
Small pelvis	15 (12.9%)
Unavailability of 24 h theatre/blood transfusion/skilled doctors and anaesthetists	1 (0.9%)
Mal-presentation/breech presentation	11 (9.5%)
Bad obstetric history	3 (2.6%)
Choice of BTL	2 (1.7%)
Placenta praevia	21 (18.1%)
Don't know	35 (30.2%)
Women counselled at discharge after previous C/S on reasons ERCD is recommended in subsequent pregnancy (*n* = 19)	
Small pelvis	13 (68.5%)
Classical uterine incision	2 (10.5%)
High risk of uterine rupture if any VBAC	2 (10.5%)
BTL would also be offered	2 (10.5%)
Counselling doctor preferred mode of delivery (perception of the participant)	
None	44 (21.8%)
Elective repeat caesarean section	107 (53%)
Trial of labour	51 (25.2%)
Level of provider at ANC KNH	
Senior house officer	174 (86.1%)
Consultant obstetrician	28 (13.9%)

patient occupation (p = 0.795).The following correlates were, however, significantly associated with the preferred mode of delivery: counselling doctor preferred mode of delivery ($p < 0.001$), women preferred mode of delivery before attending KNH ($p < 0.001$) and level of care provider (p = 0.02) (Table 8).

No association with preferred mode of delivery was found in terms of estimated foetal birth weight at the time of decision (p = 0.372) and knowledge on risks associated with repeat CS as compared to TOLAC (p = 0.482). However, knowledge of women regarding overall chances of success of TOLAC ($p < 0.001$), risk of uterine rupture in TOLAC ($p < 0.001$) and women's knowledge on recovery from vaginal delivery against

Table 6 Decision or choice of TOLAC and ERCD before attending KNH ANC and after counseling

Before KNH-ANC visit (TOLAC)	After ANC visit (TOLAC)		
	Yes	No	Total
Yes	58	28	86 (42.6%)
No	8	108	116
Total	66 (32.8%)	136	
Before KNH-ANC visit (ERCD)	After ANC visit (ERCD)		
	Yes	No	
Yes	91	4	95 (47%)
No	45	62	107
Total	136 (67.2%)	66	

repeat caesarean delivery ($p < 0.001$) were significantly associated with the preferred mode of delivery (Table 9).

Discussion

The study findings show that few women chose TOLAC and even fewer were making an informed decision. Most women preferred repeat caesarean delivery before attending ANC at KNH and this was significantly associated with the patient's choice after ANC counseling. Equally, women's mode of delivery was significantly linked with the preference of the counselling doctor and their qualification. Women appear to know little about their mode of delivery.

However, this study did not establish an association between preferred mode of delivery and women's demographic characteristics (age, educational level, marital status, occupation, parity) and number of antenatal visits.

A small number of women chose TOLAC probably because of inadequate information and influence of the counselling doctor from ANC. A recent study published by Sarah and collaborators has demonstrated the same findings [6]. The majority of the women did not make an informed decision at KNH and this was probably because of lack of adequate information provided in ANC or largely due to poor women counselling. This study proposes minimum criteria for an informed decision in a woman with one previous caesarean delivery attending KNH. No similar studies involving clear criteria to determine whether they are making informed decisions have been performed.

However, worldwide the practice of obstetrics and gynecology has always faced special ethical questions in the implementation of informed consent [2]. More studies need to be done for a generalization of the proposed criteria. Most of the women did not know the overall chances of success (60-80%) and the risks of uterine rupture (<1%) with TOLAC. These findings are different from the study done by Sarah and collaborators in USA

Table 7 Minimum criteria for a woman with one previous caesarean delivery to make an informed decision on mode of delivery at KNH

Criteria	*N* (%)
Women informed on mode of delivery (available options) (*n* = 202)	
TOLAC	61 (30.2%)
ERCD	126 (62.4%)
Both	0
Women's knowledge on factors influencing mode of delivery (*n* = 116)	
Classical scar as a reason for ERCD	7 (6%)
Small pelvis as a reason for ERCD	15 (12.9%)
Big baby as a reason for ERCD	21 (18.1%)
Current medical or obstetric complications as a reason for ERCD	30 (25.9%)
Adequacy of facility for delivery (A 24 h-theater…)	1 (0.9%)
Women's knowledge on success and risk of uterine rupture in TOLAC (*n* = 202)	
Patient knowledge on overall chance of TOLAC success	65 (32.2%)
Patient knowledge on risk of uterine rapture in TOLAC	64 (31.7%)
Reasons of previous caesarean as factor of success for TOLAC	60 (29.7%)
Women's knowledge on risks of ERCD over TOLAC (*n* = 163)	
Increased blood loss	124 (76.1%)
High risk of infection	106 (65.0%)
Complication of anaesthesia	36 (22.1%)
Injury to organ	5 (3.1%)
Recovery is longer	140 (85.9%)
Consent form signed and documented in the patient file (*n* = 202)	23 (11.4%)

Table 8 Antenatal and obstetric correlates associated with the preferred mode of delivery amongst one previous caesarean delivery women attending KNH ANC

Parameters	ERCD *n* = 136	TOLAC *n* = 66	*P*-value
Women's parity			
1	104 (76.5%)	49 (74.2%)	0.286
2-3	28 (20.6%)	17 (25.8%)	
> 3	4 (2.9%)	0	
Number of ANC visits at the time of recruitment			
< 3	35 (26.3%)	19 (30.2%)	0.574
≥ 3	98 (73.7%)	44 (69.8%)	
Counselling doctor preferred mode of delivery			
None	29 (21.3%)	15 (22.7%)	0.001
Repeat caesarean section	107 (78.7%)	0	
Vaginal delivery	0	51 (77.3%)	
Women's preferred mode of delivery before attending KNH			
Trial of labour	28 (20.6%)	58 (87.9%)	0.001
Elective repeat c/s	91 (66.9%)	4 (6.1%)	
Not sure	14 (10.3%)	3 (4.5%)	
Any	3 (2.2%)	1 (1.5%)	
Level of provider at ANC KNH			
Senior house officer	123 (90.4%)	51 (78.5%)	0.020
Consultant	13 (9.6%)	14 (21.5%)	

[6] and the difference is probably due to Sarah's questionnaire administered to the women at admission and not immediately during the antenatal visits.

There was a significant correlation with women's preferred mode of delivery before attending ANC KNH and chosen mode of delivery after ANC counseling ($p < 0.001$). This was probably due to alternative sources of information and poor antenatal education regarding both modes of delivery. Most factors influencing mode of delivery in women not counselled on mode of delivery during antenatal visits were identified as friend advice and internet information. No similar study has shown the alternative source of information besides health providers counselling on decision making. In this study majority of the senior house officers were offering repeat caesarean delivery due to probably less experience and lack of standard guidelines in management of a woman with one previous caesarean delivery.

According to Wells (2010), physicians that did not offer VBAC were also more likely to be practicing <10 years, have been involved in a law suit related to caesarean delivery or have experienced uterine rupture with maternal or foetal complications [8]. Most inexperienced providers tend to have bias towards informed consent of patients with one previous caesarean delivery. In addition, some patients having limited understanding of pregnancy and child birth would be easily influenced by the most senior doctors. However some challenges associated with informed consent are to be remembered: information that may be considered necessary or desirable in formally educated urban populations may be of little relevance in less formally educated or rural populations, or vice versa. Also, in some cultures it might not be customary to provide certain forms of information, such as describing uncertainty about the effectiveness of the treatment, or information about possible alternative treatments.

Some of the providers therefore apply the dictum of Craigin: "Once a caesarean, always a caesarean" [9]. Because informed consent laws and principles do not specify the amount of information that must be disclosed, physicians might find it useful to know what they have to disclose.

In literature, advanced maternal age, single marital status and less than 12 years education are associated with a reduced likelihood of successful TOLAC [10]. In addition, this study found a limited documentation in patient's files. Proper documentation is a useful tool in

Table 9 Women's knowledge correlates associated with the preferred mode of delivery amongst one previous caesarean delivery patients attending KNH ANC

Parameters	ERCD *n* = 136	TOLAC *n* = 66	*P*-value
Women's knowledge regarding the risks of uterine scar rupture			
Very low (<1%) but increased with number of c/s	17 (26.6%)	47 (73.4%)	0.001
Very high (>50%)	27 (93.1%)	2 (6.9%)	
Don't know	92 (84.4%)	17 (15.6%)	
Women's knowledge regarding overall chances of success of TOLAC			
Very high (>50%)	12 (8.8%)	53 (80.3%)	0.001
Very low (<25%)	40 (29.4%)	0	
Don't know	84 (61.8%)	13 (19.7%)	
Women's knowledge on recovery from vaginal delivery against repeat C/S			
Same	-	1 (1.5%)	0.001
Longer for repeat C/S	103 (75.7%)	63 (95.5%)	
Longer for a vaginal delivery	2 (1.5%)	0	
I don't know	31 (22.8%)	2 (3%)	
Estimated foetal birth weight in Kg clinically or by U/S at the time of the decision of mode of delivery			
< 3.5	10 (7.4%)	5 (7.6%)	0.372
≥ 3.5	4 (2.9%)	-	
Not documented	122 (89.7%)	61 (92.4%)	
Women's awareness on risks associated with repeat C/S than TOLAC			
Increased blood loss	76 (26.6%)	48 (32%)	0.482
High risk of infection	65 (22.7%)	41 (27.3%)	
Complication of anaesthesia	26 (9.1%)	10 (6.8%)	
Rupture in case of big baby	8 (2.8%)	2 (1.3%)	
Injury to organs	3 (1%)	2 (1.3%)	
Recovery is longer	96 (33.6%)	44 (29.3%)	
Limb numbness	12 (4.2%)	3 (2%)	

informed consent. Without proper documentation a patient may not get adequate and relevant information. Researchers have also shown that the patients may not accurately remember all the facts disclosed in a discussion [11, 12] In practice, there is no consent form for TOLAC patients available in Kenya. Few patients signed the consent form for ERCD while none did for TOLAC. Consent forms should be available at the moment of decision to prove that the patient was given information, understood and consented.

Some of the main limitations of this study are the small sample size and lack of standardization in women counselling. However, this study has two major strengths: it is original and proposes minimum criteria for an informed decision in women with prior caesarean delivery attending KNH. Data was obtained from an institution offering VBAC and the population was not only more educated but also more urbanized and middle class than the average across the country. The results may therefore represent a better informed population suggesting wider knowledge gaps throughout the country. This study should be considered as a preliminary evaluation of current practice and patterns. It is intended therefore, to provoke further interest in the subject of making informed decisions by women with previous caesarean deliveries.

Conclusions and recommendations

Conclusions

There is overall lack of information on both modes of delivery while doctor's preference affects patient's decision. There is lack of documentation in patient's files as well on minimum proposed criteria for informed decision at KNH.

Recommendations

Develop a standard protocol and policy for management of women with a previous caesarean section attending KNH. Need for training of providers using such a protocol on the importance of documentation.

Abbreviation

ANC: Antenatal Clinic; C/S: Cesarean Section; ERC: Ethics Research Committee; ERCD: Elective Repeat Cesarean Delivery; KNH: Kenyatta National Hospital; MD: Medical Doctor; MMed: Master in Medicine; RCD: Repeat Cesarean Delivery; RCOG: Royal College of Obstetricians and Gynecologists; SPSS: Statistical Package for Social Science; TOL: Trial of Labor; TOLAC: Trial of Labor after Cesarean Delivery; USA: United States of America; VBAC: Vaginal Birth after Cesarean Delivery

Acknowledgements

We wish to thank the Research program Kenyatta National Hospital for providing financial support. Also acknowledged is KNH- Reproductive Health Department for allowing the study to be conducted in the Antenatal clinic. Thanks and appreciation to Dr. Anne Marie Biraboneye, Dr. Humphrey Kunda, Dr. Jessica Uwera, Dr. Louise Kpoto and Dr. David Thuo who ploughed through several preliminary versions of the study findings, making critical suggestions and posing challenging questions. Last but not least, lots of thanks to all women who attended KNH ANC during the period of data collection, this work would not have been feasible if they did not consent.

Funding

The Research program Kenyatta National Hospital provided only the financial support during data collection and no incentive given to the authors as well to the study participants.

Authors' contributions

PBS Conception and design; Acquisition of data; Analysis and interpretation of data; Drafting and revising the article and; Approval of the final version and Accountable for all aspects of the work. OO Design and acquisition of data; Analysis and interpretation of data; Drafting and revising the article; Approval of the final version and Accountable for all aspects of the work. JVR Drafting the article and revising it critically; Approval of the final version and Accountable for all aspects of the work. SW Interpretation of data; Approval of the final version and Accountable for all aspects of the work. KL Analysis and interpretation, Approval of the final version and Accountable for all aspects of the work. JK Revising the first draft, Approval of the final version and Accountable for all aspects of the work.

Competing interests

The authors declare that they have no competing interests.

Author details

[1]Department of Obstetrics and Gynaecology, Jeanne de Navarre Hospital Center, Château-Thierry, France. [2]Department of Obstetrics and Gynaecology, University of Nairobi, Nairobi, Kenya. [3]Athena Institute, VU University Amsterdam, Amsterdam, The Netherlands. [4]Department of Obstetrics and Gynaecology, University of Nairobi, Nairobi, Kenya. [5]Kenya Medical Research Institute, Nairobi, Kenya. [6]Department of research and programs, Kenyatta National Hospital, Nairobi, Kenya.

References

1. Wells EC, Cunningham GF. Choosing the route of vaginal delivery. www.uptodate.com. Accessed 4 Aug 2014.
2. ACOG. Updates of ethical decision making in obstetrics and gynaecology in ethics obstetrics and gynaecology. 2004.
3. Paul S, Appelbaum M. Assessment of patients 'competence to consent to treatment. N Engl J Med. 2007;357:1834.
4. Michael S, Anthony B, Jillann F, et al. The guide to informed decision-making in healthcare. 1st ed; 2012. https://www.health.qld.gov.au/consent/documents/ic-guide.pdf consulted August 2014.
5. Torri DM. Use of calculators for predicting successful of labour after caesarean delivery. Up-to-date. 2014.
6. Sarah N, Matalon S, Rosenn B, et al. Trial of labour versus repeat: are patients making an informed decision? Am J Obstet Gynecol. 2012;207:204.
7. The American Academy of Pediatrics and the American College of Obstetricians and Gynecologists. Guidelines for Perinatal Care. J Contin Educ Heal Prof. 2007;8(2):111.
8. Wells C. Vaginal birth after delivery: views from a private practitioner. Semin Perinatol. 2010;34:245.
9. Edwin C. Conservatism in obstetrics. New York Medical Journal. 1916;104:1.
10. Srinivas SK, Stamilio DM, Samuel MD, et al. Vaginal birth after caesarean delivery: does maternal age affect safety and success? Paediatr Perinat Epidemiol. 2007;21:114.
11. Robinson G, Meray A. Informed consent: recall by patients tested postoperatively. Ann Thorac Surg. 1976;22:209.
12. Herz DA, Looman JE, Lewis SK. Informed consent: is it a myth. Neurosurgery. 1992;30:453.

Cesarean section to prevent mother-to-child transmission of hepatitis B virus in China

Mei Yang[1†], Qin Qin[2,3†], Qiong Fang[1], Lixin Jiang[1] and Shaofa Nie[3*]

Abstract

Background: Hepatitis B virus (HBV) is predominantly transmitted through mother-to-child transmission (MTCT). To date, it remains unclear whether the method of parturition affects MTCT of HBV. In order to clarify whether cesarean section, when compared with vaginal delivery, could reduce the risk of MTCT of HBV in China, we conducted this meta-analysis.

Methods: A systematic literature search was performed of the PubMed (Medline), Embase, ISI Web of Science, China Biological Medicine Database, China National Knowledge Infrastructure, and VIP Database for Chinese Technical Periodicals databases for articles written in English or Chinese through July 2015.The reference lists of relevant articles were also scrutinized for additional papers. Randomized controlled trials, cohort studies, or case-control studies investigating the effect of delivery mode on MTCT of HBV were included.

Results: This analysis involved 28 articles containing 30 datasets. The data encompassed 9906 participants. The MTCT rate of HBV was 6.76% (670 of 9906) overall, with individual rates of 4.37% (223 of 5105) for mothers who underwent cesarean section and 9.31% (447 of 4801) for those who underwent vaginal delivery. The summary relative risk (RR) was 0.51 (95%CI: 0.44–0.60, $P < 0.001$), indicating a statistically significant decrease in HBV vertical transmission via cesarean section compared with vaginal delivery. The heterogeneity among studies was moderate with an I^2of29.3%.Publication bias was not detected by the Egger's and Begg's tests, and the funnel plot was symmetric. In the subgroup analyses, maternal hepatitis B e antigen status and follow-up time did not affect the significance of the results, but hepatitis B immune globulin (HBIG) administration to mother and infant did.

Conclusions: Cesarean section could reduce the risk of MTCT of HBV in comparison to vaginal delivery in China. However, owing to several limitations of our meta-analysis, future well-designed randomized controlled trials with adequate statistical power, might be a more appropriate next step.

Keywords: Cesarean section, Hepatitis B virus, Mother-to-child transmission, Meta-analysis

Background

Hepatitis B is a potentially life-threatening liver infection caused by hepatitis B virus (HBV). It is a major global health problem. It can cause chronic infection and puts people at high risk of death from cirrhosis and liver cancer. According to the World Health Organization, an estimated 240 million people have chronic hepatitis B infection [1]. More than 780,000 people die every year due to complications of hepatitis B infection, including cirrhosis and liver cancer [2]. Hepatitis B prevalence is highest in sub-Saharan Africa and East Asia, where 5–10% of the adult population is chronically infected. The infected population of China accounts for one-third of the infected population worldwide [3].

HBV is predominantly transmitted through mother-to-child transmission (MTCT). In China, 30–50% of HBV carriers are infected through vertical transmission [3, 4]. Since the introduction of universal screening of pregnant women, combined with passive and active immunoprophylaxis, the

* Correspondence: sf_nie@mails.tjmu.edu.cn
†Equal contributors
[3]Department of Epidemiology and Biostatistics, School of Public Health, Tongji Medical College, Huazhong University of Science and Technology, 13 Hangkong Road, Wuhan 430030, China
Full list of author information is available at the end of the article

MTCT rate of HBV has declined significantly. Passive immunoprophylaxis consists of the administration of hepatitis B immune globulin (HBIG) at birth, and active immunoprophylaxis is performed by the administration of the hepatitis B vaccine according to the standard 3-dose schedule. Although HBIG and vaccines given at birth are able to reduce transmission in most cases, in 10% to 20% of cases of infected mothers, transmission still occurs, especially from mothers with high viral loads and who are positive for hepatitis B e antigen (HBeAg) [5, 6].

Previous studies demonstrated that cesarean section might reduce the risk of MTCT for some viruses, such as human immunodeficiency virus and herpes simplex virus [7–9]. Numerous studies in China have sought to examine the relationship between delivery mode and rate of MTCT of HBV [10–16]. However, the effect of different delivery modes on MTCT of HBV remains unclear. To elucidate the question of whether cesarean section, as compared to vaginal delivery, may reduce the risk of MTCT of HBV, we conducted this meta-analysis.

Methods

Search strategy

A systematic literature search was performed of the PubMed (Medline), Embase, ISI Web of Science, China Biological Medicine Database, China National Knowledge Infrastructure, and VIP Database for ChineseTechnical Periodicals databases for articles written in English or Chinese through July 2015.The following search terms were used:"hepatitis B virus" or "HBV,", "mother-to-child transmission" or "vertical transmission", "cesarean section" or "vaginal delivery" or "natural delivery" or "delivery mode". We also scrutinized the reference lists of relevant articles included in our analysis and previous systematic reviews and meta-analyses for additional papers. We did not contact the authors of the primary studies for additional information.

Study selection

Studies were included in this meta-analysis if they satisfied the following criteria:

1) Studies were randomized controlled trials, cohort studies, or case-control studies; 2) the participants were pregnant mothers with chronic HBV infection, defined as maternal blood positive for HbsAg; 3) the intervention of interest was cesarean section and the comparison was vaginal delivery; 4) the outcome was vertical transmission of HBV, defined as infant HBsAg and/or HBV DNA positivity. Reviews, editorials, case reports/series, overlapping studies, and duplicates were excluded. We also excluded studies with patients co-infected with hepatitis C virus, hepatitis D virus, and/or human immunodeficiency virus. If the same population was studied in more than one study, we included the study with the largest sample size.

Quality assessment

Our study used a 9-score system based on the Newcastle-Ottawa Scale (NOS) to assess the original study quality. The maximum score of 9 points could be assigned to a study that had the highest methodological quality, with 4, 2, 3 scores respectively being assigned to selection of study groups, comparability of study groups, assessment of outcomes, and adequacy of follow-up. Studies with scores of 0–3, 4–6, or 7–9 were regarded as low, moderate, and high quality, respectively (Table 1).

Data extraction

Two authors (MY and QQ) independently conducted the data extraction process using a standard extraction form. When discrepancies arose, a third author (QF) was consulted. The following information was extracted from each study: first author's name, publication year, study area, study design, number of infants born by cesarean section or by vaginal delivery, number of infants positive for HBV born by cesarean section or by vaginal delivery, percentage of mothers positive for HBeAg (HBeAg+), intervention administered (HBIG and/or antiviral treatment), percent age of infants who received HBIG, percent age of infants who received the HBV vaccine as scheduled, and the follow-up time of the study.

Statistical analysis

In this meta-analysis, the relative risk (RR) and 95% confidence interval (CI) of HBV MTCT in cesarean section compared to vaginal delivery were considered as the effect size for all studies. Any results stratified by maternal HBeAg status were treated as two separate reports.

The heterogeneity between studies was assessed using the Cochran Q test and I^2 statistic [17]. For the I^2 metric, I^2 values of 25, 50, and 75% represent low, moderate, and high degrees of heterogeneity, respectively [18]. The fixed effect model (Mantel-Haenszel method) was applied to pool the effect when heterogeneity level was low; otherwise, the random effect model described by DerSimonian and Laird was utilized [19].

Subgroup analyses were conducted according to maternal HBeAg status, maternal HBIG administration and/or antiviral treatment, infant immunoprophylaxis status with HBIG, and follow-up time. Sensitivity analysis was performed by omitting one study at a time to examine the influence of each individual study on the overall relative risk. Publication bias was evaluated by Egger's regression test [20], Begg's adjusted rank correlation test [21], and visual inspection of the funnel plot. All tests were two-sided and $P < 0.05$ was considered

Table 1 Quality assessment of included studies

Studies	Selection				Comparability	Outcome			Total scores
	Representativeness of the exposed group	Selection of the unexposed group	Ascertainment of exposure	Outcome of interest not present at start of study	Control for important factor or additional factor	Outcome assessment	Follow-up long enough for outcome to occur	Adequacy of follow-up of cohorts	
Wang Qingtu, 2001 [45]	1	1	1	1	2	1	–	–	7
Wang Jianshe, 2002 [16]	1	1	1	1	2	1	1	1	9
Wang Lan, 2004 [44]	1	1	1	1	–	1	1	1	7
Wang Yuan, 2005 [43]	1	1	1	1	2	1	1	1	9
Gu Jie, 2006 [42]	1	1	1	1	2	1	1	1	9
Qian Yanhua, 2006 [41]	1	1	1	1	1	1	1	1	8
Fan Yi, 2007 [40]	1	1	1	1	2	1	1	1	9
Chen Jing1, 2007 [38]	1	1	1	1	1	1	1	1	8
Chen Jing2, 2007 [38]	1	1	1	1	1	1	1	1	8
Li Jijun1, 2007 [39]	1	1	1	1	1	1	1	1	8
Li Jijun2, 2007 [39]	1	1	1	1	1	1	1	1	8
Chen Hong, 2008 [37]	1	1	1	1	1	1	1	1	8
Liu Xia, 2008 [36]	1	1	1	1	–	1	1	1	7
Liu Honge, 2009 [35]	1	1	1	1	1	1	1	1	8
Zhang Qingying, 2009 [34]	1	1	1	1	2	1	1	1	9
Zhu Yunxia, 2010 [32]	1	1	1	1	2	1	1	1	9
Yang Peifang, 2010 [33]	1	1	1	1	2	1	1	1	9
Yang Xiaomei, 2011 [30]	1	1	1	1	2	1	1	1	9
Zhang Weili, 2011 [31]	1	1	1	1	1	1	1	1	8

Table 1 Quality assessment of included studies *(Continued)*

Huang Liu, 2012 [29]	1	1	1	1	2	1	1	1	9
Guo Zhen, 2013 [15]	1	1	1	1	2	1	1	1	9
Wang Ling, 2013 [28]	1	1	1	1	2	1	1	1	9
Hu Yali, 2013 [14]	1	1	1	1	2	1	1	1	9
Yin Yuzhu, 2013 [12]	1	1	1	1	2	1	1	1	9
Pan Calvin Q., 2013 [13]	1	1	1	1	1	1	1	1	8
Zhang Lei, 2014 [11]	1	1	1	1	2	1	1	1	9
Wang Lina, 2014 [26]	1	1	1	1	2	1	1	1	9
Li Weiru, 2014 [25]	1	1	1	1	2	1	1		9
Huang Dan, 2014 [27]	1	1	1	1	2	1	1	1	9
Liu Cuiping, 2015 [10]	1	1	1	1	2	1	1	1	9

statistically significant. All statistical analyses were conducted with Stata 11.0 (StataCorp, College Station, TX).

Results

The flow diagram for literature research and study selection is shown in Fig. 1. After screening the title and/or abstract of 1489 potentially relevant articles, 166 articles were evaluated in detail. Of these, 3 articles [22–24] were excluded for not having been conducted in China. Finally, 28 publications [10–16, 25–45] were eligible for inclusion in the meta-analysis.

Table 2 displays the main characteristics of the identified studies on the effect of delivery mode on MTCT of HBV. All included articles were published in the period between 2001 and 2015. Among the articles, 2 were case-control studies. All of the others were retrospective cohort studies. Seven were published in English, and the others were published in Chinese. Two articles reported the results grouped by maternal HBeAg status. Six studies were conducted exclusively in HBeAg + mothers, two were conducted solely in HBeAg-mothers, eight did not specify this information, and the remaining studies had mixed HBeAg + and HBeAg- populations (HBeAg + range from 3.83% to 67.19%). Two studies were conducted among pregnant women who all received HBIG administration, nine were conducted among those without HBIG administration, 15 did not specify, and four had mixed populations (HBIG range from 21.93 to 80%). One study was conducted with 7.81% of the mothers having received antiviral therapy, 14 were conducted among those who had not received antiviral therapy, and the remaining did not report whether antiviral therapy had been administered. Infants were tested for HBV within 24 h of birth before immunoprophylaxis in 6 studies. Among the studies with a follow-up period of more than 1 month, all infants received the hepatitis B vaccine in 24 studies. With regard to HBIG administration in infants in these 24 studies, 17 studies were conducted with 100% administration, 3 did not report this information, and 4 studies had a range from 53.3 to 84.34%.

Meta-analysis

This analysis involved 28 articles with 30 datasets comprising 9906 participants. The MTCT rate of HBV was 6.76% (670 of 9906) overall, with individual rates of 4.37% (223 of 5105) for mothers who underwent cesarean section and 9.31% (447 of 4801) for those who

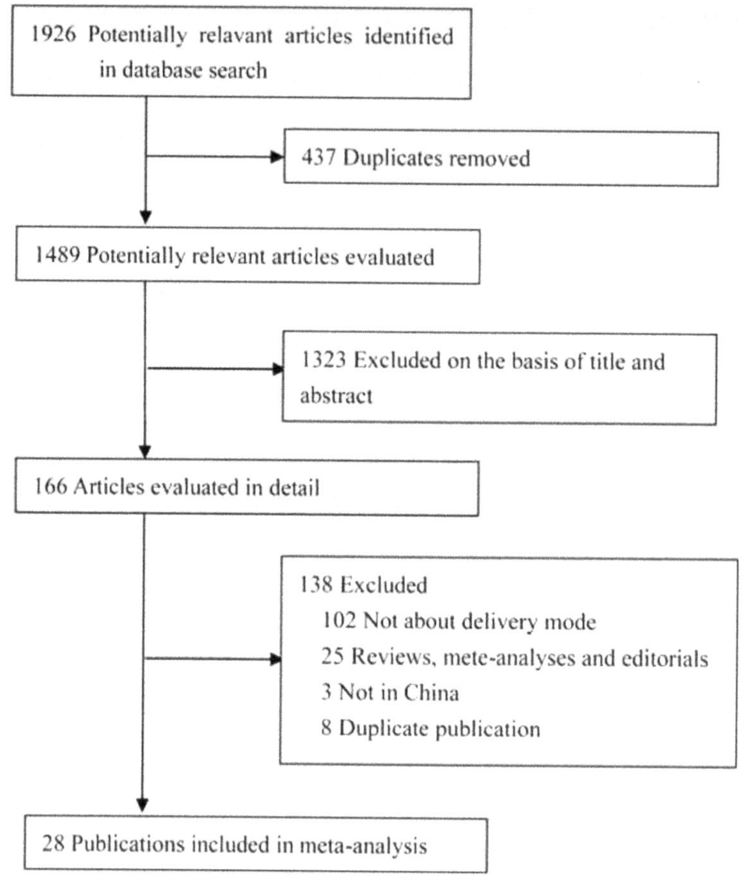

Fig. 1 The flow diagram for literature research and study selection

underwent vaginal delivery. The study-specific RRs and the pooled estimate are shown in Fig. 2. The summary RR was 0.51 (95%CI: 0.44–0.60, $P < 0.001$), indicating a statistically significant decrease in HBV vertical transmission with cesarean section, as compared to vaginal delivery. The heterogeneity among studies was moderate with I^2of29.3% ($P_{heterogeneity} = 0.069$). In the sensitivity analysis, the pooled RRs were similar before and after removal of each study, indicating the robust stability of the current result. Publication bias was not detected by Egger's ($P = 0.452$) and Begg's ($P = 0.254$) tests, and the funnel plot was symmetric (Fig. 3).

Subgroup analyses were conducted to examine the stability of the primary result (Table 3). Significant results did not differ substantially by maternal HBeAg status and follow-up time. As for the stratified analyses by maternal HBIG administration, the risk of MTCT of HBV was significantly decreased in the cases of cesarean section when compared to vaginal delivery among pregnant women without HBIG administration and those where HBIG administration had not been specified, but not among those with HBIG administration (100% or mixed). A significant effect of cesarean section on the MTCT of HBV was found in those studies where either 100% or a smaller percentage of infants had been administered HBIG, as well as in studies where administration of HBIG to infants had not been reported. With regard to infant vaccination, the significant effect of cesarean section did not differ among infants who received vaccination and those whose vaccination status was unknown.

Discussion

In this meta-analysis, we found that cesarean section could significantly reduce the risk of MTCT of HBV in China. The significant effect was not affected by maternal HBeAg status and follow-up time, but was influenced by both maternal and infant HBIG administration. Our results are consistent with the findings of two previous meta-analyses [46, 47]; however, one only included 4 studies and another included 10 studies worldwide. In the meta-analysis reported by Chang et al. [46], most of the included studies were performed in China, but some Chinese articles were excluded owing to the lack of available translations. We were able to take full advantage of Chinese databases and include 28 studies

Table 2 Characteristics of identified studies in this meta-analysis

			Study	Newborns		HBV+ newborns		Mothers		Infants		
Author	Year	Area	design	Caesarean	Vaginal	Caesarean	Vaginal	HBeAg + (%)	Intervention	HBIG	Vaccine	Follow-up
Wang Qingtu	2001	Shandong	RC	38	84	4	28	100	NR	NR	NR	1 h
Wang Jianshe	2002	Shanghai	RC	117	184	13	17	36.54	NR	100%	1, 2 and 7 months	12 months
Wang Lan	2004	Shandong	RC	61	183	11	61	100	NR	75.82%	0, 1 and 6 months	1 month
Wang Yuan	2005	Jiangsu	RC	58	42	1	0	22	100% HBIG	100%	0, 1 and 6 months	2 month
Gu Jie	2006	Ningxia	RC	64	85	2	5	34.9	No	100%	0, 1 and 6 months	12 months
Qian Yanhua	2006	Jiangsu	RC	26	24	0	2	NR	80% HBIG	80%	0, 1 and 6 months	12 months
Fan Yi	2007	Guangdong	RC	92	103	2	9	4.1	NR	100%	0, 1 and 6 months	6 months
Chen Jing1	2007	Tianjin	RC	176	53	27	13	100	NR	NR	NR	1 h
Chen Jing2	2007	Tianjin	RC	112	68	3	10	0	NR	NR	NR	1 h
Li Jijun1	2007	Gansu, Jiangsu	RC	12	49	4	19	100	NR	NR	0, 1 and 6 months	3–9 years
Li Jijun2	2007	Gansu, Jiangsu	RC	74	184	5	28	0	NR	NR	0, 1 and 6 months	3–9 years
Chen Hong	2008	Beijing	RC	112	180	4	5	4.45	No	NR	0, 1 and 6 months	6 months
Liu Xia	2008	Tianjin	RC	153	54	14	15	NR	NR	NR	NR	2 h
Liu Honge	2009	Guangdong	RC	86	123	2	9	3.83	NR	100%	0, 1 and 6 months	1 month
Zhang Qingying	2009	Shanghai	RC	166	52	1	7	NR	No	100%	0, 1 and 6 months	6 months
Zhu Yunxia	2010	Beijing	RC	114	102	5	6	100	No	100%	0, 1 and 6 months	7 months
Yang Peifang	2010	Shanghai	RC	32	36	0	1	19.1	No	100%	0, 1 and 6 months	12 months
Yang Xiaomei	2011	Guangdong	RC	33	49	4	7	NR	NR	100%	0, 1 and 6 months	6 months
Zhang Weili	2011	Shanghai	RC	508	127	17	5	NR	NR	100%	0, 1 and 6 months	3 months
Huang Liu	2012	Guangdong	RC	122	168	9	17	NR	NR	NR	NR	24 h
Guo Zhen	2013	Shanxi	CC	584	549	29	72	36.19	NR	NR	NR	24 h
Wang Ling	2013	Sichuan	RC	112	148	7	16	NR	100% HBIG	100%	0, 1 and 6 months	6 months
Hu Yali	2013	Jiangsu	RC	285	261	7	6	24.73	NR	53.30%	0, 1 and 6 months	5–7 years
Yin Yuzhu	2013	Guangdong	RC	692	668	12	9	34.76	39.70% HBIG	100%	0, 1 and 6 months	12 months
Pan Calvin Q.	2013	Beijing	RC	496	673	7	23	54.5	No	100%	0, 1 and 6 months	7–12 months
Zhang Lei	2014	Multicenter	RC	221	194	17	22	100	21.93% HBIG	84.34%	0, 1 and 6 months	8-12 months
	2014	Guangdong	RC	149	122	6	9	34.32	No	100%		7–12 months

Table 2 Characteristics of identified studies in this meta-analysis *(Continued)*

Wang Lina											0, 1 and 6 months	
Li Weiru	2014	Guangdong	RC	120	120	2	12	NR	No	100%	0, 1 and 6 months	6 months
Huang Dan	2014	Hubei	RC	86	64	4	8	18.67	No	100%	0, 1 and 6 months	6 months
Liu Cuiping	2015	Sichuan	CC	204	52	4	6	67.19	7.81% antiviral; 43.36% HBIG	100%	0, 1 and 6 months	6–12 months and/or 1–3 years

performed in China in this meta-analysis, making it the largest and most robust meta-analysis to date.

The mechanism of MTCT of HBV remains unclear. Most MTCTs likely occur perinatally by microperfusion of maternal blood to the fetal circulation during the uterine contractions and tearing of the placenta at birth. Other possible modes of infection include swallowing amniotic fluid, vaginal secretions, or exposure to maternal blood during vaginal delivery [13]. Elective cesarean section results in the least amount of placental contraction and has been speculated to involve the least maternal-fetal transfusion [15]. It also limits direct contact of the fetus with infected secretions or blood in the maternal genital tract.

Several limitations of our meta-analysis should be acknowledged. Despite demonstrating the efficacy of cesarean section for preventing MTCT of HBV, the conclusion of this study must be considered with great caution. Firstly, the included studies were retrospective cohort and case-control studies, not randomized controlled trials. Some bias and confounding factors could not be well controlled in the retrospective studies. Secondly, the data on maternal HBV DNA level in the included studies were lacking, making it difficult to reach conclusions. The maternal HBV DNA level was

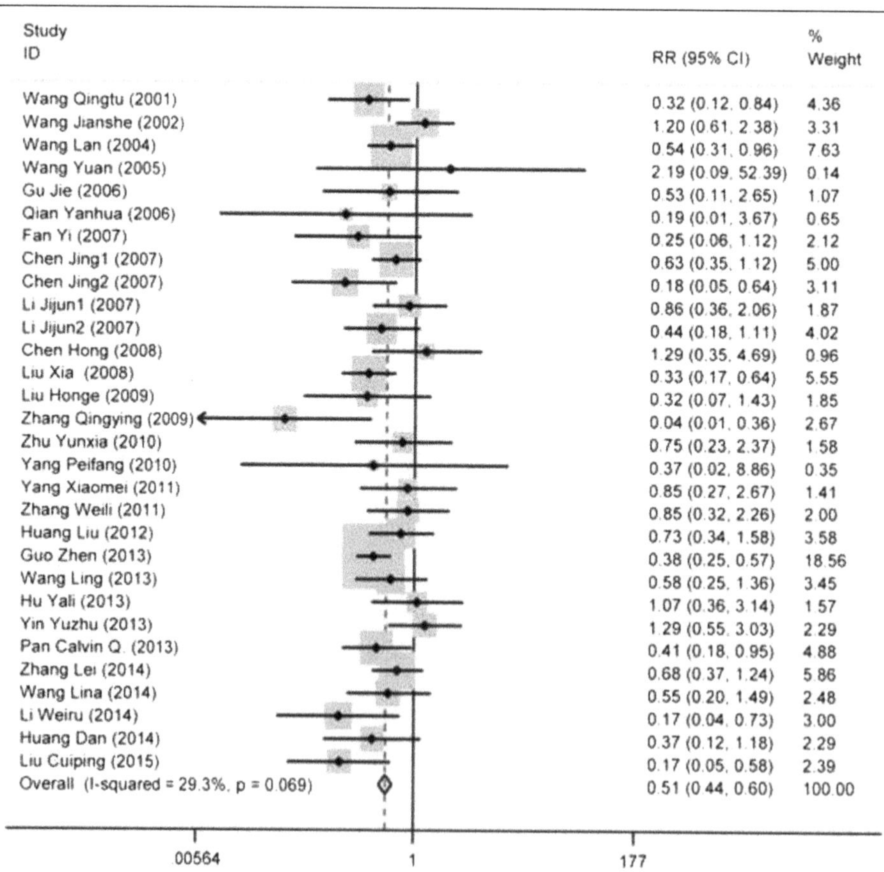

Fig. 2 The forest plot of the efficacy of caesarean section versus vaginal delivery for preventing hepatitis B virus vertical transmission

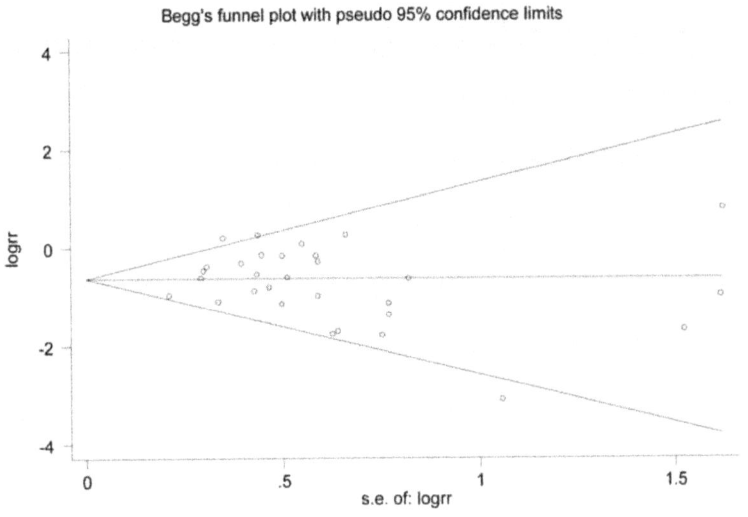

Fig. 3 Funnel plot of publication bias

Table 3 Subgroup analyses on the effect of delivery mode on the risk of hepatitis B virus vertical transmission

Characteristic	No. of reports	RR (95% CI)	*P* for test	I^2(%)	*P* for heterogeneity
All studies	30	0.51 (0.44–0.60)	<0.001	29.3	0.069
Maternal HbeAg status					
HBeAg+	6	0.59 (0.44–0.78)	<0.001	0.0	0.731
HBeAg-	2	0.33 (0.16–0.68)	0.003	21.1	0.260
Mixed	14	0.53 (0.42–0.68)	<0.001	40.3	0.059
Not reported	8	0.45 (0.32–0.63)	<0.001	43.2	0.090
Maternal HBIG administration					
Yes (100%)	2	0.63 (0.28–1.44)	0.276	0.0	0.427
No	9	0.44 (0.27–0.72)	0.001	22.1	0.247
Mixed	4	0.54 (0.23–1.30)	0.169	61.2	0.052
Not reported	15	0.54 (0.42–0.70)	<0.001	32.9	0.105
Infant HBIG administration					
Yes (100%)	17	0.55 (0.42–0.71)	<0.001	36.9	0.064
Mixed	4	0.63 (0.43–0.92)	0.017	0.0	0.594
Not reported	9	0.45 (0.35–0.57)	<0.001	29.7	0.182
Infant vaccine					
0–1-6 months	23	0.55 (0.44–0.67)	<0.001	14.1	0.268
1–2-7 months	1	–	–	–	–
Not reported	6	0.41 (0.32–0.54)	<0.001	23.7	0.256
Follow-up time					
≥ 1 month	24	0.58 (0.48–0.71)	<0.001	22.7	0.157
≤ 24 h	6	0.41 (0.32–0.54)	<0.001	23.7	0.256
Region					
EDA	22	0.55 (0.45–0.67)	<0.001	34.8	0.056
CLDA	2	0.38 (0.26–0.56)	<0.001	0.0	0.978
WUDA	3	0.43 (0.23–0.80)	0.008	26.6	0.256
Mixed	3	0.63 (0.40–0.97)	0.037	0.0	0.573

Abbreviations: *HBeAg* hepatitis B e antigen, *HBIG* hepatitis B immune globulin, *RR* relative risk, *CI* confidence interval, *EDA* eastern developed areas, *CLDA* central less developed areas, *WUDA* western or undeveloped areas

considered as the most important independent risk factor for vertical transmission by many studies [5, 48, 49]. Thirdly, although we found the significant effect did not differ by maternal HBeAg status, in most of the studies we included, the authors did not report maternal HBeAg status, or the participants had mixed HBeAg statuses. HBeAg positivity had a close relationship with HBV DNA level. Finally, HBIG administration and antiviral therapy in pregnant women were not reported in most studies. The results may have been affected by the lack of these data. In addition, owing to missing clinical details on hepatitis B, varying study quality, and study heterogeneity, it would be difficult to justify a randomized trial of cesarean section, which is currently an unproven and invasive intervention. A detailed, well-designed observational study, where all infants receive HBIG and vaccination and all mothers experience perinatal hepatitis B care, might be a more appropriate next step.

Conclusions

Our meta-analysis found that cesarean section could reduce the risk of MTCT of HBV in comparison to vaginal delivery in China. Whether elective cesarean section can be recommended for clinical practice as a preventive measure against MTCT of HBV should be considered with caution. Future well-designed randomized control trials with adequate statistical power will be needed to confirm our findings.

Abbreviations

CLDA: Central less developed areas; EDA: Eastern developed areas; HBeAg: Hepatitis B e antigen; HBIG: Hepatitis B immune globulin; HBV: Hepatitis B virus; MTCT: Mother-to-child transmission; NOS: Newcastle-Ottawa Scale; WUDA: Western or undeveloped areas

Acknowledgments

We acknowledge Li Liu for her assistance with identifying and screening the abstracts of studies obtained from the searched databases.

Funding

This work was supported by the Health Public Welfare Project of Futian District (FTWS2015048) and the National Natural Science Foundation of China (NSFC81172752). The funders had no role in study design, data collection and analysis, decision to publish, or preparation of the manuscript.

Authors' contributions

MY, QQ, and SFN were responsible for the design and concept of the manuscript. MY, QQ, QF, and LXJ were responsible for the literature search and retrieving data, and MY and QQ were responsible for analyzing the data. All authors were responsible for writing the manuscript. All authors read and approved the final manuscript.

Competing interests

The authors declare that they have no competing interest.

Author details

Futian District Center for Disease Control and Prevention of Shenzhen China, Futian District, Shenzhen 518000, China. [2]Department of Health Prevention and Care, Zhongshan Hospital, Xiamen University, Xiamen 361004, China. [3]Department of Epidemiology and Biostatistics, School of Public Health, Tongji Medical College, Huazhong University of Science and Technology, 13 Hangkong Road, Wuhan 430030, China.

References

1. World Health Organization. http://www.who.int/mediacentre/factsheets/fs204/en/. Updated July 2015.
2. Lozano R, Naghavi M, Foreman K, Lim S, Shibuya K, Aboyans V, Abraham J, Adair T, Aggarwal R, Ahn SY, et al. Global and regional mortality from 235 causes of death for 20 age groups in 1990 and 2010: a systematic analysis for the global burden of disease study 2010. Lancet. 2012;380(9859):2095–128.
3. Cui Y, Jia J. Update on epidemiology of hepatitis B and C in China. J Gastroenterol Hepatol. 2013;28(Suppl 1):7–10.
4. Lv N, Chu XD, Sun YH, Zhao SY, Li PL, Chen X. Analysis on the outcomes of hepatitis B virus perinatal vertical transmission: nested case-control study. Eur J Gastroenterol Hepatol. 2014;26(11):1286–91.
5. Pan CQ, Han GR, Jiang HX, Zhao W, Cao MK, Wang CM, Yue X, Wang GJ. Telbivudine prevents vertical transmission from HBeAg-positive women with chronic hepatitis B. Clin Gastroenterol Hepatol. 2012;10(5):520–6.
6. Tran TT. Hepatitis B and pregnancy. Curr Hepat Rep. 2009;8(3):91–5.
7. Legardy-Williams JK, Jamieson DJ, Read JS. Prevention of mother-to-child transmission of HIV-1: the role of cesarean delivery. Clin Perinatol. 2010; 37(4):777–85. ix
8. Sauerbrei A, Wutzler P. Herpes simplex and varicella-zoster virus infections during pregnancy: current concepts of prevention, diagnosis and therapy. Part 1: herpes simplex virus infections. Med Microbiol Immunol. 2007;196(2):89–94.
9. Read JS, Newell MK. Efficacy and safety of cesarean delivery for prevention of mother-to-child transmission of HIV-1. Cochrane Database Syst Rev. 2005; 4:CD005479.
10. Liu CP, Zeng YL, Zhou M, Chen LL, Hu R, Wang L, Tang H. Factors associated with mother-to-child transmission of hepatitis B virus despite immunoprophylaxis. Inter Med (Tokyo, Japan). 2015;54(7):711–6.
11. Zhang L, Gui X, Wang B, Ji H, Yisilafu R, Li F, Zhou Y, Zhang L, Zhang H, Liu X. A study of immunoprophylaxis failure and risk factors of hepatitis B virus mother-to-infant transmission. Eur J Pediatr. 2014;173(9):1161–8.
12. Yin Y, Zhou J, Zhang P, Hou H. Identification of risk factors related to the failure of immunization to interrupt hepatitis B virus perinatal transmission. Chin J Hepatol. 2013;21(2):105–10.
13. Pan CQ, Zou HB, Chen Y, Zhang X, Zhang H, Li J, Duan Z. Cesarean section reduces perinatal transmission of hepatitis B virus infection from hepatitis B surface antigen-positive women to their infants. Clin Gastroenterol Hepatol. 2013;11(10):1349–55.
14. Hu Y, Chen J, Wen J, Xu C, Zhang S, Xu B, Zhou YH. Effect of elective cesarean section on the risk of mother-to-child transmission of hepatitis B virus. BMC Pregnancy Childbirth. 2013;13:119.
15. Guo Z, Shi XH, Feng YL, Wang B, Feng LP, Wang SP, Zhang YW. Risk factors of HBV intrauterine transmission among HBsAg-positive pregnant women. J Viral Hepat. 2013;20(5):317–21.
16. Wang J, Zhu Q, Zhang X. Effect of delivery mode on maternal-infant transmission of hepatitis B virus by immunoprophylaxis. Chin Med J. 2002; 115(10):1510–2.
17. Higgins JP, Thompson SG, Deeks JJ, Altman DG. Measuring inconsistency in meta-analyses. BMJ (Clinical research ed). 2003;327(7414):557–60.
18. Higgins JP. Commentary: heterogeneity in meta-analysis should be expected and appropriately quantified. Int J Epidemiol. 2008;37(5):1158–60.
19. Lau J, Ioannidis JP, Schmid CH. Quantitative synthesis in systematic reviews. Ann Intern Med. 1997;127(9):820–6.
20. Egger M, Davey Smith G, Schneider M, Minder C. Bias in meta-analysis detected by a simple, graphical test. BMJ (Clinical research ed). 1997; 315(7109):629–34.
21. Begg CB, Mazumdar M. Operating characteristics of a rank correlation test for publication bias. Biometrics. 1994;50(4):1088–101.
22. Wen WH, Chang MH, Zhao LL, Ni YH, Hsu HY, Wu JF, Chen PJ, Chen DS, Chen HL. Mother-to-infant transmission of hepatitis B virus infection: significance of maternal viral load and strategies for intervention. J Hepatol. 2013;59(1):24–30.

23. Dwivedi M, Misra SP, Misra V, Pandey A, Pant S, Singh R, Verma M. Seroprevalence of hepatitis B infection during pregnancy and risk of perinatal transmission. Indian J Gastroenterol. 2011;30(2):66–71.
24. Lee SD, Tsai YT, Wu TC, Lo KJ, Wu JC, Yang ZL, Ng HT. Role of caesarean section in prevention of mother-infant transmission of hepatitis B virus. Lancet. 1988;2(8615):833–4.
25. Li W, Huang P, Jian Y. The impact of delivery mode on the mother-to-child transmission of hepatitis B virus. China Foreign Med Treat. 2014;4(12):51–2.
26. Wang L, Li X, Yin B. Effect of delivery mode on hepatitis B virus mother-to-child transmission. Med Front. 2014;19:253–4.
27. Huang D. Effect of delivery mode on hepatitis B virus mother-to-child vertical transmission. Med Recapitulate. 2014;20(11):2099–100.
28. Wang L. Research on effect of delivery mode on hepatitis B virus mother-to-child transmission. J Guangxi Med Univ. 2013;30(1):188–90.
29. Huang L, Fan H, Ji B, Ye M. Research about the efficacy of delivery mode on maternal-infant transmission of hepatitis B virus. New Med. 2012;43(4):247–9.
30. Yang X, Gan T, Liu Z, Zhang N: Effects of delivery mode and HBV DNA loads on the mother-to-child transmission of hepatitis B virus. Hainan Med J. 2011;22(1):20-22.
31. Zhang W, Zhao J, Li W. Influencing factors of mother-infant vertical transmission of hepatitis B virus. Chin J Contemp Pediatr. 2011;13(8):644–6.
32. Zhu Y, Zou H, Chen Y, Zhang H, Duan Z. Effect of different delivery modes on mother-to-infant transmission of hepatitis B virus. J Shanxi Med Univ. 2010;41(6):495–7.
33. Yang P. Effect of delivery mode on mother-to-child vertical transmission of hepatitis B virus. Hebei Med J. 2010;32(3):318–9.
34. Zhang Q, Zhao J, Jiang P. Effect of delivery mode on maternal-infant transmission of hepatitis B virus. Chin J Clin Med. 2009;16(4):570–1.
35. Liu H, Fan H. Research on the relationship between maternal-infant transmission of hepatitis B viru and delivery mode. Chin J Mod Drug Appl. 2009;3(10):30–1.
36. Xia L, Jinyu H. Clinical study on the relationship between delivery styles of pregnant women with high capacity of HBV and HBV infection of two hour-old newborns. Mod Prev Med. 2008;35(4):790–1.
37. Chen H, Ren J, Liu X. Influence of different delivery patterns on mother-to-child vertical transmission of HBV. Chin J Woman Child Heahh Res. 2008; 19(3):214–6.
38. Chen J, Zhang P. Effect on HBV mother-infant transmission in infectiousness and labor presentation. Med Innov Res. 2007;4(27):8–9.
39. Li J, Wang F, Zheng H, Liang X. Influence of the different labor types to the HBV mother-to-infant transmission. Chin J Vaccines Immunization. 2007; 13(4):306–8.
40. Fan Y, Xiao X, Li A, Tang X. Influence of delivery mode on maternal-infant transmission of hepatitis B virus. Guangdong Med J. 2007;28(2):252–3.
41. Qian Y. Influence of labor types on the effect of interdicting mother-infant HBV transmission. Occup Health. 2006;22(17):1332–4.
42. Gu J, Wang Y, Zhao L. Effect of delivery mode on interdicting maternal-infant transmission of hepatitis B virus. Ningxia Med J. 2006;28(11):858–9.
43. Wang Y, He C, Huang W, Cai X, Yao J. Clinical research on factors associated with mother-to-child transmission of hepatitis B virus after combined immunization. Matern Child Health Care China. 2005;20(13):1655–7.
44. Wang L, Hu W, Wang Q, Qi h. Relationship between delivery mode and maternal-infant transmission of hepatitis B virus. Cent Plains Med J. 2004;31(9):10–1.
45. Wang Q, Xiu X, Guo Y, Tao H. Effect of different delivery modes on interdicting maternal-infant transmission of hepatitis B virus. Shandong Med J. 2001;41(22):44–5.
46. Chang MS, Gavini S, Andrade PC, McNabb-Baltar J. Caesarean section to prevent transmission of hepatitis B: a meta-analysis. Can J Gastroenterol Hepatol. 2014;28(8):439–44.
47. Yang J, Zeng XM, Men YL, Zhao LS. Elective caesarean section versus vaginal delivery for preventing mother to child transmission of hepatitis B virus–a systematic review. Virol J. 2008;5:100.
48. Zou H, Chen Y, Duan Z, Zhang H, Pan C. Virologic factors associated with failure to passive-active immunoprophylaxis in infants born to HBsAg-positive mothers. J Viral Hepat. 2012;19(2):e18–25.
49. Han GR, Cao MK, Zhao W, Jiang HX, Wang CM, Bai SF, Yue X, Wang GJ, Tang X, Fang ZX. A prospective and open-label study for the efficacy and safety of telbivudine in pregnancy for the prevention of perinatal transmission of hepatitis B virus infection. J Hepatol. 2011;55(6):1215–21.

18

A randomized controlled double blind trial comparing the effects of the prophylactic antibiotic, Cefazolin, administered at caesarean delivery at two different timings (before skin incision and after cord clamping) on both the mother and newborn

Chinta Annie Jyothirmayi[1], Ajay Halder[2], Bijesh Yadav[3], Santosh Thomas Samuel[4], Anil Kuruvilla[1] and Ruby Jose[2*]

Abstract

Background: Caesarean delivery (CD) increases the risk of postpartum infection by 5 to 20 fold. Prevention of surgical site infection (SSI) is the goal of antibiotic prophylaxis. This study was carried out to assess the optimum timing for prophylactic antibiotic administration and to assess the amount of the antibiotic crossing the placental barrier.

Methods: Eligible mothers were recruited, after informed consent, once the decision for CD was made. Each mother received two injections, one prior to skin incision and one after cord clamping, (one being the study drug Cefazolin, and the other, a placebo) based on the randomization code. Demographic, maternal and neonatal monitoring data until discharge from hospital, and at the 6 weeks postpartum visit were collected. Levels of the prophylactic antibiotic were measured from the cord blood in every 8th neonate. The objective of the study was to compare the effects of the prophylactic antibiotic, intravenous Cefazolin 1 g, administered at Caesarean delivery (CD) at two different timings (before skin incision and after cord clamping) on both the mother and newborn. The secondary outcomes that were followed up were the number of maternal and neonatal readmissions. An appropriate test for significance, Fisher's exact test was used to find the association between risk variables and outcome.

Results: The total numbers of mothers enrolled were 1106, of whom 553 mothers received antibiotic prior to skin incision (pre-incision) and 543 mothers received antibiotic after cord clamping (post-incision). The pre-incision group had significantly less febrile illness (RR = 0.48, 95% CI: 0.29 - 0.80) and SSI (RR = 0.14, 95% CI: 0.04 - 0.53) when compared with the post- incision group. The post-incision group significantly had >7 days hospital stay when compared to the 4-7 days stay of the pre-incision group ($p = 0.005$).There were no differences in any of the neonatal outcomes. The quantity of the antibiotic in the cord blood was only 2-3%.

(Continued on next page)

* Correspondence: rubyjose1@gmail.com
[2]Department of Obstetrics and Gynecology Unit IV, Christian Medical College, Vellore, India
Full list of author information is available at the end of the article

(Continued from previous page)

Conclusions: Pre incision prophylactic antibiotic protected the mother from SSI and febrile illness and decreased the hospital stay significantly.

Keywords: Prophylactic antibiotic, Caesarian delivery, Pre-incision, Post-incision

Background

Caesarean delivery (CD) is considered an important risk factor for postpartum infection. When compared to women who deliver vaginally, those delivered by (CD) face a 5 to 20 fold increase in risk of infection [1]. Prevention of surgical site infection (SSI) by decreasing the burden of microorganisms at the surgical site during the operative procedure is the goal of antibiotic prophylaxis [1]. The efficacy of antibiotic prophylaxis for reducing SSI is well known [2].

Prophylactic antibiotics are expected to work in conjunction with the antiseptic measures taken before and during surgery [3, 4]. It is suggested that antibiotic given 30 min to 1 h before skin incision will cause adequate bactericidal concentration in the system before inoculation. Prophylactic antibiotics act mainly by destroying the bacteria and slowing production of bacterial proteases, thus preventing the attachment of bacteria to the mucosal surfaces. The greatest therapeutic effect occurs when antibiotics are administered just before or coincident when maximal bacterial contamination and tissue trauma occurs.

At CD, in our Institution, the prophylactic antibiotic was being administered after cord clamping, so that it did not reach the foetal circulation. Concerns of masking signs of sepsis in babies, developing resistance to antibiotics and masking organisms in blood culture because of the transplacental transfer of the drug was the main reason for administration of the drug after cord clamping. However, recent studies suggested that, giving the drug prior to skin incision would significantly decrease the incidence of maternal infection without causing harm to the baby [5, 6]. Administration of IV antibiotics prior to skin incision definitely showed a decrease of 9% in the rate of maternal infections with no increase in the rate of neonatal sepsis, duration of hospital stay for the infant or any complications secondary to the administration of antibiotic to the mother [7].The objectives of the study were:

1. To compare the effects of the prophylactic antibiotic, intravenous Cefazolin1gm, administered at Caesarean delivery (CD) at two different timings(30 min to 1 h) before skin incision and immediately after cord clamping) on both the mother and newborn.
2. To quantify the amount of antibiotic that has crossed the placental barrier in to the cord blood.

Methods

This randomized controlled double blinded trial was carried out at the Christian Medical College and Hospital (CMCH), Vellore in the Departments of Obstetrics and Gynaecology and Neonatology, over a period of 7 months from March 2013 to September 2013. CMCH is a tertiary care centre situated in Vellore, in South India, and has around 15,000 deliveries a year, catering mostly to women from the surrounding 2 states of Tamil Nadu and Andhra Pradesh.

All mothers more than or equal to 37 completed weeks of gestational age who had a decision made for CD (elective and emergency)were included in the study, after informed consent from each participant. The study was cleared by the Institutional Review Board and the Ethics Committee of Christian Medical College, Vellore. [IRB Min no. 8084 dated 21.11.2012]. The Clinical Trials Registry India (CTRI) was [CTRI/2016/03/006710 dated, 04/03/2016].

Mothers with known allergy to Cephalosporin or Penicillin, those who received antibiotics within a week prior to CD, those with altered liver or renal functions and those on antiepileptic medication were excluded from the study. Babies with known major congenital anomalies were not included as well. Women undergoing CD were randomized to receive both single dose of IV Cefazolin 1 g and placebo. As per the randomization, every mother was given IV Cefazolin1gm either 30 min to 1 h, prior to skin incision, with placebo administered within a minute after cord clamping or placebo administered 30 min to 1 h prior to skin incision and Cefazolin 1 g IV, within a minute after cord clamping. The randomization covers with the blinded drugs were opened in the Operation Theatre (OT).The medications were administered by the Anaesthetist appropriately as per the randomisation. Cord blood was collected in every 8th neonate to estimate the amount of antibiotic levels in the neonate. The cord blood (5 ml) was collected soon after delivery of the baby in a blood collecting test tube, centrifuged and the serum was refrigerated for analysis. The drug level (Cefazolin) was analysed by a developed and validated High Pressure Liquid Chromatography (HPLC) with Ultra violet protection method in the clinical pharmacological unit. Thus, the investigator, the patient and the Labour Room personnel were blinded to the drug used. After CD, all the outcomes listed below were assessed until discharge from hospital and at the first postpartum visit at 6 weeks and noted. In addition, basic demographic and obstetric data were noted as well. The primary maternal outcomes assessed were the presence of SSI, endometritis, UTI and length of hospital stay. The primary outcomes assessed for the neonate were incidence of early and late onset sepsis, oral thrush, increased frequency of stools, necrotizing enterocolitis (NEC) and length of hospital stay. The secondary outcomes in the mother and the neonate that were followed up were the number of readmissions and maternal / neonatal death due to sepsis until 6 weeks postpartum.

The sample size to compare the effect of IV Cefazolin on the mother and infant on infections was found to be 600 in each arm with 90% power, at 5% level of significance, an anticipated difference of 9% in each group and with a 20% loss to follow-up.

Permutated Block Randomization of sizes 2, 4 and 6 was done for treatment allocation using SAS 9.1.3. Pre numbered or coded identical containers for the antibiotics and the placebo prepared by pharmacy which were administered serially to patients. Randomization was done according to computer generated blockrandomization.1200 mothers planned for CD were recruited into the study, but only 1106 of those could be analysed. Five hundred fifty three mothers received the antibiotic prior to skin incision and placebo after cord clamping referred to as Pre-incision group in the study. The remaining 543 received placebo prior to skin incision and IV Cefazolin after cord clamping referred to as Post-incision in the study.

Operational definitions

Surgical site infections (SSI)

Evidence of clinical signs and symptoms of infection with or without microbiological evidence, based on the CDC definition that describes three levels of SSI [8].

Endometritis

Inflammation of the inner layer of the uterus, diagnosed clinically by the presence of pyrexia, uterine tenderness, sub involution of the uterus and foul smelling lochia along with or without microbiological evidence.

Urinary tract infections (UTI)

Presence of clinical symptoms of dysuria, increased frequency of micturition and pyrexia along with or without microbiological evidence.

Early on set neonatal sepsis

Presence of any or a combination of features of sepsis namely hypo or hyperthermia, poor feeding, lethargy, dusky extremities, tachypnea or apnea within the first 72 h of life.

Late onset neonatal sepsis

Presence of the above features after the first 72 h of life until the first 1 week of life.

Oral thrush

Presence of white plaque like rash on buccal mucosa caused mainly by fungal organism giving rise to difficulty in feeding.

Necrotizing enterocolitis (NEC)

Necrosis of the gut seen as temperature instability, poor feeding, lethargy, .vomiting, abdominal distension, feed intolerance, sometimes with bloody stools.

Length of hospital stay

Defined as the number of days, the day mother is admitted into the hospital and for the neonate, the day neonate is born, until mother/neonate is discharged from hospital.

Maternal and neonatal readmission

Any admission to the same hospital or any other facility after first discharge from hospital.

Neonatal deaths due to sepsis

Death following sepsis which has been confirmed by positive growth on blood culture/high C reactive protein levels with leukocytosis or leucopoenia or thrombocytopenia.

All maternal outcomes were assessed by the Consultant Obstetrician who was assigned to the post- operative ward, who had a minimum of 4 years of clinical experience. All newborns were assessed by the Registrar/ Neonatologist on duty, who assigned the APGAR score as well. If the Neonatologist or Registrar was not available on site in an emergency, the Labour room Registrar assessed the APGAR score. Sepsis in the neonate was assessed by a Consultant Neonatologist with a minimum of 4 years of clinical experience.

All monitoring details were collected by the Principal Investigator.

Statistical methods

Data entry was done into EpiData software in the Neonatal department. Analysis was done using SPSS 16 software. All categorical variables were summarized using frequencies and percentages and continuous variables were using mean and standard deviation. The association between risk variables and the primary outcome (Pre-incision and Post-incision) were tested using Fisher's exact test. Adverse effects with IV Cefazolin, though thought to be unlikely were monitored and all data were submitted to the institutional Data Safety Monitoring Board for review at the end of the trial.

Results

One thousand two hundred mothers were recruited but details of only 1106 mothers could be used for analysis over the study period of 7 months. Ninety four mothers could not be included after randomization, as the drug numbers were inadvertently missed. Among 1106 mothers recruited for the study, 553 mothers received IV Cefazolin prior to skin incision and 543 mothers received antibiotics after cord clamping. Ten mothers were excluded at the end of the study for the following reasons; 1 mother developed allergy to IV Cefazolin, 3 neonates died (not due to sepsis) and 6 neonates had congenital anomalies (undiagnosed antenatally). The scheme of patient recruitment presented in Fig. 1.

Demographic data of the mothers and neonates

The demographic data for mothers and neonates are presented in Table 1. There were no differences in demographic characteristics of the mothers and neonates across the two groups. However, on the whole there were more mothers who underwent emergency caesarean delivery (75.7%) than elective (24.3%).

The mean (SD) gestational age of the mothers at delivery was 38.5(1.8). Of the 1096 mothers, 479 (43.5%) were primiparas and 622 (56.5%) were multiparas. Emergency CDs were done on 834 (75.7%) and the rest were elective CDs 267 (24.3%). Hypertensive disease complicated 194 (17.6%), Diabetes was present in 159 (14.4%), and hypothyroidism in 16 (1.5%). The indications for CD was mostly for previous CD in 371(33.7%), non reassuring fetal heart status in 348 (31.6%), labour dysfunction (arrest of dilatation, failed Induction) in 108 (9.8%), transverse or oblique lie of the fetus in 106 (9.8%), scar rupture in 28 (2.5%) and cord prolapse in 2(0.2%).

There were 553 neonates in the Pre-incision group and 543 in the Post-incision group, of whom 557 were male and 539 were female babies. The mean (SD) birth weight of the babies was 3 kg (0.65). There were 12 (2.2%) and 7 (1.3%) of neonates weighing 1-2 kg in Pre-incision and Post-incision respectively. Babies weighing more than 4 kg were less than 2% in both groups.

The mean (SD) APGAR scores of the babies at birth were 8 (1).Most of the newborns, 524 (94.9%) in the Pre-incision group and 527 (97.1%) in the Post-incision group had started feeds within 12 h after birth. Some of the newborns, 23 (4.2%) in the Pre-incision and 10 (1.8%) in Post-incision groups started feeds in 12 to 24 h. The reasons for the delay in.

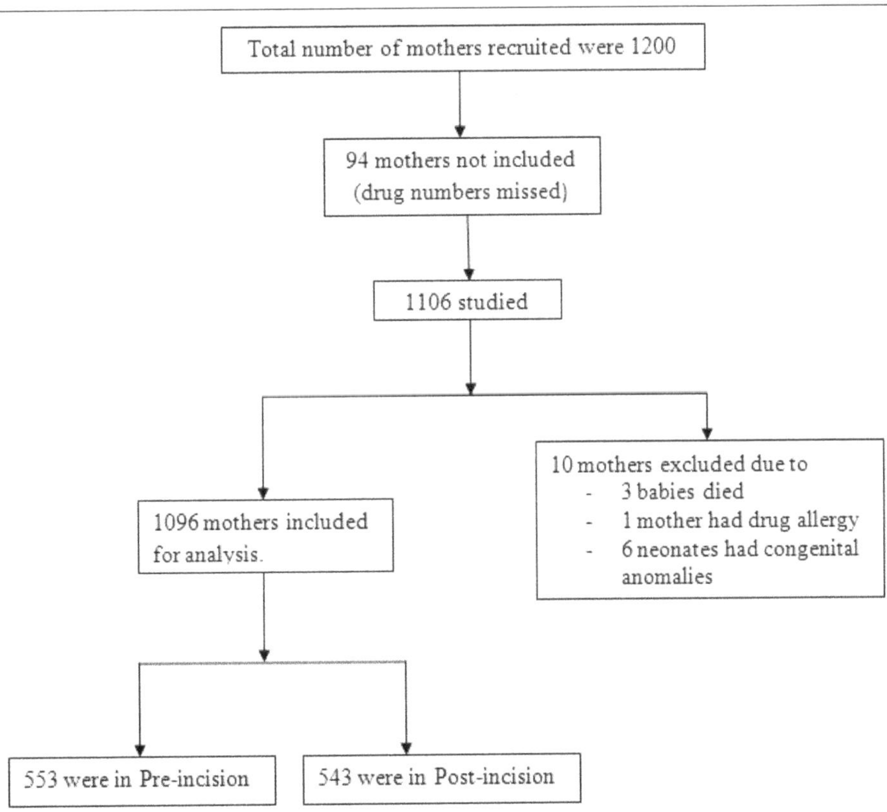

Fig. 1 The scheme of patient recruitment

Table 1 Demographic Variables of Mothers and Neonates

Variables	Pre incision		Post incision		*P* value
	n	%	n	%	
Parity:					
Primiparous	252	45.6	224	41.3	0.15
Multiparous	301	54.4	319	58.7	
Risk Factors:					
Hypertension	98	17.7	96	17.7	
Diabetes	86	15.6	71	13.1	0.63
Hypothyroidism	9	1.6	7	1.3	
None	360	65.1	369	68.0	
Type of CD:					
Elective	131	23.7	136	25.0	0.60
Emergency	422	76.3	407	75.0	
Indication for CD:					
Fetal distress	165	29.8	181	33.3	
Abnormal lie	56	10.1	50	9.2	
Cord Prolapse	1	0.2	1	0.2	0.41
Previous Caesarean	179	32.4	190	35.0	
Arrest of dilatation	55	9.9	52	9.6	
Failed Induction	81	14.6	57	10.5	
Scar rupture	16	2.9	12	2.2	
Sex of baby:					
Male	279	50.5	278	51.2	0.80
Female	274	49.5	265	48.8	
APGAR at 5 min:					
Normal	535	96.7	522	96.1	0.58
Abnormal	18	3.3	21	3.9	
Feeds in hours:					
< 12	524	94.9	527	97.1	
12-24	23	4.2	10	1.8	0.08
> 24	5	0.9	6	1.1	

commencing feeds were, due to transfer of the baby to the nursery either for tachypnea, grunting or hypoglycaemia requiring IV fluids.

Results of the primary maternal outcomes

The outcome data for mothers and neonates are presented in Table 2.The primary maternal outcomes that were assessed were, the presence of post operative infectious morbidity comprising of SSI, endometritis, UTI and length of hospital stay. When considering the primary maternal outcomes, the mothers who received prophylactic antibiotics pre incision, had less post operative complications such as febrile illness and SSI.

The pre-incision group had significantly less febrile illness (RR = 0.48, 95% CI: 0.29 – 0.80) and SSI (RR = 0.14, 95% CI: 0.04 – 0.53) compared with the post incision group. The total number of UTI's was 16 (2.9%) in the Pre-incision group and 21 (3.9%) in the Post incision group which was not significant. Hospital stay of more than 7 days which indirectly revealed that delay was probably due to some infectious morbidity was 11 (2%) in the Pre-incision versus 28 (5.2%) in the Post-incision group. The post-incision group compared to the pre-incision group had significant more mothers with a length of stay >7 compared to having a length of stay of 4-7 days (RR = 0.55, 95% CI: 0.33 – 0.91, p = 0.005). The pre incision group had a lower risk of a positive growth of significant micro organisms in blood culture than the post incision group (RR = 0.47 95% CI: 0.33 – 0.67).Blood culture reported significant growth in 23 (4.2%) mothers in the Pre-incision and in 70 (12.9%) mothers in the Post-incision group, signifying increased rate of infections in the post incision group. Readmission rates after discharge from hospital were similar in both groups.

Results of the primary outcomes in the neonate

The primary outcomes assessed for the neonate were incidence of early and late onset sepsis, oral thrush, increased frequency of stools, and length of hospital stay. There were no neonates with oral thrush or NEC in either group. Admissions of the neonates to the NICU were for various reasons, for example, low APGAR at birth, transient tachypnea of newborn, hypoglycaemia, meconium aspiration and dysmorphism. The numbers of admissions to NICU were more from the Pre-incision group, 23 (4.2%) as compared to the Post-incision group 17 (3.1%), but this was not statistically significant (p = 0.42). Most of the neonates 528 (95.7%) and 508 (93.6%) stayed in hospital 4 to 7 days in the Pre-incision and Post-incision groups respectively. Blood culture was found positive in 58 (10.5%) in the Pre-incision and 66 (12.2%) in the Post-incision group which was not statistically significant (P = 0.39). Proven sepsis by other tests was present in 5 (0.95%) in both groups. None of the babies had any other immediate complications.

Results of the secondary outcomes in the mother and newborn

There were no maternal deaths or readmissions after discharge and the percentage of infants who had weight gain at 6 weeks was similar. As for the newborns, the readmission rates were similar 17 (3.1%) and 26 (4.8%) in both groups respectively and weight gain at 6 weeks were similar. There were no neonatal deaths due to sepsis at the postpartum visit.

The cord blood level of Cefazolin in 19 of Group 1 (Pre-incision) babies had <1 mg/dl. Forty three babies had cord blood level of Cefazolin between 1 and 10 mg/

Table 2 Outcome Variables of Mothers and Neonates

Variables	Pre incision		Post incision		RR	95% CI	P value
	n	%	n	%			
Mothers							
Hospital days:							
1-3	2	0.4	5	0.9	0.56	0.17 – 1.80	0.28
4-7	539	97.6	510	93.9	1.00		
> 7	11	2.0	28	5.2	0.55	0.33 – 0.91	0.005
Gestational Age:							
< =37	136	25.0	126	23.2	1.05	0.92 – 1.20	0.48
> 37	407	75.0	418	76.8	1.00		
Blood culture:							
Yes	23	4.2	70	12.9	0.47	0.33 – 0.67	<0.001
No	529	95.8	473	87.1	1.00		
Proven sepsis:							
Yes	8	1.4	8	1.4	0.99	0.60 – 1.62	0.97
No	544	98.6	535	98.5	1.00		
Post op Complications;							
Febrile illness	11	2.0	32	5.9	0.48	0.29 – 0.80	0.005
SSI	2	0.4	25	4.6	0.14	0.04 – 0.53	<0.001
Endometritis	5	0.9	14	2.6	0.49	0.23 – 1.05	0.02
UTI	16	2.9	21	3.9	0.81	0.56 – 1.18	0.24
None	518	93.8	451	83.1	1.00		
Readmission:							
Yes	7	1.3	11	2.0	0.77	0.43 – 1.39	0.35
No	543	98.2	532	98.0	1.00		
Neonates							
NICU Admission:							
Yes	23	4.2	17	3.1	1.15	0.87 – 1.50	0.42
No	530	95.8	526	96.9	1.00		
Hospital days:							
1-7	528	95.7	508	93.6	1.00		
> 7	24	4.3	35	6.4	0.80	0.58 – 1.09	0.14
Weight of Baby (Kg):							
1-2	12	2.2	7	1.3	1.23	0.86 – 1.75	0.36
2-3	271	49.0	257	47.3	1.00		
3-4	246	47.7	269	49.5	0.93	0.82 – 1.05	0.26
> 4	6	1.1	10	1.8	0.73	0.39 – 1.38	0.32
Blood culture:							
Yes	58	10.5	66	12.2	0.91	0.75 – 1.12	0.39
No	495	89.5	477	87.8	1.00		
Neonates							
Proven Sepsis:							
Yes	5	0.95	5	0.95	0.99	0.53 – 1.85	0.99
No	547	99.1	538	99.1	1.00		

Table 2 Outcome Variables of Mothers and Neonates *(Continued)*

Variables	Pre incision		Post incision		RR	95% CI	P value
	n	%	n	%			
Weight gain at review:							
Yes	540	97.8	526	96.9	1.22	0.79 – 1.90	0.35
No	12	2.2	17	3.1	1.00		
Readmission:							
No	533	96.9	517	95.2	1.28	0.83 – 1.87	0.16
Yes	17	3.1	26	4.8	1.00		

RR Relative Risk

dl, 60 babies had levels between 10 and 20 mg/dl, and 17 babies had levels between 20 and 30 mg/dl. The maternal blood levels however were not checked.

The toxic level of the drug in the blood is not known. However the study showed that on an average, only 2-3% of the drug administered to the mother reached the baby. This may suggest that the drug may not cause harm to the baby since very little amount reaches the baby once administered to the mother, although the study was not powered for this outcome.

Discussion

Infectious morbidity for the mother, consisting primarily of endomyometritis and wound infection remains a leading cause of post operative complications. Infectious morbidity following CD remains among the top five causes of mortality in mothers' worldwide, causing a huge burden to the society [9].

In the study by Sullivan et al. [7], on 357 women, decreased total infectious morbidity in the study group was found (RR = 0.4, 95% CI = 0.18 to 0.87). There was a decreased endometritis risk as well in the pre incision group (RR = 0.2, 95% CI = 0.15 to 0.94).There was no increase in neonatal sepsis (P = 0.99), sepsis work up (P = 0.96) or increased hospital stay (P = 0.17). In the present study, the results were almost similar in that, the incidence of SSI was decreased and duration of hospital stay was decreased with antibiotics given Pre-incision than after cord clamping. Unlike the study by Sullivan et al. [7], in the present study, the incidence of endometritis was similar in both groups. Administration of prophylactic cefazolin prior to skin incision resulted in a decrease in both endometritis and total post caesarean infectious morbidity, compared with administration at the time of cord clamping. This dosing did not result in increased neonatal septic workups or complications.

The decrease in SSI in the study by Owens et al. [10], compares well with the present study, though the incidence of endometritis does not. There was a

3.9% decrease in the incidence of wound infections and 3.6% decrease in endometritis in the group which received antibiotics prior to skin incision as compared to a 2.2% decrease in the incidence of wound infection and 2.5% decrease in the incidence of maternal endometritis in the other group and this was statistically significant (p = 0.03) [10].

Baasqee et al. [11], reporting on 2313 women and 2345 newborns showed that preoperative administration was associated with a significant 41% reduction in the rate of endometritis compared with intra operative administration (RR = 0.59, 95% CI = 0.37-0.94). In the preoperative group, there were non-significant reductions in the rates of wound infection (RR 0.71,95% CI = 0.44-1.14), maternal febrile morbidity (RR = 0.94, 95% CI = 0.46-1.95), neonatal sepsis (RR = 0.81, 95% CI = 0.47-1.41), neonatal septic work-up (RR = 0.93, 95% CI = 0.71-1.21) and neonatal intensive-care unit admission (RR = 0.92, 95% CI = 0.65-1.28). There were non-significant increases in the rates of maternal pyelonephritis (RR = 1.09, 95% CI = 0.49-2.43) and neonatal pneumonia (RR = 3.36, 95% CI = 0.55-20.47).

This was different from the present study, which did not reveal decrease in the incidence of endometritis.

Faribaet al. [12], in their study on 410 patients found no difference in the incidence of postpartum endometritis (RR = 0.34, 95% CI = 0.04 to 3.24), which was similar to the present study. There was no difference in the incidence of wound infection (RR = 3.06, 95% CI = 0.13 to 74.69) and total puerperal morbidity (RR = 1.02, 95% CI = 0.47 to 2.22), unlike the present study. There was no difference in the incidence of neonatal sepsis (RR = 0.34, 95% CI = 0.04 to 3.24), septic workup (RR = 0.41, 95% CI = 0.08 to 2.07), or intermediate NICU admission (RR = 0.73, 95% CI = 0.24 to 2.26), which was similar to the present study.

Small *et al.* [13], in the Cochrane database publication, concluded that endometritis was reduced by two thirds to three quarters and a decrease in wound infection was also identified. Prophylactic antibiotics given to all women undergoing elective or non-elective cesarean section is clearly beneficial for women but there is uncertainty about the consequences for the baby. In the present study, infectious morbidity was definitely decreased and no adverse effect was found for the neonate.

The limitations of the study were that, though the sample size calculated was 1200 mothers, the actual numbers fell short. The study was powered only for the main maternal outcomes.

The operational definitions for some of the maternal and neonatal outcomes were based on clinical signs and symptoms, and not on any laboratory tests.

Conclusion

Intravenous antibiotics can be administered to mothers prior to skin incision for Caesarean section and this decreases the incidence of the overall postoperative infectious morbidity in the mother. No significant adverse effects were seen in neonates when intravenous Cefazolin was administered prior to skin incision, although the present study was not powered for neonatal morbidity.

Abbreviations

CD: Cesarean delivery; CMCH: Christian Medical College and Hospital; CTRI: The Clinical Trials Registry India; IRB: Institutional Review Board; NEC: Necrotizing enterocolitis; NICU: Neonatal intensive care unit; OT: Operation theatre; RR: Relative Risk; SSI: Surgical site infection; UTI: Urinary tract infection

Acknowledgements

All the contributions by the authors to the research work were voluntary and we acknowledge the cooperation from all 3 obstetric units in recruiting patients and the Labour room Registrars and Consultants.

Funding

Not applicable.

Authors' contributions

All the authors read and approved the final version of the manuscript. CAJ: Was the Principal investigator of the study and collected all data. AH: Was involved in designing the methods of data abstraction and verified the results. BY: Was involved in data analyses and interpretation and also involved in data abstraction supervision, quality control assurance. STS: Involved in drafting the background section along with CAS. AK: Implementation of the study, guidance in writing up. RJ: Provided leadership in phrasing the research question. Involved in designing the methods of data abstraction and verified the results. Drafted the discussion section, reviewed and approved the overall manuscript.

Competing interests

All other authors declare that they have no competing interests.

Author details

[1]Department of Neonatology, Christian Medical College, Vellore, India. [2]Department of Obstetrics and Gynecology Unit IV, Christian Medical College, Vellore, India. [3]Department of Biostatistics, Christian Medical College, Vellore, India. [4]MLL Hospital, Madanapalle, Chittoor, Andhrapradesh, India.

References

1. Declercq E, Barger M, Cabral HJ, Evans SR, Kotelchuck M, Simon C, Weiss J, Heffner LJ. Maternal outcomes associated with planned primary cesarean births compared with planned vaginal births. Obstet Gynecol. 2007;109:669–77.
2. Armson BA. Is planned cesarean childbirth a safe alternative? CMAJ. 2007; 176:475–6.
3. Bratzler DW, Dellinger EP, Olsen KM, Perl TM, Auwaerter PG, Bolon MK, Fish DN, Napolitano LM, Sawyer RG, Slain D, Steinberg JP, Weinstein RA, American Society of Health-System Pharmacists, Infectious Disease Society of America, Surgical Infection Society, Society for Healthcare Epidemiology of America. Clinical practice guidelines for antimicrobial prophylaxis in surgery. Am J Health-Syst Pharm. 2013;70:195–283.
4. Classen DC, Evans RS, Pestotnik SL, Horn SD, Menlove RL, Burke JP. The timing of prophylactic administration of antibiotics and the risk of surgical-wound infection. N Engl J Med. 1992;326:281–6.

5. Francis C, Mumford M, Strand ML, Moore ES, Strand EA. Timing of prophylactic antibiotic at cesarean section: a double-blinded, randomized trial. J Perinatol. 2013;33:759–62.
6. Baaqeel H, Baaqeel R. Timing of antibiotic prophylaxis for caesarean section. BJOG Int J Obstet Gynaecol. 2013;120:778–9.
7. Sullivan SA, Smith T, Chang E, Hulsey T, Vandorsten JP, Soper D. Administration of cefazolin prior to skin incision is superior to cefazolin at cord clamping in preventing postcesarean infectious morbidity: a randomized, controlled trial. Am J Obstet Gynecol. 2007;196(455):e1–5.
8. Health Protection Agency. Surveillance of Surgical Site Infection in England: October 1997–September 2005. London: Health Protection Agency. p. 2006.
9. Reichman DE, Greenberg JA. Reducing surgical site infections: a review. Rev Obstet Gynecol. 2009;2:212–21.
10. Owens SM, Brozanski BS, Meyn LA, Wiesenfeld HC. Antimicrobial prophylaxis for cesarean delivery before skin incision. Obstet Gynecol. 2009;114:573–9.
11. Baaqeel H, Baaqeel R. Timing of administration of prophylactic antibiotics for caesarean section: a systematic review and meta-analysis. BJOG Int J Obstet Gynaecol. 2013;120:661–9.
12. Nokiani FA, Akbari H, Rezae M. Timing of prophylactic antibiotic administration in term cesarean section: A randomized clinical trial. Iran J Clin Infect Dis. 2009;4:71–6.
13. Smaill FM, Gyte GM. Antibiotic prophylaxis versus no prophylaxis for preventing infection after cesarean section. Cochrane Database Syst Rev. 2010;(1):1-198.

19

Trend of caesarean deliveries in Egypt and its associated factors: evidence from national surveys, 2005–2014

Rami H. Al Rifai

Abstract

Background: The continued rise in caesarean section (c-section) deliveries raises a major public health concern worldwide. This study assessed the trend of c-section deliveries and examined factors associated with a rise in c-section deliveries among the Egyptian mothers, from 2005 to 2014, by place of delivery.

Methods: This study utilized the 2005, 2008, and 2014 Egypt Demographic and Health Surveys (EDHS). The EDHS reported on the mode of delivery for the last birth occurred within five years preceding each survey including place of delivery and sociodemographic information for a total sample of over 29,000 mothers in the three surveys. To document trend of c-section, the EDHS-2005 was set as a reference in two binary logistic regression models; among all mothers together and for mothers stratified by place of delivery (public or private). *P*-value for the trend was assessed by entering the year of the survey as a continuous variable. The study followed STROBE statement in reporting observational studies.

Results: Institutional-based c-sections increased by 40.7 points from EDHS-2005 to EDHS-2014 (aOR, 3.46, 95%CI: 3.15–3.80, $P_{trend} < 0.001$). Compared to mothers with low socioeconomic status (SES), mothers with high SES had higher odds (aOR, 1.78, 95%CI: 1.25–2.54, $P = 0.001$) for c-section, but only in EDHS-2005. The adjusted trend of c-sections was found to be 4.19-time (95%CI: 3.73–4.70, $P < 0.001$) higher in private sector while that in public sector it was 2.67-time (95%CI: 2.27–3.13, $P = 0.001$) higher, in EDHS-2014 relative to EDHS-2005. This increase in the private sector is explained by significant increases among mothers who are potentially at low risk for c-sections; mothers aged 19-24 years vs. ≥35 years (aOR: 0.31, 95%CI: 0.21–0.45, in EDHS-2005 vs. 0.43, 95%CI: 0.33–0.56, in EDHS-2014, $P < 0.001$); primigravida mothers vs. mothers with ≥4 children (aOR: 1.62, 95%CI: 1.12–2.34, in EDHS-2005 vs. 3.76, 95%CI: 2.94–4.80 in EDHS-2014); and among normal compared to high risk birth weight babies (aOR: 0.79, 95%CI: 0.62–0.99 in EDHS-2005 $P < 0.05$ vs. 0.83, 95%CI: 0.65–1.04 in EDHS-2014, $P > 0.05$).

Conclusions: Results showed a steady rise in c-sections in Egypt that has reached an alarming level in recent years. This increase appears to be associated with a shift towards delivery in private health care facilities. More vigilance of c-section deliveries, particularly in the private sector, is warranted.

Keywords: Egypt, Caesarean section delivery, Maternal health, Maternal delivery

Correspondence: rrifai@uaeu.ac.ae
Institute of Public Health, College of Medicine and Health Sciences, United Arab Emirates University, Al-Ain, United Arab Emirates

Background

Caesarean section (c-section) delivery is a major surgical operation aimed at saving lives [1]. Globally, the proportion of c-sections, one of the most common surgeries, continues to rise particularly in high- and middle-income countries [1]. Caesarean sections should be performed when vaginal delivery poses a risk to the mother or baby as in case of prolonged labor, fetal distress, or fetal malpresentation. The World Health Organization (WHO) underscores the importance of focusing on the needs of the pregnant mothers and discourages performing c-sections with no need. Caesarean delivery without a medical need places mothers and their babies at-risk of short- and long-term health consequences [1]. It is associated with increased risk of blood transfusion, hysterectomy, maternal and child death [2–4], uterine rupture, placenta accreta, and placenta previa [5, 6]. It also costs more and requires longer hospitalization than vaginal delivery [7].

The WHO has considered a population-based rate of c-sections between 10 and 15%, as an ideal rate that was associated with a notable decline in maternal mortality ratio (MMR) and neonatal mortality rate (NMR) [1]. In 2008, half of 137 countries have exceeded this recommended threshold [8]. In 23 out of 24 countries, proportion of c-sections without medical indication ranged between 0.01% and 2% [3]. Caesarean section rate varied across different countries, worldwide. The rate was between 20% and 22.5% in the United Kingdom and Canada. In Italy and South America, c- section rate was as high as 85% [9–11]. In Saudi Arabia, the c-section rate increased by 80%, from 10.6% to 19.1%, between the years 1997 and 2006 [12]. Private practice has contributed to the increased c- section rate internationally. In Rome, the rate of c-section delivery was reported to be approximately 44%; 85% of all birth in some private clinics of Rome were c-section [13]. In Jordan, a neighboring country to Egypt, between 2002 and 2012, the c-section deliveries increased significantly over time, from 18.2% in 2002 to 30.3% in 2012; an increase by 70% in c-sections was in the private hospitals [14].

Health services in Egypt are provided by three sectors based on the financing source: the public, the parastatal, and the private sector. The public sector covers the government and quasi-governmental hospitals (parastatal). Public hospitals receive funding from the Ministry of Finance while the government ministries have a controlling share of decision making in parastatal hospitals [15]. Public hospitals include a total of 1,048 inpatient facilities with more than 80,000 beds. The private sector has a total of 2,024 inpatient facilities with a total of 22,647 beds that accounts for approximately 16% of the total inpatient bed capacity in Egypt [15].

In the past two decades, there were significant achievements in matters related to maternal health in Egypt. Home-based deliveries declined by over 60% [16], medically assisted births rose sharply from 35% in 1988 to 92% in 2014, and 90% of mothers received antenatal care (ANC) services from a trained provider [16]. The MMR declined from 174/100,000 live births in 1992 to 54/100,000 in 2010 [17]. However, over the last two years, the MMR has slightly increased to 57/100,000; 23.5% of these mortalities delivery were initiated in a private clinic [17]. The NMR was 14/1,000 births during the five-year period prior to 2014 [16].

The last study tracking changes in c-sections in Egypt was reported in 2004 [18]. According to which, based on data from two Egyptian Demographic and Health Surveys (EDHS), the institutional-based proportion of c-sections increased from 13.9% in 1988 to 22% in 2000 [18]. Birth delivery in the private sector was associated with this increase [18]. However, this study did not explore the change in c-section rate among mothers who are potentially at low risk for c-section. Although EDHS is a non-institutional-based survey, it is reported that the DHS data on c-section deliveries are sufficiently reliable for national and global monitoring purposes since the recall bias on reporting a major surgical procedure is very low [19]. With the increased access to healthcare services in Egypt, represented by a decline in home-based deliveries and an increase in ANC services [16], the specific objectives of this study are: to (1) assess the trend of c-section deliveries and (2) to identify factors associated with the over time change in c-sections in Egypt, from 2005 to 2014, with a focus on the role of place of delivery in performing c-sections, particularly for mothers who are potentially at low risk for c-section delivery.

Methods

Data sources

The EDHS survey aimed at providing national estimates with special emphasis on maternal and child health [16]. Employing a standardized and rigorous sampling and data collection methodology, the survey collected information from a nationally representative sample of Egyptian individuals with a large sample size [16]. Details related to sampling design, sample size, study instruments, data collection, how informed consent was obtained, and other related methodology are described elsewhere [16]. The EDHS data are accessible from the Measure DHS website [20]. The STROBE statement for reporting observational studies was followed [21] (STROBE checklist can be found in the Additional file 1).

Study population

For the purpose of this study, the 2005, 2008, and 2014 EDHS ever-married women databases were merged based on established guidelines for managing DHS data [22]. All mothers who replied by “yes” or “no” to the question "*Has your last baby born in the past five years, including this year, was delivered by a c-section or normal/vaginal delivery?*" were included in the analysis, leaving a final sample of 29,489 mothers (weighted sample of 29,107) after excluding five women with missing data and 28,269 women who did not report giving birth within the prior five years (Fig. 1).

Study variables

Sociodemographics

Specific information collected in the EDHS that reported [14, 18, 23] or could potentially have an influence on the mode of birth delivery was characterized. Sociodemographic characteristics included mother's age at last birth (≤18, 19–24, 25–29, 30–34, and ≥35 years). Mother's socioeconomic status (SES) was defined based on composite scores of the mother's education level and household's wealth status. This was performed to address the problem of multicollinearity between education and income [24]. First, mothers were dichotomized according to their education level as either with "low education" (primary or below) or with "high education" (secondary or above) and trichotomized them according to their wealth status into tertiles: poor, middle, or rich. Details related to the EDHS wealth index can be found elsewhere [16]. Then, based on the sum of scores of education and wealth variables, mothers with low SES (poor and with low education), middle SES (either poor or with low education), and high SES (non-poor and with high education) were identified [24].

Mothers were categorized according to their lifetime parity into primigravida, multipara with 2–3, or multipara with ≥4 births. Female genital mutilation (FGM) status was reported in a binary variable (yes or no). Body mass index (BMI) (kg/m^2) was calculated as the ratio of the weight in kilograms divided by height squared (m^2) data that were collected at the time of survey. Mother's BMI was trichotomized into normal (BMI = 18.5–24.9 kg/m2), underweight (BMI <18.5 kg/m2), or overweight/obese (BMI ≥25 kg/m2) [25]. Maternal BMI has been linked to increased risk of adverse pregnancy outcomes leading to c-section delivery. Underweight and overweight/obese mothers were defined as a "high-risk" group for c-section. Underweight mothers are more likely to have underweight babies and pre-term delivery [26] while overweight/obese mothers are more likely to have overweight babies, preeclampsia, macrosomia, and gestational diabetes [27–30].

Spatial characteristics

Spatial characteristics included place of residence (rural or urban) and geographical region (urban governorates, urban or rural-lower Egypt, and urban or rural-upper Egypt).

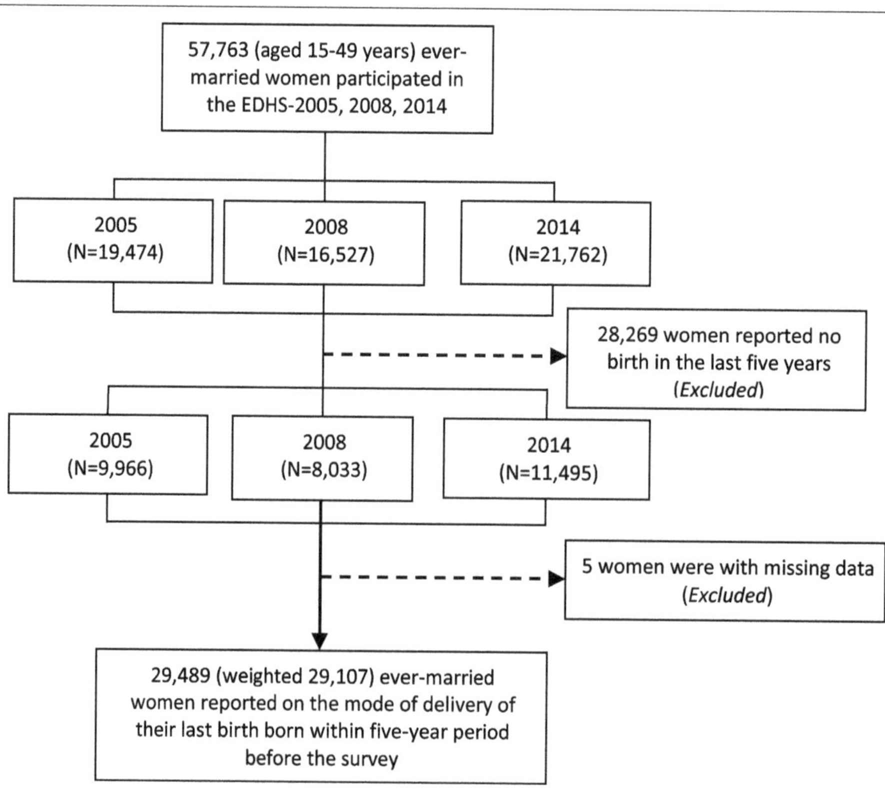

Fig. 1 Sample selection, unweighted numbers

Newborn characteristics

Mothers were categorized according to the birth weight as mother with: normal (2,500–3,999 g), low (<2,500 g), or high (≥4,000 g) birth weight baby. According to the birth multiplicity of the last birth born within the 5 years prior to the EDHS survey, mothers were categorized into two groups (singleton or multiple births). Mothers reported singleton or normal birth weight (2,500 to 3,999 g) babies were categorized as "low risk" while multiple or low/high birth weight (<2,500 g or ≥4,000 g) babies were categorized as a "high risk" group for c-section [14, 23]. Low/high birth weight or multiple births are main obstetric variables to increase risk of c-section [23, 31]. The mode of last birth delivery in relation to mode of delivery of the previous birth occurred within the five years of survey was categorized into vaginal after c-section, repeated c-section, repeated vaginal, or c-section after vaginal. Primigravida mothers were also included within this variable.

Institutional characteristics

According to the number of ANC visits made by mother during her last pregnancy, mothers were categorized into four groups (no visits, 1–3, ≥4, or don't know/missing). Place of birth delivery was categorized into: home, public sector including parastatal health care facilities, or private sector.

Statistical analyses

Frequency of mothers for each survey and their percentage distribution per each measured characteristic for all births and for institutional-based births were calculated, by survey round. Also, the proportion of institutional-based c-sections for each measured characteristic by survey round were recorded and assessed the over time trend of c-sections for each measured category's item by chi-square tests for trend.

The crude and adjusted trend of c-sections utilizing the EDHS-2005 as a reference in binary and multivariable logistic regression models for all institutional-based deliveries, and stratified by place of delivery, after merging the datasets were subsequently investigated. This stratification was done to examine the role of place of delivery on the over time trend of c-sections in Egypt. In the binary logistic regression models, *P*-value for the trend was assessed for each model by entering the year of the survey as a continuous variable.

The quantitative association between institutional-based c-sections and each measured characteristic for each survey separately was also investigated. The crude (ORs) and adjusted odds ratios (aORs) and their respective 95% confidence intervals (CIs) were reported. To adjust for any potential confounding effect, all covariates were entered under analysis simultaneously in multivariable models.

A place of delivery-stratified multivariable logistic regression analysis was performed to quantify the association between institutional-based c-sections and the measured characteristics for each survey round. This was performed to understand which factors were associated with increased trend of c-sections in Egypt, stratified by place of delivery.

The sampling weights available in the EDHS databases were applied in all of performed statistical calculations. The data were analyzed using IBM SPSS version 22.0 (IBM Corp., Armonk, NY, USA) [32]. *P*-values <0.05 were considered statistically significant.

Results

The three EDHSs were based on a nationally representative sample of 57,763 ever-married women aged 15 to 49 years, of which, 29,107 mothers reported on the mode of delivery of their last birth born within five years preceding each survey (Fig. 1).

Table 1 presents descriptive characteristics of all mothers and mothers who reported institutional-based delivery by survey round. The table shows that the institutional-based last birth occurred at mother's age of ≥35 years or ≤18 years declined slightly from 11.4% to 10.2% and from 4.9% to 3.7%, from EDHS-2005 to EDHS-2014, respectively. Percentage of mothers with low SES who reported institutional-based birth declined by 4.9 percentage points mainly for an increase by 3.9 percentage points for the favor of mothers with a medium SES. Percentage of primigravida or mothers with ≥4 children declined from 28.2% to 24.3% and from 21.7% to 20.7%, respectively. Percentage of overweight mothers increased from 76.2% to 79.6%. Over the study period, percentage of institutional-based normal birth weight babies increased by 13.6 percentage points. Institutional-based c-sections increased from 32.4% in EDHS-2005 to 61.8% in EDHS-2014. Repeated c-sections increased by 10 percentage points along a slight increase in c-sections after vaginal delivery by only 1.1 percentage points. Birth delivery declined in public sector by 11.8 percentage points for the favor of the private sector.

Proportion of c-sections by year showed that the population-based trend of c-sections increased exponentially from 17.8% in 2000 to 59.7% in 2014 that further increased from 26.6% to 67.3% when the analysis was limited to the institutional-based deliveries, during the same study period (Fig. 2).

Table 2 shows the over time changes in proportion of institutional-based c-sections. From EDHS-2005 to EDHS-2014, proportion of c-sections increased among mothers in each measured characteristic within each measured category. Largest increases were among

Table 1 Descriptive characteristics of all mothers ($N = 29,107$) and mothers with the last institutional-based ($N = 22,194$) birth occurred within five years prior to each survey, by survey round

	EDHS-2005		EDHS-2008		EDHS-2014	
	All births *N* = 9823	Institutional births *N* = 6517	All births *N* = 7893	Institutional births *N* = 5713	All births *N* = 11,391	Institutional births *N* = 9964
	%	%	%	%	%	%
Socio-demographic						
Age at last birth, years						
≥ 35	11.7	11.4	11.1	11.2	10.5	10.2
30–34	18.2	18.3	16.6	16.4	19.1	18.8
25–29	29.2	30.3	30.6	31.2	32.9	33.2
19–24	36.0	35.1	36.8	36.3	33.8	34.1
≤ 18	4.9	4.9	4.9	4.8	3.7	3.7
Socioeconomic status						
Low	28.4	18.7	24.6	16.6	16.7	13.8
Medium	26.2	24.5	25.1	23.5	29.6	28.4
High	45.4	56.8	50.1	60.0	53.7	57.9
Lifetime parity						
Multipara with ≥4 children	27.5	21.7	23.7	19.2	23.1	20.7
Multipara with 2–3 children	48.7	50.1	49.7	50.2	54.2	55.0
Primigravida	23.8	28.2	26.6	30.6	22.7	24.3
FGM[a]						
No	3.9	4.9	4.7	5.7	8.6	9.2
Yes	96.0	95.1	95.3	94.3	91.4	90.7
Missing	0.01					
BMI						
Normal 18.5–24.9 (low risk)	25.7	22.3	28.7	25.5	19.8	19.3
Underweight <18.5 (high risk)	0.6	0.5	0.6	0.4	0.3	0.3
Overweight ≥25 (high risk)	72.7	76.2	70.1	73.4	79.0	79.6
Missing	1.0	1.1	0.6	0.7	0.8	0.8
Spatial						
Residence						
Urban	38.1	48.0	38.1	45.3	31.8	34.3
Rural	61.9	52.0	61.9	54.7	68.2	65.7
Region						
Urban governorates	14.8	19.7	16.4	20.4	10.8	11.8
Urban-Lower Egypt	10.0	13.1	10.1	12.0	9.4	10.4
Rural-Lower Egypt	31.1	32.2	34.3	35.4	39.0	40.2
Urban-Upper Egypt	12.6	14.4	10.8	11.9	11.1	11.5
Rural-Upper Egypt	30.1	19.4	27.3	18.8	28.8	25.2
Frontier governorates	1.2	1.1	1.4	1.5	0.9	0.9
Newborn characteristics						
Birth weight						
Normal (2,500–3,999 g)	30.5	39.0	35.1	43.5	49.4	52.6
High risk (<2,500, ≥4,000 g)	8.7	10.8	8.1	10.1	13.5	14.1
Not weighted/Missing	60.8	50.2	56.8	46.3	37.1	33.3

Table 1 Descriptive characteristics of all mothers ($N = 29{,}107$) and mothers with the last institutional-based ($N = 22{,}194$) birth occurred within five years prior to each survey, by survey round *(Continued)*

	EDHS-2005		EDHS-2008		EDHS-2014	
	All births $N = 9823$	Institutional births $N = 6517$	All births $N = 7893$	Institutional births $N = 5713$	All births $N = 11{,}391$	Institutional births $N = 9964$
	%	%	%	%	%	%
Birth multiplicity						
Singleton birth	97.6	97.0	97.9	97.4	97.8	97.6
Multiple birth	2.4	3.0	2.1	2.6	2.2	2.4
Delivery mode						
Vaginal	78.5	67.6	70.8	59.7	45.9	38.2
C-section	21.5	32.4	29.2	40.3	54.1	61.8
Delivery mode in relation to the previous[b]						
Primigravida	66.0	69.0	69.0	70.5	66.2	66.8
Vaginal after caesarean	0.5	0.4	0.4	0.4	0.4	0.3
Repeated caesarean	5.2	7.8	6.9	9.5	15.6	17.8
Repeated vaginal	27.0	20.9	22.2	17.5	15.2	12.1
Caesarean after vaginal	1.3	1.9	1.5	2.1	2.6	3.0
Institutional						
Antenatal care visits						
No visits	28.5	18.3	25.8	17.1	9.7	7.3
1–3	10.1	8.3	6.9	6.0	7.1	6.1
≥4	60.7	72.8	66.5	76.2	82.8	86.2
Don't know/missing	0.7	0.6	0.8	0.7	0.4	0.4
Place of delivery						
Home	33.6	0.0	27.6	0.0	12.5	0.0
Public sector	26.9	40.6	27.2	37.6	25.2	28.8
Private sector	39.5	59.4	45.2	62.4	62.3	71.2
Missing		4		3		

Weighted numbers and percentages
BMI: body mass index
[a] female genital mutilation, [b] previous birth occurred within past five years

mothers aged ≤18 years (34.1 points), primigravida mothers (34.4 points), mothers with normal BMI (31.4 points), normal birth weight (30.1 points) or singleton babies (29.5 points), and in the private sector (32.6 points). Of the 6158 institutional-based c-sections performed in EDHS-2014, 77.3% were performed in the private sector.

The multivariable analysis revealed a 3.46-time (95% CI: 3.15–3.80) increase in trend of c-sections in EDHS-2014 relative to EDHS-2005. The further place of delivery-stratified multivariate analysis showed that this increase in trend of c-sections was higher in private sector (aOR, 4.19, 95% CI: 3.73–4.70) than in public sector (aOR, 2.67, 95% CI: 2.27–3.13) (Table 3).

Table 4 shows the results of bivariate and multivariable logistic regression of association between institutional-based c-section and measured characteristics by survey round. As the table shows, relative to mothers aged ≥35 years, in EDHS-2014, the trend of c-section among

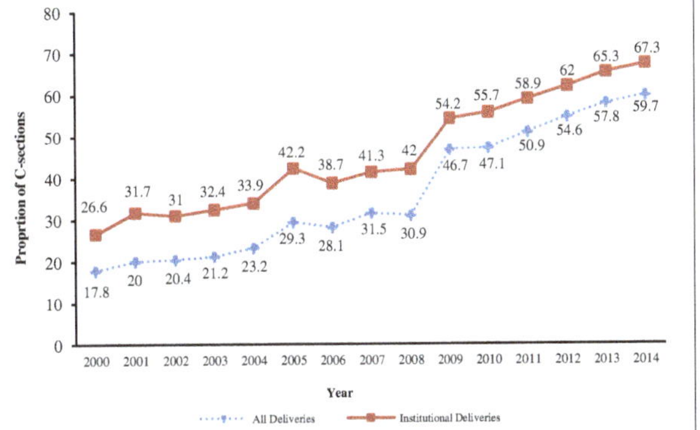

Fig. 2 Trend in c-section deliveries in Egypt, 2000–2014

Table 2 Institutional-based proportion of c-section deliveries among mothers with a last birth occurred within five years prior to each survey, by survey round

	EDHS-2005 N = 6517 C-section, %	EDHS-2008 N = 5713 C-section, %	*P-value*[a]	EDHS-2014 N = 9964 C-section, %	*P-value*[b]	Absolute difference (% in 2014–% in 2005
Socio-demographic						
Age at last birth						
≥ 35	37.2	44.3	0.007	62.4	<0.001	25.2
30–34	35.5	43.1	<0.001	62.4	<0.001	26.9
25–29	33.6	42.3	<0.001	61.5	<0.001	27.9
19–24	29.2	37.1	<0.001	61.8	<0.001	32.6
≤ 18	25.8	33.6	0.038	59.9	<0.001	34.1
P-value[b]	<0.001	<0.001		0.903		
Socioeconomic status						
Low	22.7	33.5	<0.001	51.6	<0.001	28.9
Medium	29.2	35.2	0.001	57.9	<0.001	28.7
High	37.0	44.2	<0.001	66.1	<0.001	29.1
P-value[b]	<0.001	<0.001		<0.001		
Lifetime parity						
Multipara with ≥4 children	27.3	33.3	0.001	52.2	<0.001	24.9
Multipara with 2–3 children	32.9	40.8	<0.001	61.8	<0.001	28.9
Primigravidas	35.6	43.9	<0.001	70.0	<0.001	34.4
P-value[b]	<0.001	<0.001		<0.001		
FGM[c]						
No	44.8	53.5	0.027	68.9	<0.001	24.1
Yes	31.8	39.5	<0.001	61.1	<0.001	29.3
P-value[b]	<0.001	<0.001		<0.001		
Missing	5	0		3		
BMI						
Normal (18.5–24.9)	26.2	36.3	<0.001	57.6	<0.001	31.4
High risk (<18.5, ≥25)	34.2	41.6	<0.001	62.8	<0.001	28.6
P-value[b]	<0.001	<0.001		<0.001		
Missing	69	41		80		
Spatial						
Residence						
Urban	36.8	44.5	<0.001	65.8	<0.001	29.0
Rural	28.4	36.9	<0.001	59.7	<0.001	31.3
P-value[b]	<0.001	<0.001		<0.001		
Region						
Urban governorates	40.4	44.6	0.034	67.3	<0.001	26.9
Urban-Lower Egypt	42.0	48.8	0.008	73.6	<0.001	31.6
Rural-Lower Egypt	32.3	38.4	<0.001	65.8	<0.001	33.5
Urban-Upper Egypt	27.6	41.2	<0.001	57.8	<0.001	30.2
Rural-Upper Egypt	22.2	34.4	<0.001	50.2	<0.001	28.0
Frontier governorates	24.7	28.9	0.550	51.6	0.002	26.9
P-value[b]	<0.001	<0.001		<0.001		
Newborn characteristics						
Birth weight						
Normal (2,500–3,999)	35.1	41.4	<0.001	65.2	<0.001	30.1
High risk (<2,500, ≥4,000)	41.6	51.1	0.001	67.1	<0.001	25.5

Table 2 Institutional-based proportion of c-section deliveries among mothers with a last birth occurred within five years prior to each survey, by survey round *(Continued)*

	EDHS-2005 N = 6517 C-section, %	EDHS-2008 N = 5713 C-section, %	*P-value*[a]	EDHS-2014 N = 9964 C-section, %	*P-value*[b]	Absolute difference (% in 2014–% in 2005
P-value[b]	0.002	<0.001		0.182		
Not weighted/Missing	3272	2648		3317		
Birth multiplicity						
Singleton birth	32.0	40.1	<0.001	61.5	<0.001	29.5
Multiple birth	48.0	50.0	0.709	75.2	<0.001	27.2
P-value[b]	<0.001	0.016		<0.001		
Mode of delivery in relation to the previous birth[d]						
Primigravidas mother	32.9	40.8	<0.001	61.4	<0.001	28.5
Vaginal after caesarean	–	–	–	–	–	
Repeated caesarean	–	–	–	–	–	
Repeated vaginal	–	–	–	–	–	
C-section after vaginal	–	–	–	–	–	
Institutional						
Antenatal care visits						
No visits	18.8	30.1	<0.001	42.4	<0.001	23.6
1–3	26.7	34.1	0.019	48.6	<0.001	21.9
≥ 4	36.4	43.3	<0.001	64.4	<0.001	28.0
P-value[b]	<0.001	<0.001		<0.001		
Don't know/missing	40	41		36		
Place of delivery						
Public sector	29.4	35.4	<0.001	48.5	<0.001	19.1
Private sector	34.4	43.2	<0.001	67.0	<0.001	32.6
P-value[b]	<0.001	<0.001		<0.001		

[a] *P*-value, assessed over time differences in proportion of institutional-based caesarean delivery between EDHS-2005 and EDHS-2008, and between EDHS-2008 and EDHS-2014
[b] *P*-value, assessed differences in proportion of institutional-based caesarean delivery between each measured sub-categories in each survey
[c] female genital mutilation
[d] previous birth occurred within the past five years

mothers aged ≤18 years (aOR, 0.33, 95% CI: 0.23–0.47) or 19–25 years (aOR, 0.41, 95% CI: 0.31–0.55) was higher when it compared with c-sections in EDHS-2005 (aOR, 0.26, 95% CI: 0.16–0.50 and 0.31, 95% CI: 0.22–0.42, respectively). In EDHS-2005, mothers from high SES (aOR, 1,78, 95% CI: 1.25–2.54, $P = 0.001$) were more likely to undergo c-section relative to those with low SES, but in EDHS-2014 this observed significant difference disappeared. Among primigravida, trend of c-sections in EDHS-2014 (aOR, 5.57, 95% CI: 4.46–6.97)

Table 3 Bivariate and multivariate logistic regression for the trend of institutional-based c-section delivery among all mothers, stratified by place of delivery

Among all mothers	OR (95% CI)		aOR (95% CI)	
Survey round (Ref: EDHS-2005)				
EDHS-2008	1.41 (1.31–1.52)***		1.39 (1.25–1.54)***	
EDHS-2014	3.37 (3.20–3.60)***		3.46 (3.15–3.80)***	
Place of delivery	Public sector		Private sector	
Survey round (Ref: EDHS-2005)	OR (95% CI)	aOR (95% CI)	OR (95% CI)	aOR (95% CI)
EDHS-2008	1.32 (1.16–1.49)***	1.35 (1.13–1.61)**	1.45 (1.33–1.60)***	1.42 (1.25–1.62)***
EDHS-2014	2.26 (2.02–2.53)***	2.67 (2.27–3.13)**	2.88 (3.58–4.21)***	4.19 (3.73–4.70)***

OR: odds ratio, aOR: adjusted odds ratio (for all covariates under analysis), CI: confidence interval
P-value for the trend was assessed by entering the year of the survey as a continuous variable
*$P < 0.05$, **$P = 0.001$, ***$P < 0.001$

Table 4 Bivariate and multivariate logistic regression for the association between institutional-based c-section as dependent variable and measured characteristics by the survey round

Characteristics	EDHS-2005		EDHS-2008		EDHS-2014	
	OR (95% CI)	aOR (95% CI)	OR (95% CI)	aOR (95% CI)	OR (95% CI)	aOR (95% CI)
Socio-demographic						
Age at last birth (Ref: ≥35 yrs)						
30–34	0.93 (0.77–1.12)	0.77 (0.57–1.04)	0.93 (0.77–1.12)	0.83 (0.61–1.11)	1.00 (0.86–1.17)	0.77 (0.61–0.95)*
25–29	0.85 (0.71–1.01)	0.47 (0.35–0.65)***	0.85 (0.71–1.01)	0.72 (0.55–0.95)**	0.97 (0.84–1.11)	0.54 (0.44–0.66)***
19–24	0.70 (0.59–0.83)***	0.31 (0.22–0.42)***	0.70 (0.59–0.83)***	0.41 (0.31–0.55)***	0.98 (0.85–1.13)	0.41 (0.31–0.55)***
≤ 18	0.58 (0.44–0.78)***	0.26 (0.16–0.50)***	0.63 (0.47–0.85)***	0.37 (0.23–0.60)***	0.90 (0.71–1.15)	0.33 (0.23–0.47)***
Socioeconomic status (Ref: low)						
Medium	1.40 (1.18–1.67)***	1.55 (1.07–2.24)*	1.08 (0.91–1.29)	0.79 (0.58–1.07)	1.29 (1.13–1.47)***	0.98 (0.80–1.21)
High	2.0 (1.72–2.32)***	1.78 (1.25–2.54)**	1.57 (1.35–1.83)***	0.77 (0.57–1.04)	1.83 (1.63–2.07)***	0.97 (0.85–1.12)
Lifetime parity (Ref: multipara with ≥4 children)						
Multipara with 2–3 children	1.31 (1.14–1.50)***	1.06 (0.81–1.38)	1.38 (1.19–1.59)***	1.41 (1.08–1.84)*	2.13 (1.89–2.41)***	1.52 (1.27–1.81)***
Primigravidas	1.47 (1.23–1.71)***	2.91 (2.11–4.00)***	1.57 (1.34–1.83)***	3.88 (2.83–5.33)***	1.48 (1.34–1.64)***	5.57 (4.46–6.97)***
FGM[a] (Ref: no)						
Yes	0.57 (0.46–0.72)***	0.69 (0.51–0.94)*	0.57 (0.45–0.71)***	0.61 (0.44–0.84)**	0.71 (0.61–0.82)***	0.93 (0.76–1.13)
BMI (Ref: normal 18.5–24.9)						
High risk (<18.5, ≥25)	1.46 (1.28–1.67)***	1.27 (1.02–1.59)*	1.26 (1.11–1.42)***	1.38 (1.13–1.77)**	1.25 (1.13–1.38)***	1.44 (1.24–1.69)***
Spatial						
Residence (Ref: urban)						
Rural	0.68 (0.61–0.76)***	0.78 (0.09–6.56)	0.73 (0.66–0.81)***	0.66 (0.12–3.52)	0.77 (0.71–0.84)***	0.73 (0.19–2.68)
Region (Ref: urban governorates)						
Urban-Lower Egypt	2.07 (1.20–3.56)**	0.94 (0.73–1.21)	1.93 (1.19–3.15)**	1.08 (0.81–1.43)	1.93 (1.26–2.96)**	1.16 (0.91–1.47)
Rural-Lower Egypt	2.21 (1.27–3.83)**	0.99 (0.12–8.35)	2.29 (1.39–3.75)**	1.40 (0.26–7.61)	2.62 (1.70–4.04)***	1.08 (0.29–4.00)
Urban-Upper Egypt	1.45 (0.85–2.49)	0.50 (0.38–0.67)	1.49 (0.92–2.41)	0.90 (0.68–1.17)	1.81 (1.19–2.74)**	0.62 (0.49–0.77)***
Rural-Upper Egypt	1.17 (0.67–2.03)	0.90 (0.10–7.66)	1.68 (1.02–2.76)*	1.27 (0.23–6.92)	1.28 (0.84–1.97)	0.74 (0.20–2.75)
Frontier governorates	0.87 (0.51–1.51)	0.47 (0.18–1.22)	1.26 (0.77–2.05)	0.56 (0.25–1.25)	0.95 (0.62–1.44)	0.69 (0.33–2.74)
Newborn characteristics						
Birth weight (Ref: high risk <2,500, ≥4,000)						
Normal 2,500–3,999	0.75 (0.64–0.90)**	0.76 (0.63–0.91)**	0.67 (0.56–0.81)***	0.65 (0.54–0.79)***	0.92 (0.81–1.04)	0.86 (0.75–0.98)*
Birth multiplicity (Ref: multiple)						
Singleton	0.51 (0.38–0.68)***	0.44 (0.30–0.65)**	0.67 (0.48–0.92)*	0.50 (0.32–0.781)**	0.52 (0.39–0.70)***	0.46 (0.32–0.66)***
Previous birth c-section[b] (Ref: no)						
Yes	66.3 (44.3–99.2)***	113 (58.4–218)***	61.4 (39.6–95.1)***	114.4 (55.3–236)***	69.4 (47.9–100)***	123.3 (71.9–211)***
Primigravidas	1.87 (1.64–2.10)***	2.76 (2.23–3.41)***	1.90 (47.9–100)***	2.83 (2.30–3.49)***	2.64 (2.38–2.91)***	3.82 (3.27–4.46)***
Institutional						
ANC (Ref: no visits)						
1–3 visits	1.56 (1.24–2.00)***	1.58 (1.01–2.47)**	1.20 (0.93–1.56)	1.18 (0.76–1.85)	1.28 (1.04–1.60)*	0.87 (0.61–1.24)
≥ 4 visits	2.48 (2.11–2.90)***	1.64 (1.21–2.23)**	1.77 (1.52–2.06)***	1.51 (1.17–1.94)**	2.45 (2.10–2.90)***	1.31 (1.01–1.70)*
Place of delivery (Ref: public)						
Private sector	1.26 (1.13–1.40)***	1.36 (1.14–1.62)**	1.39 (1.26–1.55)***	1.40 (1.17–1.66)***	2.16 (1.98–2.36)***	1.96 (1.72–2.23)***

Number of cases included in multivariate models was only 12,894 (9236 children were not weighted and 64 mothers did not report on the ANC visits)
OR: odds ratio, aOR: adjusted odds ratio (for all covariates under analysis), CI: confidence interval, ANC: antenatal care
[a] female genital mutilation, [b] previous birth occurred within the past five years
$^{*}P < 0.05$, $^{**}P = 0.001$, $^{***}P < 0.001$

was higher than that in EDHS-2005 (aOR, 2.91, 95% CI: 2.11–4.00). Normal birth weight babies had higher odds undergoing c-section delivery in EDHS-2014 (aOR, 0.86, 95% CI: 0.75–0.98) compared to EDHS-2005 (aOR, 0.76, 95% CI: 0.63–0.91).

Furthermore, place of delivery-stratified multivariable logistic regression demonstrated that in private sector, mothers aged ≤18 years had less likelihood to undergo c-sections in EDHS-2005 (aOR, 0.28, 95% CI: 0.15–0.53) compared to EDHS-2014 (aOR, 0.40, 95% CI: 0.26–0.63). However, in EDHS-2014 same age group of mothers was 84% less likely to undergo c-sections in the public sector. In public sector, SES was not associated with c-section delivery in all survey rounds, but in private sector, the significant association of SES with c-section observed in EDHS-2005 disappeared in EDHS-2014. The likelihood of primigravida mothers to undergo c-section in public sector declined from 2.21-time (95% CI: 1.37–3.58) to 1.72-time (95% CI: 1.18–2.50) whereas it increased in private sector from 1.62-times (95% CI: 1.12–2.34) to 3.76-times (95% CI: 2.94–4.80), in EDHS-2005 to EDHS-2014, respectively. Normal birth weight babies were significantly at lower risk to undergo c-section in EDHS-2005, but in EDHS-2014 they had an equal likelihood with high-risk birth weight babies in both public and private sectors (Table 5).

Discussion

The study estimated trend of c-sections among Egyptian mothers sampled in 2005, 2008, and 2014. There was a substantial rise in trend of institutional-based c-sections by more than three-fold, over the study period. The private sector appears to be the driver of the rising c-sections in Egypt, a substantial increase was also observed in use of this surgical procedure in public sector. The more than 4-folds increase in c-sections in the private sector was driven by substantial increases in c-sections among mothers who are potentially at low risk for c-section delivery.

In Egypt, the nearly 60% population-based proportion of c-sections performed in 2014 greatly exceeds the threshold of 10–15% recommended by WHO [1]. A population-based proportion of c-sections >10% did not lead to health improvements for mother or newborn [33]. Although the observed over time increase in c-section rate in Egypt is in line with what has been noted in many national and international studies [12, 14, 18, 34], this over time increase places Egypt as a country with the highest c-sections performed worldwide, after Brazil (45.9%) [8]. The institutional-based proportion (67.3%) of c-sections recorded in Egypt in 2014 is 2.2-time and 2.7-time higher than that recently recorded in Jordan (30.3%) [14] and in Saudi Arabia (25%) [35], respectively. The decline in home-based deliveries by over 60% merely reflects an improvement in provided health care services in Egypt. Over the past decade, per capita total expenditure on health increased from US$75.8 in 2000 to US$123.2 in 2010 [36]. However, improving administered health care services should not justify the massive increase in c-sections. This exponential rise in c-sections indicates an overuse for this surgical procedure that might be due to many c-sections may increasingly be performed without any medical indication.

This rise in c-sections would pose further economic burden in a resource limited-setting such as Egypt, which is already burdened with different economic difficulties where 26.3% of Egyptians live below the poverty line [37]. In 2008, the WHO estimated that 253,890 unnecessary c-sections had been performed with a total cost of US$ 41,085,585 per year [38]. Referring to the obtained results, the discernible increase in c-sections in Egypt in 2014, this study assumes that the unnecessary c-sections and its associated spending at least would double the ones estimated in 2008 [38]. Furthermore, the increased c-sections would pose further unfavorable health outcomes as a result of adverse outcomes associated with c-sections [5, 6] in a country already burdened with a relatively high MMR and NMR in addition to other infectious diseases mainly hepatitis C virus that infect nearly 15% of the 15 to 59 years old Egyptian people [39]. This disease alone consumes about 20% of the Ministry of Health and Population total annual budget to treat infected individuals [40]. Rigorous institutional-based study is needed to assess the impact of this high proportion of c-sections and identify the exact medical and non-medical needs for c-section deliveries for future planning and effective policy interventions.

In the three surveys, childbearing at ≤18 years or ≥35 years, living in high SES, maternal overweight/obesity, pregnancy with high-risk birth weight or multiple babies, delivery in a private sector were found as significant factors associated with c-section delivery in Egypt except for SES in EDHS-2014. Older mothers are more likely to experience different complications during pregnancy and delivery [41–45], even in the absence of complications, and they are more inclined to have c-section, especially primigravida mothers [44]. Younger mothers are more likely to have small pelvis to deliver a fetus which necessitate a c-section [46]. Women with high SES are more likely to be educated and to have higher income who tend to delay giving birth until older age, therefore, increasing their likelihood of a c-section delivery [42]. However, the disappeared association of SES with c-sections observed in EDHS-2014 merely explains the penetration of health care services to the socially and economically disadvantaged mothers, nevertheless this should not justify the increased c-sections among this socially deprived group. Maternal overweight/obesity increases the risk of different c-section inducing factors such as preeclampsia and gestational diabetes [47].

Table 5 Place of delivery-stratified multivariate logistic regression for the association between institutional-based c-section delivery as dependent variable and measured characteristics, by the survey round

	EDHS-2005		EDHS-2008		EDHS-2014	
	Public aOR (95% CI)	Private	Public aOR (95% CI)	Private	Public aOR (95% CI)	Private
Socio-demographic						
Age at last birth (Ref: ≥35 yrs)						
30–34	0.23 (0.09–0.62)**	0.59 (0.41–0.87)**	0.70 (0.43–1.15)	0.93 (0.63–1.36)	0.75 (0.51–1.10)	0.79 (0.61–1.07)
25–29	0.33 (0.19–0.54)***	0.40 (0.28–0.56)***	0.89 (0.57–1.40)	0.66 (0.46–0.93)*	0.52 (0.36–0.74)***	0.56 (0.44–0.72)***
19–24	0.71 (0.44–1.14)	0.31 (0.21–0.45)***	0.37 (0.23–0.61)***	0.44 (0.30–0.64)***	0.39 (0.27–0.57)***	0.43 (0.33–0.56)***
≤ 18	1.23 (0.77–1.98)	0.28 (0.15–0.53)***	0.27 (0.11–0.67)**	0.43 (0.24–0.79)**	0.16 (0.07–0.35)***	0.40 (0.26–0.63)***
Socioeconomic status (Ref: low)						
Medium	1.31 (0.76–2.27)	1.71 (1.04–2.83)*	1.23 (0.74–2.06)	0.59 (0.39–0.88)**	0.86 (0.60–1.22)	1.07 (0.83–1.38)
High	1.51 (0.90–2.55)	2.04 (1.26–3.29)**	1.25 (0.76–2.05)	0.61 (0.42–0.88)**	1.11 (0.78–1.59)	0.97 (0.76–1.25)
Lifetime parity (Ref: ≥4)						
2–3	1.54 (1.05–2.26)*	1.04 (0.76–1.41)	1.41 (0.95–2.07)	2.20 (1.60–3.03)***	1.41 (1.05–1.89)*	1.82 (1.51–2.21)***
Primigravidas	2.21 (1.37–3.58)**	1.62 (1.12–2.34)*	1.50 (0.92–2.44)	3.73 (2.56–5.42)***	1.72 (1.18–2.50)**	3.76 (2.94–4.80)***
FGM[a] (Ref: no)						
Yes	0.77 (0.41–1.45)	0.68 (0.48–0.97)*	0.51 (0.24–1.06)	0.62 (0.43–0.89)*	0.81 (0.55–1.20)	0.95 (0.75–1.20)
BMI (Ref: normal 18.5–24.9)						
High risk (<18.5, ≥25)	1.14 (0.78–1.67)	1.34 (1.01–1.77)*	1.24 (0.88–1.76)	1.52 (1.19–1.92)**	1.78 (1.32–2.40)***	1.33 (1.11–1.60)**
Spatial						
Residence (Ref: urban)						
Rural	0.82 (0.60–10.9)	0.70 (0.01–36.73)	0.95 (0.10–8.69)	0.52 (0.04–7.05)	0.56 (0.08–4.04)	1.0 (0.14–6.96)
Region (Ref: urban governorates)						
Urban-Lower Egypt	1.14 (0.73–1.79)	0.91 (0.66–1.24)	0.95 (0.57–1.62)	1.13 (0.79–1.60)	1.04 (0.69–1.56)	1.19 (0.88–1.60)
Rural-Lower Egypt	1.06 (0.08–14.7)	1.07 (0.02–56.6)	1.29 (0.14–12.19)	1.56 (0.11–21.4)	1.55 (0.21–11.4)	0.74 (0.11–5.14)
Urban-Upper Egypt	0.34 (0.19–0.58)***	0.61 (0.43–0.86)**	0.96 (0.59–1.54)	0.89 (0.64–1.24)	0.62 (0.42–0.91)*	0.60 (0.45–0.80)**
Rural-Upper Egypt	0.67 (0.05–9.46)	1.18 (0.02–63.2)	1.27 (0.14–11.9)	1.32 (0.09–18.2)	1.04 (0.14–7.67)	0.51 (0.07–3.54)
Frontier governorates	0.81 (0.24–2.71)	0.25 (0.05–1.23)	0.56 (0.18–1.77)	0.62 (0.19–1.91)	0.72 (0.19–2.75)	0.68 (0.27–1.73)
Newborn characteristics						
Birth weight (Ref: high risk <2,500, ≥4,000)						
Normal (2,500–3,999)	0.63 (0.47–0.84)**	0.79 (0.62–0.99)*	0.46 (0.34–0.62)***	0.81 (0.64–1.04)	0.83 (0.66–1.05)	0.83 (0.65–1.04)
Birth multiplicity (Ref: multiple)						
Singleton	0.39 (0.20–0.75)**	0.46 (0.28–0.77)**	1.0 (0.47–0.2.11)	0.33 (0.18–0.60)***	0.57 (0.32–1.03)	0.41 (0.26–0.66)***
Previous birth C-section[b] (Ref: no)						
Yes	53.6 (25.8–120.4)***	263.3 (82.2–843)***	66.5 (25.1–176)***	236.5 (73.1–765)***	95.4 (41.7–218)***	145.3 (71.0–297)***
Primigravidas	2.61 (1.81–3.70)***	2.85 (2.19–3.72)***	1.84 (1.27–2.70)**	3.56 (2.76–4.60)***	2.48 (1.86–3.32)***	4.52 (3.75–5.45)***
Institutional						
ANC (Ref: no visits)						
1–3	0.92 (0.46–1.84)	2.33 (1.27–4.28)**	0.72 (0.30–1.74)	1.33 (0.77–2.29)	1.04 (0.58–1.84)	0.78 (0.49–1.24)
≥ 4	1.59 (1.03–2.44)*	1.71 (1.11–2.63)*	1.89 (1.29–2.77)**	1.29 (0.91–1.81)	1.44 (0.98–2.10)	1.21 (0.84–1.74)

Number of cases included in multivariate models was only 12,894 (9236 children were not weighted and 64 mothers did not report on the ANC visits)
OR: odds ratio· aOR: adjusted odds ratio (for all covariates under analysis), CI: confidence interval, ANC: antenatal care
[a] female genital mutilation, [b] previous birth occurred within the past five years
$^{*}P < 0.05$, $^{**}P = 0.001$, $^{***}P < 0.001$

One of the principal objectives of this investigation was to identify main drivers of the increased c-sections in Egypt. Study findings documented that place of delivery is a major contributor to the exponentially increased c-sections in Egypt. Although the private sector occupies only 16% of total hospitals beds in Egypt [15], the trend of c-sections increased by more than 4-time over the study period. This finding is still persistent in Egypt and in line with the previous study reported in 2004 and analyzed comparably collected data [18]. Lack of compliance with regulations by private practitioners and inadequate enforcement of the law, public's perception that medical services in private sector due to the availability of necessary medical technology and better inpatient quality care services for this surgical intervention, particularly in presence of near birth complications, as well as obstetricians' predisposition to manage their time, are suggested [18, 23] and documented factors associated with the increasing c-sections in the private sector [31, 43, 48].

The study found that this sizeable rise in proportion of c-sections in the private sector was driven by increasing c-sections among mothers who are theoretically and empirically known as not at risk of c-section including mothers who fallen in an age group of 25–29 years, mothers of normal BMI, and mothers reported normal birth weight or singleton babies. This increase contributed substantially to the overall increase in c-sections in Egypt which supports the notion that a sizeable proportion of performed c-sections might be performed unnecessarily. This is in line with what has been recently reported from nationally-representative data in Jordan [14]. According to which, the rising in c-sections from 18.2% in 2002 to 30.3% in 2012, driven primarily by substantial rises among apparently low-risk mothers; mothers with normal birth weight or singleton babies [14].

It is worth to be mentioned that encouragement of vaginal delivery is very important to curb the steady rise in c-sections in Egypt. This study observed a decline by 12.8% in repeated institutional-based vaginal deliveries among mothers reported two births in five years preceded the survey. External cephalic version (turning the fetus from a breech or transverse position into a vertex position), vaginal birth after a previous c-section, and one-on-one trained support during labor were effective psychosocial and structural strategies at reducing the likelihood of c-sections, even among those who may have a medical indication [49]. Moreover, initiatives to raise peoples' and health professionals' awareness about the adverse outcomes associated with c-section and advantages of vaginal delivery are also urgently needed. Educating mothers about risks associated with c-section, midwifery training, and establishment of birthing centers, could also help encourage mothers to deliver vaginally.

The strengths of this study are that the data were from large, randomly selected population-based three datasets collected by accredited and reliable official entities using comparable methodology. The larger sample size and high response rates provided in the study with good statistical power and objective outcome measures. However, in population-based survey, the probability of recall bias is low since mothers who had a c-section delivery would not easily forget the mode of delivery given its surgical nature, particularly for the last birth [19]. Estimates associated with c-section were adjusted for any potential confounding effect of the measured characteristics. Stratification according to the place of delivery provided more insights about the substantial contribution of the private sector to the rising c-sections in Egypt with revealing contributing factors for the increased c-sections in this sector.

Findings from this study should be interpreted in light of the following limitations. The cross-sectional design of the EDHS limits the causality pathway with regard to the factors found associated with increased c-sections. Given the nature of the household-based survey where medical records are usually unavailable, collected data did not include information about whether the c-sections were performed under medical indications such as fetal mal-presentation or based solely on maternal demand, except for the birth weight and birth multiplicity that served as the only obstetric indicators could potentially at medically necessary c-section. Despite of these limitations, this study provided evidence-based estimates on trend of c-section deliveries in Egypt and associated factors to fine-tune strategies necessary to halt the rising c-sections in Egypt.

Conclusions

Obtained results demonstrated that the proportion of c-sections in Egypt has been increasing steadily in recent years and has reached an alarming level. The proportion of c-sections documented in the last EDHS conducted in 2014 quadrupled the maximum threshold recommended by the WHO. The increase in number of birth deliveries occurred in the private sector appears to be associated with a shift towards delivery in private facilities. This increase in the private sector, particularly among mothers who were potentially at low risk of c-sections requires an urgent need to adopt critical policies and strategies that able to halt the steady rise in c-sections in Egypt and improve reproductive health and mothers and babies health outcomes. In the meantime, an in-depth institutional-based study collecting data on the exact indications associated with c-sections in Egypt is also necessary.

Abbreviations

ANC: Antenatal care; aOR: Adjusted odds ratio; CI: Confidence interval; C-section: Caesarean section; DHS: Demographic and health surveys; EDHS: Egypt Demographic and Health Surveys; MMR: Maternal mortality ratio; NMR: Neonatal mortality rate; OR: Odds ratio; SES: Socioeconomic status; STROBE: Strengthening the Reporting of Observational Studies in Epidemiology; WHO: World Health Organization

Acknowledgements

Author is very grateful to the EDHS for collecting data. In addition, he would like to acknowledge all individuals and institutions in Egypt involved in the implementation of the 2005, 2008, and 2014 EDHS. The statements made herein are solely the responsibility of the author.

Funding

This work received no specific funding . Author is grateful to the College of Medicine and Health Sciences at the United Arab Emirates University, for covering the publication fees. The statements made herein are solely the responsibility of the author.

Author's contributions

RA, conceptualized and designed the study, analyzed the data, and drafted and critically wrote the article.

Competing interests

The author declares that he has no competing interests.

References

1. World Health Organization. Statement on Caesarean Section Rates. (http://apps.who.int/iris/bitstream/10665/161442/1/WHO_RHR_15.02_eng.pdf) Accessed 12 Apr 2016.
2. World Health Organization. Cesarean section without medical indication increases risk of short-term adverse outcomes for mothers. Geneva: WHO. Available from: http://whqlibdoc.who.int/hq/2010/WHO_RHR_HRP_10.20_eng.pdf. Accessed 21 Mar 2015.
3. Souza JP, Gulmezoglu A, Lumbiganon P, Laopaiboon M, Carroli G, Fawole B, et al. Caesarean section without medical indications is associated with an increased risk of adverse short-term maternal outcomes: the 2004-2008 WHO global survey on maternal and Perinatal health. BMC Med. 2010;8:71. doi: https://doi.org/10.1186/1741-7015-8-71. PubMed PMID: 21067593; PubMed Central PMCID: PMCPMC2993644.
4. Villar J, Carroli G, Zavaleta N, Donner A, Wojdyla D, Faundes A, et al. Maternal and neonatal individual risks and benefits associated with caesarean delivery: multicentre prospective study. BMJ. 2007;335(7628):1025. doi: https://doi.org/10.1136/bmj.39363.706956.55. PubMed PMID: 17977819; PubMed Central PMCID: PMCPMC2078636.
5. Kennare R, Tucker G, Heard A, Chan A. Risks of adverse outcomes in the next birth after a first cesarean delivery. Obstet Gynecol 2007;109(2 Pt 1): 270-276. doi: https://doi.org/10.1097/01.AOG.0000250469.23047.73. PubMed PMID: 17267823.
6. Daltveit AK, Tollanes MC, Pihlstrom H, Irgens LM. Cesarean delivery and subsequent pregnancies. Obstet Gynecol 2008;111(6):1327-1334. doi: https://doi.org/10.1097/AOG.0b013e3181744110. PubMed PMID: 18515516.
7. Allen VM, O'Connell CM, Farrell SA, Baskett TF. Economic implications of method of delivery. Am J Obstet Gynecol 2005;193(1):192-197. doi: https://doi.org/10.1016/j.ajog.2004.10.635. PubMed PMID: 16021078.
8. Gibbons L, Belizan JM, Lauer JA, Betran AP, Merialdi M, Althabe F. Inequities in the use of cesarean section deliveries in the world. Am J Obstet Gynecol. 2012;206(4):331 e1-331 19. doi: https://doi.org/10.1016/j.ajog.2012.02.026. PubMed PMID: 22464076.
9. Scioscia M, Vimercati A, Cito L, Chironna E, Scattarella D, Selvaggi LE. Social determinants of the increasing caesarean section rate in Italy. Minerva Ginecol 2008;60(2):115-120. PubMed PMID: 18487961.
10. McCallum C. Explaining caesarean section in Salvador da Bahia, Brazil Sociol Health Illn 2005;27(2):215-242. doi: https://doi.org/10.1111/j.1467-9566.2005.00440.x. PubMed PMID: 15787776.
11. Nuttall C. Caesarean section controversy. The caesarean culture of Brazil. BMJ. 2000;320(7241):1074. PubMed PMID: 10836808.
12. Ba'aqeel HS. Cesarean delivery rates in Saudi Arabia: a ten-year review. Ann Saudi Med. 2009;29(3):179-183. PubMed PMID: 19448379; PubMed Central PMCID: PMCPMC2813649.
13. Giani U, Bruzzese D, Pugliese A, Saporito M, Triassi M. [Risk factors analysis for elective caesarean section in Campania region (Italy)]. Epidemiol Prev 2011;35(2):101-110. PubMed PMID: 21628753.
14. Al Rifai R. Rising cesarean deliveries among apparently low-risk mothers at university teaching hospitals in Jordan: analysis of population survey data, 2002-2012. Glob Health Sci Pract. 2014;2(2):195-209. doi: https://doi.org/10.9745/GHSP-D-14-00027. PubMed PMID: 25276577; PubMed Central PMCID: PMCPMC4168617.
15. Ministry of Health and Population (MOHP) [Egypt] E-ZA, and ORC Macro. Egypt service provision assessment survey 2002. Calverton, Maryland: Ministry of Health and Population, El-Zanaty Associates, and ORC Macro. Available from: https://dhsprogram.com/pubs/pdf/SPA5/SPA5.pdf. Accessed 20 Apr 2016.
16. Ministry of Health and Population [Egypt] E-ZaAE, and ICF International. Egypt demographic and health survey 2014. Cairo, Egypt and Rockville, Maryland, USA: Ministry of Health and Population and ICF International. 2015.
17. UNFPA. UNFPA-Egypt. Available from: http://egypt.unfpa.org/ Accessed 2 Apr 2016.
18. Khawaja M, Jurdi R, Kabakian-Khasholian T. Rising trends in cesarean section rates in Egypt. Birth. 2004;31(1):12-16. PubMed PMID: 15015988; PubMed Central PMCID: PMCPMC1457115.
19. Stanton CK, Dubourg D, De Brouwere V, Pujades M, Ronsmans C. Reliability of data on caesarean sections in developing countries. Bull World Health Organ. 2005;83(6):449-455. doi: /S0042–96862005000600013. PubMed PMID: 15976896; PubMed Central PMCID: PMCPMC2626266.
20. Measure. Demographic and Health Surveys. Measures DHS. 2010.
21. STROBE Statement—Checklist of items that should be included in reports of cross-sectional studies. Availbale from: http://www.strobe-statement.org/fileadmin/Strobe/uploads/checklists/STROBE_checklist_v4_cross-sectional.pdf. Accessed 20 Nov 2015.
22. Rutstein S, Rojas G. Guide to DHS statistics. Demographic and Health Surveys ORC Macro, Calverton, Maryland. 2006. Available from: http://citeseerx.ist.psu.edu/viewdoc/download?doi=10.1.1.431.8235&rep=rep1&type=pdf. Accessed 22 Mar 2016
23. Khawaja M, Al-Nsour M. Trends in the prevalence and determinants of caesarean section delivery in Jordan: evidence from three demographic and health surveys, 1990–2002. World Health Popul 2007;9(4):17-28. PubMed PMID: 18567949.
24. Rahman M, Nakamura K, Kizuki M. Socioeconomic differences in the prevalence, awareness, and control of diabetes in Bangladesh. J Diabetes Complicat 2015;29(6):788-793. doi: https://doi.org/10.1016/j.jdiacomp.2015.04.011. PubMed PMID: 25981122.
25. Organization WH. Physical status: the use and interpretation of anthropometry. Geneva, Switzerland: WHO (http://whqlibdoc.who.int/trs/WHO_TRS_854.pdf). Accessed 30 March, 2015.
26. Hoellen F, Hornemann A, Haertel C, Reh A, Rody A, Schneider S, et al. Does maternal underweight prior to conception influence pregnancy risks and outcome? In Vivo 2014;28(6):1165-1170. PubMed PMID: 25398817.
27. Leung TY, Leung TN, Sahota DS, Chan OK, Chan LW, Fung TY, et al. Trends in maternal obesity and associated risks of adverse pregnancy outcomes in a population of Chinese women. BJOG 2008;115(12):1529-1537. doi: https://doi.org/10.1111/j.1471-0528.2008.01931.x. PubMed PMID: 19035989.

28. Liu Y, Dai W, Dai X, Li Z. Prepregnancy body mass index and gestational weight gain with the outcome of pregnancy: a 13-year study of 292,568 cases in China. Arch Gynecol Obstet 2012;286(4):905-911. doi: https://doi.org/10.1007/s00404-012-2403-6. PubMed PMID: 22695822.
29. Zhang Y, Wang ZL, Liu B, Cai J. Pregnancy outcome of overweight and obese Chinese women with gestational diabetes. J Obstet Gynaecol 2014; 34(8):662-665. doi: https://doi.org/10.3109/01443615.2014.920787. PubMed PMID: 24911378.
30. Ding XX, Xu SJ, Hao JH, Huang K, Su PY, Tao FB. Maternal pre-pregnancy BMI and adverse pregnancy outcomes among Chinese women: results from the C-ABCS. J Obstet Gynaecol 2016;36(3):328-332. doi: https://doi.org/10.3109/01443615.2015.1050652. PubMed PMID: 26492517.
31. Gomes UA, Silva AA, Bettiol H, Barbieri MA. Risk factors for the increasing caesarean section rate in Southeast Brazil: a comparison of two birth cohorts, 1978-1979 and 1994. Int J Epidemiol 1999;28(4):687-694. PubMed PMID: 10480697.
32. Corporation. I. IBM SPSS statistics for windows, version 22.0. Armonk, New York: IBM Corporation; 2013. 2013.
33. Souza JP, Betran AP, Dumont A, de Mucio B, Gibbs Pickens CM, Deneux-Tharaux C, et al. A global reference for caesarean section rates (C-model): a multicountry cross-sectional study. BJOG 2016;123(3):427-436. doi: https://doi.org/10.1111/1471-0528.13509. PubMed PMID: 26259689.
34. Subedi S. Rising rate of cesarean section–a year review. Journal of Nobel Medical College. 2012;1(2):72–6.
35. Wahabi H, Fayed A, Esmaeil S, Alzeidan R, Elawad M, Tabassum R, et al. Riyadh mother and baby multicenter cohort study: the cohort profile. PLoS One. 2016;11(3):e0150297. doi: https://doi.org/10.1371/journal.pone.0150297. PubMed PMID: 26937965; PubMed Central PMCID: PMCPMC4777404.
36. World Health Organization. Country statistics and global health estimates by WHO and UN partners. Egypt: WHO statistical profile. Last updated: January 2015. Available from: http://www.who.int/gho/countries/egy.pdf?ua=1. Accessed 10 May 2016.
37. UNDP. UNDP human development report 2015, Egypt central Agency for Public Mobilization and Statistics – CAPMAS. 2015.
38. Luz Gibbons JMB, Jeremy A Lauer, Ana P Betrán, Mario Merialdi and Fernando Althabe. The Global Numbers and Costs of Additionally Needed and Unnecessary Caesarean Sections Performed per Year: Overuse as a Barrier to Universal Coverage. World Health Report (2010) Background Paper, 30. Available from: http://www.who.int/healthsystems/topics/financing/healthreport/30C-sectioncosts.pdf. Accessed 10 Jan 2016.
39. El-Zanaty FaAW. Egypt demographic and health survey 2008. Cairo, Egypt: Ministry of Health, El-Zanaty and Associates, and Macro International. 2009.
40. World Health Organization. World Hepatitis Day – July 28, 2012. MMWR: Morbidity & Mortality Weekly Report 61: 1/3p. 2012.
41. Bell JCD, Graham WJ, Penney GC, Ryan M, Hall MH. Do obstetric complications explain high caesarean section rates among women over 30? A retrospective analysis. Br Med J. 2001;322:894–5.
42. Mishra US, Ramanathan M. Delivery-related complications and determinants of caesarean section rates in India. Health Policy Plan 2002;17(1):90-98. PubMed PMID: 11861590.
43. Padmadas SS, Kumar S, Nair SB, Kumari A. Caesarean section delivery in Kerala, India: evidence from a National Family Health Survey. Soc Sci Med 2000;51(4):511-521. PubMed PMID: 10868667.
44. Peipert JF, Bracken MB. Maternal age: an independent risk factor for cesarean delivery. Obstet Gynecol 1993;81(2):200-205. PubMed PMID: 8423950.
45. Webster LA, Daling JR, McFarlane C, Ashley D, Warren CW. Prevalence and determinants of caesarean section in Jamaica. J Biosoc Sci 1992;24(4):515-525. PubMed PMID: 1429779.
46. Nour NM. Health consequences of child marriage in Africa. Emerg Infect Dis. 2006;12(11):1644-1649. doi: https://doi.org/10.3201/eid1211.060510. PubMed PMID: 17283612; PubMed Central PMCID: PMCPMC3372345.
47. Leddy MA, Power ML, Schulkin J. The impact of maternal obesity on maternal and fetal health. Rev Obstet Gynecol. 2008;1(4):170-178. PubMed PMID: 19173021; PubMed Central PMCID: PMCPMC2621047.
48. Platt MJ, Marshall A, Pharoah PO. The effects of assisted reproduction on the trends and zygosity of multiple births in England and Wales 1974-99. Twin Res 2001;4(6):417-421. PubMed PMID: 11780931.
49. Walker R, Turnbull D, Wilkinson C. Strategies to address global cesarean section rates: a review of the evidence. Birth 2002;29(1):28-39. PubMed PMID: 11843787.

20

Improving the care pathway for women who request Caesarean section: an experience-based co-design study

Sara L. Kenyon[1*], Nina Johns[2], Sandhya Duggal[1], Ruth Hewston[3] and Nicola Gale[4]

Abstract

Background: Maternal request for Caesarean section is controversial and yet the NICE Caesarean section Guideline recommends that that if this is requested, following discussion of the risks and benefits, women should be supported in their choice. There was a desire to improve the pathway at Birmingham Women's NHS Foundation Trust.

Methods: Experience-based co-design methodology uses service user and clinicians experiences collected using qualitative methods to jointly re-design services. Firstly semi-structured interviews were conducted to elicit the views and experiences of health care professionals and women who requested Caesarean section (with and without medical indication). Analysis identified key themes arising from the health care professionals' interviews and 'touch points' (key moments or events related to the experience of care) arising from the interviews with women.. Separate workshops were then held with each group to ensure these resonated and to identify key areas for service improvement. At the first joint workshop a pathway using 'audio clips' demonstrating women's agreed 'touch points' prompted discussion and joint working began to change the pathway. A final second workshop was held to agree changes to the pathway.

Results: Interviews were conducted with health care professionals ($n = 22$, 10 consultant obstetricians and 12 midwives) and women ($n = 15$). The women's 'touch points' included repetition of request, delay in the decision for Caesarean section to be made, feeling judged, and that information was poor with similar findings identified from the health care professionals. Joint working resulted in a revised pathway for women who request Caesarean section.
Changes to the pathway for women as a result of the work include written information about 'The way your baby may be born' which is given to the woman followed by a discussion about mode of birth around the 16 week appointment. If the woman wishes to have a Caesarean section, referral is made to appropriate health care professionals (e.g., Consultant Midwife, counsellor) only if support and information would be useful. If Caesarean section is requested, woman is referred to a consultant obstetrician for an appointment at 20/40, with a decision by 28/40. Recording this in the notes minimises repeated challenge described by women. Final consent and timing of Caesarean section remain as recommended.

Conclusion: This has resulted in changes to the pathway agreed by a co-design process and which are acceptable to both health care professionals and women. Use of such methodologies should be considered more frequently when implementing service change.

Keywords: Maternal request for Caesarean section, Experience based co-design, Qualitative methods, Interviews

* Correspondence: s.kenyon@bham.ac.uk
[1]Institute of Applied Health Research, University of Birmingham, Edgbaston, Birmingham B15 2TT, UK
Full list of author information is available at the end of the article

Background

In England the rates of Caesarean section have risen from 9 % of births in 1980 to 25.4 % in 2013 (http://www.birthchoiceuk.com/Professionals/BirthChoiceUKFrame.htm?http://www.birthchoiceuk.com/Professionals/statistics.htm). Indications for the procedure vary, but one possible contributor to this rise may be an increase in maternal requests for Caesarean section [1], although the exact extent to which women request Caesarean section in the absence of clinical indications is not clear, with studies suggesting it varies from 0.3 to 14 % [2].

While it is widely accepted that matters such as place of birth, method of pain relief, position in labour or presence of a birth partner are accepted matters of maternal choice, there is controversy surrounding whether the woman should have the right to choose to have her baby by Caesarean section [3]. Reasons for this decision include fear of childbirth [4], avoidance of the pain of labour and of the risk of damage to the perineum, previous birth experiences [5] as well as convenience of a planned birth [6].

Recent evidence has suggested that, while support and control are important determinants of satisfaction with the birth experience [7, 8] fulfilment of the request for either Caesarean section or vaginal birth does not guarantee a positive birth experience [9]. A recent review [2] has found few studies that addressed women's own perceptions of their role in decision making, which is perhaps surprising. There has been an increasing drive for better understanding of patient experience, and more meaningful patient involvement in service design and improvement [10], although efforts have sometimes been limited by failure to engage in depth with patients' subjective experiences [11]. Experience Based Co-Design [12] utilises in depth accounts of experiences from service users to re-design services. The method has been used and developed in the healthcare setting over the last 10 years and is an approach to improving services that combines participatory design and user experience to bring about quality improvement. As such it provides an established research methodology for enabling Trusts to fulfil their statutory duties and involve patients and the public in improving services (https://www.england.nhs.uk/wp-content/uploads/2013/09/trans-part-hc-guid1.pdf). In-depth interviews are used to elicit the views of both health care professionals and service users. This methodology has been used successfully in a variety of health care settings including emergency departments [13], breast and lung cancer services [14] and mental health services [15]. This is the first evidence of its use within maternity care.

Context

The UK National Institute of Health and Care Excellence (NICE), in its practice recommendations in 2004 [16], stated that when a woman requested Caesarean section in the absence of an identified medical reason the request should be explored, discussed and recorded but that, while an individual clinician had the right to decline such a request, the women's decision should be respected and she should be offered referral for a second opinion. The recent update of the Caesarean section Guideline [17] has continued the controversy by stating more strongly that, for women requesting Caesarean section, if after discussion and offer of support, a vaginal birth is still not an acceptable option, she should be offered one and that an obstetrician unwilling to perform a Caesarean section should refer the women to an obstetrician who will. The current recommendation also states that the overall risks and benefits of Caesarean section compared with vaginal birth should be discussed, but the evidence available upon which to base a decision is very low quality, includes only relatively short term outcomes and does not include the risks to future fertility or further pregnancies or the health of the baby.

Since publication of the recent update of the Caesarean section Guideline in 2011, there is a desire to explore more fully the experiences and opinions of both women and health care professionals involved at Birmingham Women's NHS Foundation Trust (BWNFT). This has come from a desire to improve the pathway for all those involved and from the belief that numbers of women requesting Caesarean section following the update had risen. The Maternity and Child Health team of the West Midlands Collaboration for Leadership in Applied Health Research and Care (CLAHRC) programme is based at the University of Birmingham and undertake research in close partnership with local health services, with the aim of improving services and outcomes for patients within five years (though often much sooner than this).

Methods

Objective

This article documents an experience-based co-design project that was undertaken as collaboration between Birmingham Women's NHS Foundation Trust, the University of Birmingham and women who had used the BWNFT service.

Study design

Experience-based co-design methodology uses service user and clinicians experiences collected using qualitative methods to jointly re-design services. Our approach to was formed by the free to access online toolkit published in August 2012, incorporating several case studies which were developed through collaboration between quality improvement practitioners and academics, and disseminated through the King's Fund charity (http://www.kingsfund.org.uk/projects/ebcd). This gave detail in 16 sections to the process which involved eliciting the views of health care professionals and patients to 'co-design' service improvement. The toolkit suggests using non participant observation and semi structured qualitative interviews with staff and patient with separate workshops to discuss findings. Film clips are used to demonstrate the views of patients along the care pathway at a joint workshop, following which small co-design groups to work on different issues and a final celebration/review event is held. An overview of the experience based co-design process is presented in Fig. 1.

Research team and study oversight

The core team consisted of SK (researcher with a clinical midwifery background), NG (sociologist and methodological specialist), SD (research fellow), NJ (obstetrician) and RH (service user/mother) offering a range of perspectives on the project. In addition to this, the project advisory group consisted of another obstetrician, another service user and two midwives. Permission for the study was obtained from the NRES Committee West Midlands - Black County (12/WM/0270). The study took place between January and December 2013 and was sponsored by BWNFT and permission was also obtained from their Research and Development Department.

Participant selection

The experiences of both clinical staff and women who had experienced the maternal request for Caesarean section pathway were sought. Health care professionals included a sample of community midwives (who see women in the antenatal period), the Consultant Midwife (who sees women during their decision process for maternal request for Caesarean section and consultant obstetricians (who have to agree to the request for Caesarean section). Consultant obstetricians and the Consultant Midwife were identified by NJ (the lead obstetrician for Delivery Suite). The Community Midwifery Manager identified a sample of community midwives through the individual team leaders. Women were identified using the electronic systems at BWNFT by NJ and were sent a letter informing them about the study and asking them to contact the University team if they were prepared to be interviewed about their experiences. Exclusion criteria were women who gave birth by any other mode, women under 16 years old or women who were not fluent in spoken English.

Information about the study was sent to all those identified, and if a reply slip was returned following one reminder, responders were contacted to arrange an interview. All participants gave informed consent. Once a reply slip had been received from women we contacted NJ to find out whether or not the woman concerned had a clinical indication for Caesarean section. This enabled us to purposely/purposefully sample women who had, and did not have, a clinical indication, and enabled us to explore any differences between the two groups. Once participants had responded to the letter, SD telephoned them to discuss the project further and to arrange an interview if they agreed.

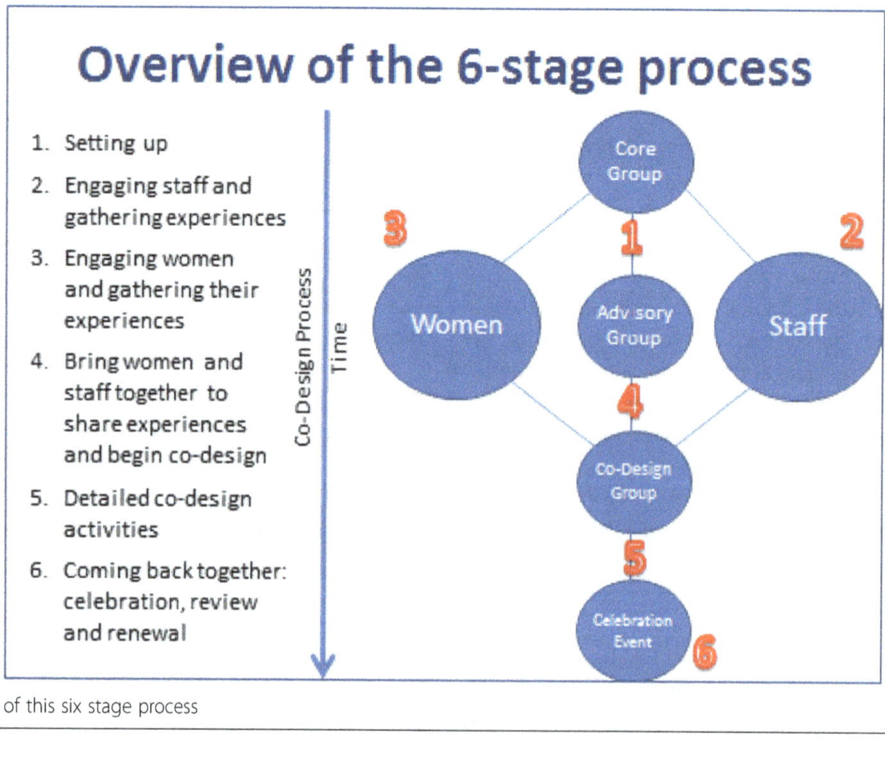

Fig. 1 An overview of this six stage process

The Research and Development Department of BWNFT collected women's baseline characteristics (age, ethnicity, parity, whether they speak English and postcode). The researchers informed them of those who responded and they provided the characteristics listed above for the responders and non-responders. This enabled us to explore differences between the groups.

Setting

Interviews for clinical staff were undertaken at their place of work. Interviews for women took place at their home to facilitate women to be able to open up and talk freely in a safe environment. The women's, staff and joint workshops were all held in meeting rooms in the BWNFT.

Data collection

Due to limited time and resources, we opted to focus on collecting interview data from staff and women using the services. Members of the project team and advisory group were familiar with the services, through working there or having used the service, and we used their experience in lieu of non-participant observation to help orientate ourselves to the service. This is a common adaptation of the Experience-Based Co-Design approach [18].

SD conducted all the interviews and took written consent from participants before interviews commenced. Interviews were digitally audio recorded, rather than video recorded as recommended by the Kings Fund guidance, for reasons of resource and of increased anonymity for participants. Again this is a common adaptation of the Experience-Based Co-Design method [18]. The interviews were semi-structured using a topic guide with broad topic areas (background, experience of pregnancy, choice to have a Caesarean section, views on risks and benefits of Caesarean section, interaction with health care professionals, interactions with family and peers, experience of antenatal and postnatal care, reflections and future plans) but the emphasis was to elicit individuals' own perspectives freely. The topic guide was developed from a literature review, discussions within the project team and refined as necessary during the first few interviews.

The interviews with women aimed to explore women's experiences of requesting a Caesarean section, with and without clinical indications, and to discuss the reasons for that decision and their experiences of the health care systems in place currently. The interviews were able to explore in more depth the reason for their decision, how health care professionals responded to their request, whether this affected their antenatal experiences and those since birth and their bonding experiences.

During the interviews the health care professionals were encouraged to discuss their thoughts and feelings around Caesarean section for maternal request, with and without medical indications, how they managed such cases in practice, and included discussion of any perceived changes as a result of the recently issued NICE guidance.

Data analysis

The audio-recorded interviews were transcribed by a recognised professional transcription service. Transcripts were reviewed for accuracy and were anonymised by the research team before analysis. The transcripts were read and coded independently by two of the researchers (NG and SD) and the emerging themes were discussed in team meetings. N-Vivo software was used to manage the dataset and the Framework method was used to managed and analyse the qualitative data, which involves comparing data across and within cases [19]. 'Touchpoints' were identified: 'the key moments and places ... where people come into contact with the services and where their subjective experience is shaped, and therefore where the desired emotional and sensory connection needs to be established' [12]. These are a key part of the experience-based co-design process as they are key moments or events that stand out for those involved as crucial to the women's experience of care and are used to help inform and structure the co-design meetings. The process of identifying touchpoints was undertaken collaboratively by the core team who read a selection of transcripts independently to identify the key touchpoints. These were compared and discussed in the Advisory Group meeting to ensure consistency of approach.

Use of an established method (in this instance the Framework method [19]) of analysing the interview data increases the rigour of finding. Ensuring the reliability and face validity of findings, through feeding back at various stages to participants and inviting comment, is integral within the co-design process. Findings from the in-depth interviews are corroborated by the individual group workshops, and a summary sent to all those interviewed (if they could not attend the workshop) for comment. Overall, processes and results were guided and agreed at each stage by the multidisciplinary Advisory Group with adoption by the Maternity Trust of the new pathway (through the Trust routine processes) ensuring findings were seen as validated.

The co-design process

Invitations were sent to all the women who had been interviewed to participate in the workshops. For the health care professionals, all relevant workshops were widely advertised within the Trust to encourage not just staff who had agreed to be interviewed to attend.

First, workshops were held with the women and the health care professionals separately so the findings could be shared and to ensure these resonated with the separate groups. In the health care professionals' workshop, data were presented to the participants and discussions included topics such as the issues of working with women and professional differences of opinion. In the women's workshop, data from the women's interviews were presented and the group agreed the key 'touchpoints' along the pathway that would be presented at the joint meeting. Each group also identified their top three priority areas for service improvement.

A joint workshop was then held during which women and health care professionals worked together to make plans for the redesign of services. The workshop was facilitated by the researchers (SK, NG and SD). The workshop opened with a brief introduction to the project by SK. Audio clips from the women's interviews were used to illustrate each touchpoint (additional written consent was obtained from the women concerned to use audio clips of them in the joint workshop). Following the workshop the group had an open and frank discussion about their responses to the audio tape. Then the group split into smaller working groups (each had at least one service user, one midwife and one obstetrician) to explore potential solutions to the problems identified. Action points were agreed and these were undertaken over the next couple of months.

The group reconvened at a celebration event, which was also attended by the chief executive of the hospital. The following were agreed: changes to the pathway, a new leaflet for women regarding possible mode of birth, and changes to the leaflet for women having elective Caesarean section. Plans for both the short and longer term were also agreed.

Storage of data

Digital recordings were stored in an electronic file, which only the research team had access to. Only those required to transcribe the recordings listened to them. Once transcribed and checked for accuracy the digital files were destroyed. In line with current practice the transcripts will be stored for 15 years. All data will be stored and archived in line with the BWNFT policies.

Results

Participants

In total, 70 women were identified from the electronic systems at BWNFT for an 18 month period and were sent information about the study, and 27 women responded. Three did not wish to be involved, 24 responded that they were happy to be interviewed, and interviews were actually undertaken with 15 women (nine women interviewed had a medical indication for the Caesarean section and six without a medical indication).

The baseline characteristics of the women interviewed shows they were more likely to have had a second baby, be European and have a professional occupation than those who were invited to be interviewed. The women invited were most commonly from the least deprived areas (based on Index of Multiple Deprivation score from their post code) but this was not the case for those interviewed, who were most commonly in the third quintile. Those interviewed were similar in age to those invited (33 years) and none required an interpreter (Table 1).

Of the health care professionals, 19 obstetricians at BWNFT were sent information about the study, 14 responded that they were happy to be interviewed, and 10 obstetricians were actually interviewed. Of those interviewed the average age was 46.3 years. Six were Obstetricians and four were Obstetrician/Gynaecologists, five male and five female and all had over 15 years' experience.

Interviews were undertaken with 11 community midwives who responded to a request from their Team Leaders. The Consultant Midwife was also interviewed. The midwives interviewed were White British, except for one who was Iranian. Their average age was 49 years and average number of years as a midwife was eleven-this varied between two and 31 years. Eleven were Band 6 and one Band 8; one had a Diploma, 10 a Degree and one a Masters. All the midwives were female.

Health care professionals workshop

There were 17 participants with a mix of community and hospital midwives, midwifery managers, student and research midwives (15 in total) as well as obstetric consultants (two). A description of the study was given, followed by a summary of the findings from the health care professionals' interviews.

The pathway for women requesting a Caesarean section was seen as relatively simple when described by staff, as shown in Fig. 2.

Discussions included how staff values and experiences influenced the pathway for women and how these issues could be changed to improve the current service. Three issues in the pathway were identified by the group as a priority for discussing in the joint workshop:

Information provided to women

The interviews identified variation in verbal information given to women (alongside the standard leaflets):

> *"I think for women, unfortunately, it's a case of who you see" (O4)*

Some of the health care professionals spoke about managing and concealing their personal feelings and opinions about maternal requests for Caesarean section.

Table 1 Baseline characteristics of women

Baseline Characteristics	Women interviewed		All women invited	
	$n = 15$	21 %	$n = 70$	100 %
Parity				
First baby	0	0 %	13	19 %
Second baby or higher	10	67 %	37	53 %
Unknown	5	33 %	20	29 %
Maternal age at CS (years) – median (std)	33 (5.54)		33 (5.22)	
Ethnicity				
Africa	0	0 %	2	3 %
Asia	0	0 %	11	16 %
Caribbean	0	0 %	2	3 %
European	13	87 %	49	70 %
Other	2	13 %	6	9 %
Index of multiple deprivation quintile				
1	2	13 %	22	31 %
2	3	20 %	15	21 %
3	6	40 %	18	26 %
4	1	7 %	7	10 %
5	3	20 %	8	11 %
Occupational classification				
1 - Managers and Senior Officials	1	7 %	5	7 %
2 - Professional Occupations	4	27 %	12	17 %
3 - Associate Professional and Technical Occupations	1	7 %	6	9 %
4 - Administrative and Secretarial Occupations	1	7 %	4	6 %
5 - Skilled Trades Occupations	0	0 %	1	1 %
6 - Personal Service Occupations	0	0 %	1	1 %
7 - Sales and Customer Service Occupations	0	0 %	1	1 %
8 - Process, Plant and Machine Operatives	0	0 %	0	0 %
9 - Elementary Occupations	1	7 %	1	1 %
Not in formal employment	0	0 %	2	3 %
Unknown	7	47 %	37	53 %
Interpreter required for mother				
Yes	0	0 %	0	0 %
No	15	100 %	70	100 %
Reason for Caesarean section				
Medical indication	9	60 %	35	50 %
No medical indication	6	40 %	35	50 %

> *"You can have your own thoughts in your head, and at the back of my head I might be thinking 'Oh my God, you want a section just because it fits in with your life, how selfish!' but I'm not going to put that across to the lady. I would still talk about it and not laugh her off and still give her the same pathway as I would for anybody" (M5)*

It was agreed that the discussion should include quality of information, inconsistency of information, lack of research based information, and the bias of health care professionals in what information is shared.

Timing of the discussion about mode of birth

The health care professionals also spoke about the importance of timing in relation to when to talk to women about their choices and options.

> *"Some women will say it as soon as they walk in through the door. So at the first visit, 'I'm not having a vaginal birth.' Other women won't say anything and they worry, worry, worry, and then they'll say this two weeks before their due date, and then you've got no time to work with them to try and sort it out. They are by far and away the most difficult ones. The ones that come in right at the start and say, 'I'm not happy about a vaginal birth, I want a section' then you've then got the rest of the pregnancy to be able to work with them. But it's very variable when they bring it up" (O4)*

This felt frustrating to health care professionals in terms of the extent to which they were able to provide good care:

> *"We usually go through ... Are you happy with what's happening? Are you happy with where you've booked your delivery? Some of them feel they can't discuss home delivery at booking because they think we are against home deliveries. And you get to the birth plan talk and she'll suddenly say 'I'm hoping on a home delivery' and I'm like 'Why didn't you say that in the beginning?' Do you know what I mean? You'll get to the 36 weeks talk and it's all about 'I want a Caesarean section', so why didn't you say that in the beginning" (M1)*

It was agreed that the timing of discussion and information giving for women should be discussed at the joint workshop. This included inconsistency of timing of information, when discussion is begun in late pregnancy, the rush to make suitable preparation for birth and the need for early discussion and so time to plan for appropriate referrals where necessary and for birth.

The role of the consultant midwife

The role of the Consultant Midwife was discussed and the part she played in the process explored. She

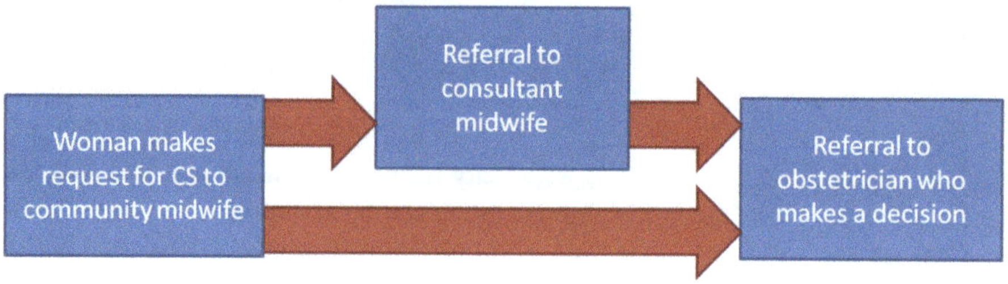

Fig. 2 Pathway for women requesting CS as described by healthcare professionals

was seen as the centre of the system as obstetricians refer onto her when a woman requested a Caesarean section:

> *"The doctor says, 'Okay, you can have a caesarean section, but you've got to go and see [the Consultant Midwife] first.' It's nothing more than a tick box exercise. The patient knows that as long as they sit there quietly, and not upset [the Consultant Midwife] and just listen to what she's got to say, that they're going to be able to come back and have their elective caesarean section. So we may as well not have wasted [the Consultant Midwife's] time" (O8)*

It is, unsurprisingly, a stressful role, as the Consultant Midwife herself explained:

> *"I felt very much that I had been if you like caught out in the middle ... she then got her Caesarean section and it was almost like "oh there, there, sorry I made you go through that, I'll do your section for you", and actually I felt unsupported and quite vulnerable ... having if you like, explored it what I considered to be appropriately with her, trying to get her to explain her fears so I can try and help manage them"*

It was agreed that this would be discussed at the joint workshop and would include the inconsistent and complex process for women requesting Caesarean section without medical indication, the central role of Consultant Midwife in the pathway for women and the conflicting role of Consultant Midwife (persuading women to change their minds and try for a vaginal birth vs the need to support women in their choice).

Other themes that emerged from the discussion included the way that a woman's decision to have Caesarean section was recorded, the need for women to repeat reason for the Caesarean section request to each health care professionals who cares for them and the lack of detailed recording of discussion between women and health care professionals when requesting Caesarean section.

Women's workshop

There were three women and four researchers present at the women's workshop.

As a result of the 15 interviews conducted with women who had requested Caesarean section, the current pathway that women had experienced in practice was documented and is illustrated in Fig. 3. This pathway was used as a basis for discussion of the key touchpoints by the women in this workshop.

The women identified three priorities for discussion at the joint workshop:

Information available to them

The women felt that good quality information on the risks and practicalities was missing and this included both short and long-term risks and benefits of elective Caesarean section (written information was related to Caesarean section generally and not specifically for women requesting caesarean and verbal information from midwives and consultants varied), information on the internet, and practical information given in advance of the operation.

It was also agreed that there was a lack of information about what the Caesarean section surgery experience is like and of the risk information comparing vaginal birth, emergency and elective Caesarean section and that these areas.

Delayed decision making

The effect a delayed decision had on experience of pregnancy was to cause unnecessary anxiety:

> *"the impression you get from the midwives, that normal delivery is the best thing for everyone ... 'Oh, we can talk about that later. We can talk about that later.' And I think if it's, you know, I think when you're pregnant the end, like, last bit is, kind of, praying on your mind from the moment you find out about it, really" (W1)*

The need to repeatedly defend their decision to have a Caesarean section

Women felt they had to continually repeat and defend their decision to each different healthcare professional

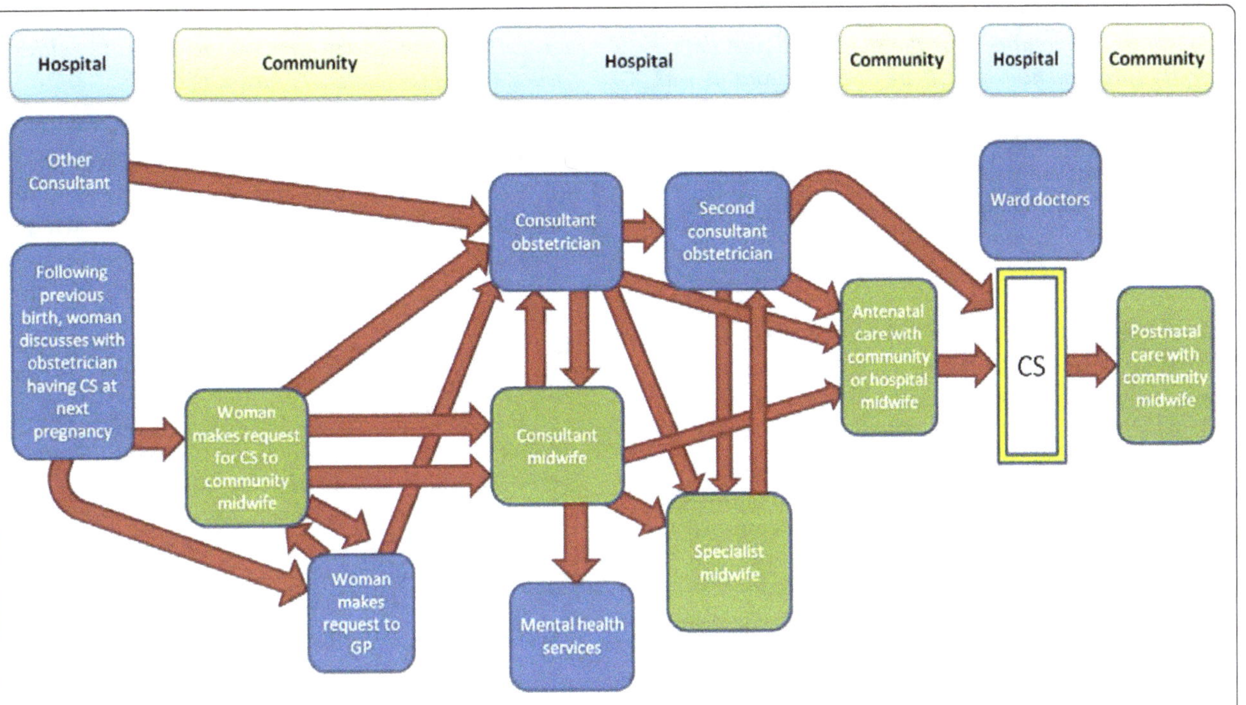

Fig. 3 Pathway for women requesting Caesarean section as described by the women interviewed

they saw and that 'no-one was listening'. They also felt that long term risk information was used to 'ram home risks'.

> *"I had a very traumatic meeting and I was made to feel like it was the worst decision I could possibly make ... I'd been very aware of the 50,000 list of risks and the one positive ... I kept going back to the same consultant who kept trying to talk me out of it. In the end we had to be firm in our decision" (W6)*

Women felt that those health care professionals were, at all stages, judging or stereotyping them, when in fact their decision was a carefully thought through, and sometimes very difficult, decision.

> *"This midwife was lovely until I said I was having a* Caesarean section *... a complete attitude change ... I explained to her the reasons and she was very dismissive from that point" (W6)*

Joint Workshop

This was attended by 15 people (five women, two obstetricians, four midwives and four researchers). A presentation was given describing the study to date and a pathway for women was demonstrated using audio clips to describe the 'touch points' as agreed at the women's workshop. Additional consent was obtained from the women for use of audio clips from their interviews. The following touchpoints were identified:

Making the request to the community midwife

Some women found that discussing their request for Caesarean section with their community midwife could be a difficult experience. In these cases they found there was little clarity on the process, little information given to them to help make the decision and some felt that their midwife was judging them for their decision, which compromised the relationship.

> *"I mean I didn't see, unfortunately I didn't see the same midwife, it was a different one every single time, so the midwives that I went to obviously check your blood pressure and your weight and things like that, they were "your decision". They all said it was your decision, your decision, your decision. And then obviously when I went to the clinic they said "Oh it's the consul- obviously it's the consultant's decision to make that". (W2)*

Making the request to the consultant obstetrician

If a woman was given an appointment with one of the BWNFT consultants who was not personally supportive of maternal request for Caesarean section, the experience could be frustrating and distressing. The women often had to ask for a second opinion.

"When I had my 12 week scan appointment I'd got a consultant appointment at the same time and I'm pretty sure I mentioned it there and then and he was having none of it. He really brushed it aside, made me feel like it was quite a silly request and I came away feeling frustrated because I'm a 30 plus year old woman, I know my own mind, I'm not silly about unnecessary medical procedures and he made me feel very small. (W12)

Making the request to the consultant midwife

If women were sent to discuss their decision with the Consultant Midwife when they already sure that they had made the right decision, they could find the consultation unnecessary, and sometimes upsetting if they felt that they were being pressurized into changing their mind, rather than the supportive process that was intended.

W12: "It was fine in itself, she was a perfectly nice lady, I just knew it was something that I had to do to get to the next step in the process of them saying yes to the elective section. So it was kind of like we talked for an hour but to me there was no point, she wasn't going to say anything that made me change my mind. It was interesting in that when we went through, because I myself got all of my medical notes, I paid for them so I could just read everything because obviously it traumatised me quite a lot and I needed to see everything especially when I found out I was pregnant the third time. And she did go through that and find a few things that I hadn't either found or didn't understand because of the medical jargon so from that aspect that was useful. There were certain things that the doctors did to try and stop the bleeding that I'd got questions about and she answered those so I suppose yeah looking back it was useful in some ways but it didn't make any difference to my decision".

Mental health services

Only one participant was referred to the mental health services and she felt that it was an inappropriate referral.

"It was quite difficult, my partner was there and there were a lot of questions about everything, going back to my childhood, whether my parents are divorced, remarried, have children of their own, which I'm not really sure how that comes into me deciding whether I want a C-section or not. So I found that quite difficult just because it was probing into my life in general and even though my husband has known my family for years and knows everything, to have to answer the questions it felt very difficult. And at the end of it she said that she couldn't support my request on medical grounds so basically I wasn't, it sounds awful but basically I wasn't crazy, there are no mental health issues, it was more anxiety based. (W12)

Antenatal care

During the antenatal care the women received, they found that they had to repeatedly come out as having requested a Caesarean section and felt that they were required to defend that decision repeatedly. This

W4: "I think it added to the stress. I think the, kind of, what seemed to be always questioning, and this, kind of, whole laying it on thick, but, you know, the repetitiveness about the risks and the problems and the major abdominal surgery, just adds to the stress [okay], you know. And I didn't really feel I did have a choice, or, when I say I didn't feel I had a choice, I felt it, you know, I really needed to have a caesarean, because the benefits outweighed the risks, really".

Postnatal care in the community

The feelings of being judged for their decision continued after the birth sometimes in social situations, but also in interactions with health care professionals.

"One of the generic checks when they're a certain age, I don't know if it was 8 week check or 12 week check or something and I took him to the doctors and the doctor was asking about his birth and I said it was an elective and he said oh I'm surprised they let you get away with that. And that really, really annoyed me so I'll never see that particular doctor again and I just thought I don't know how you can make a judgement when you have no clue about like my previous history and nobody just let me get away with anything, I had to fight tooth and nail to do it. So yeah, but that's the only negative comment that I've had".(W12)

There was then discussion of the topics prioritised by the individual health care professionals and Women's group which were strikingly similar and are detailed in Table 2.

After the pathway was shared with illustrative audio clips playing at each touchpoint, there was an open discussion of responses and reactions and some of the staff were quite shocked and moved by the experiences of the women. This produced a feeling of commitment in the room about making changes and three small co-design groups (each with at least one woman, one midwife, one obstetrician and one researcher) were then formed to discuss the following prioritized topics:

Table 2 Agreed priorities taken to joint workshop from health care professionals and Women

Priorities taken to joint workshop from health care professionals	Priorities taken to joint workshop from women
1. Quality of information for women	1. Agreement of Caesarean section decision:
o Inconsistency of information	o A clear agreement to be made between health care professionals and women about the decision for a Caesarean section
o Lack of research based information	o Decision for Caesarean section to be made earlier in pregnancy
o Bias of health care professionals in what information is shared	o Flexibility around the decision, an opportunity to change mind at any point
2. Timing and discussion and information giving	2. Repetition of Caesarean section request and referrals:
o Inconsistency of timing of information	o Repeated discussion of Caesarean section request with health care professionals
o When discussion is begun in late pregnancy, the rush to make suitable preparation for delivery	o Multiple referrals and subsequent repetition of request
o Need for early discussion and so time to plan for appropriate referrals where necessary and for delivery	
3. Referrals and role of consultant midwife o Inconsistent and complex process for	3. Information about Caesarean section: o Lack of information about what the
o women requesting caesarean section without medical indication	o Caesarean section surgery experience is like
o Central role of consultant midwife in the pathway for women requesting CS	o Lack of risk information comparing vaginal birth, emergency and elective Caesarean section
o Consultant midwife conflicting role: persuading women to change their minds and try for a vaginal delivery vs the need to support women in their choice	
4. Recording decision – repetition of request from women	
o Women requesting Caesarean section often need to repeat their reason for the request to each HCP who cares for them	
o There appears to be a lack of detailed recording of discussion between women and health care professionals when requesting Caesarean section	

- When the decision should be made that a Caesarean section was the agreed mode of birth and how that would be recorded
- How the pathway for women might be revised to reduce number and variation in the number of referrals
- What information should be given to women and when

These topics were discussed within the multidisciplinary groups, action points were agreed for health care professionals and researchers to undertake over the following weeks.

Final workshop

The results were discussed at the final workshop in December 2013, which was attended by 13 people (three women, five midwives, one obstetrician, the chief executive and three researchers). Here the revised pathway was agreed as were information leaflets regarding 'The way that your baby may be born' and 'Elective or Planned Caesarean Section' leaflets (Table 3).

Changes to the pathway for women included

- 'Information about the way your baby may be born' given to woman with information that there will be a discussion about mode of birth around 16 week appointment
- Not all women being referred to the Consultant Midwife but only those for whom support and information would be useful
- Seeing consultant obstetrician at 20 weeks for discussion of the risks and benefits
- Decision made 24-28weeks and recorded in notes
- Re-confirmation rather than challenging decision at subsequent antenatal appointments

At the meeting plans were made to take forward the ideas for interactive BWNFT website information on Caesarean section and to add BWNFT photos, Qs and As, possible short-term link to YouTube (visualise theatre/ experience of Caesarean section) and longer term plan to video going to theatre but these have not currently been taken forward. We also intended to submit grant proposal for detailed leaflet outlining comparison of short and long term risks for all types of births

Table 3 New pathway for women who request Caesarean Section

The new pathway is as follows;
• At booking-leaflet titled 'Information about the way your baby may be born' given to woman with information that there will be a discussion about mode of birth around 16 week appointment • At 16 weeks - Community Midwife discusses type of birth the woman is considering; *If woman requests caesarean section*: o Assess and consider individual to see whether an appointment with health care professionals for support and information would be useful (e.g., Consultant Midwife, counsellor) Examples include previous traumatic or difficult birth, de-brief, anxious/tocophobia, undecided. Following that consultation if Caesarean section requested refer to Consultant Obstetrician. o If woman has decided on Caesarean section, make referral for consultant obstetrician appointment at 20/40 • At 20 week appointment with consultant obstetrician-detailed discussion re mode of birth: o Risks and benefits explained o Detailed documentation of discussion and current preferences o Book appointment for 24–28 • At 24–28 weeks appointment with same obstetrician o Make decision / agreement / consent about type of birth and document clearly in hospital and hand held records the final decision for type of birth that is planned (possible use of sticker or proforma in casenotes) o Discuss plans for what happens if woman goes into spontaneous labour prior to date for elective Caesarean section, including differing risks and benefits depending on stage in labour and emergency vs elective Caesarean section o Give *Elective Caesarean section leaflet* • At every subsequent antenatal appointment re-confirm (not challenge) decision (e.g., 'Are you happy with the plan made?') which provides opportunity for woman to change her mind but not to be repeated challenged about her decision. If booked for Caesarean section and changes her mind an appropriate plan for birth will be made dependent on individual circumstances • If previously midwife led care, then woman will remain under shared care but all other appointments (except 36/40) can be in the community • Sign consent form (if not already signed) at 36/40 and book Caesarean section for 39/40

but could not identify a suitable funding source. Such a leaflet has recently been published by the Royal College of Obstetricians and Gynaecologists (https://www.rcog.org.uk/en/patients/patient-leaflets/choosing-to-have-a-caesarean-section/).

Conclusions and discussion

This methodology has been both challenging and rewarding to use but we are confident that it has resulted in an improved pathway for women requesting Caesarean section, together with a new leaflet discussing 'The way your baby may be born' and an update to the information in the leaflet for women having an elective Caesarean section. One of the most notable features of the study was the marked similarity between the issues in the pathway identified by the women and the health care professionals as a priority to deal with. This was not something that we expected and meant that topics taken forward were easy to agree.

Experience-based co-design requires commitment and engagement and can be challenging [18]. In this context, an added challenge was the professional tensions between the midwifery model of care and the medical model. Evidence suggests that while obstetricians opinions have changed over time [20], with more accepting that women should be able to make an informed choice, the views of midwives are embedded in a 'culture of normality', in which normal birth is promoted and valued [21] and that women choosing an elective Caesarean section is at odds with this. It made the healthcare professional workshop all the more important because it gave an opportunity for those issues to be aired and discussed, before engaging with the women's stories and experiences. Attempts to improve the pathway for women requesting a Caesarean section are likely to come up against cultural, professional and organisational challenges. Culturally, Caesarean section occupies a tenuous position in the public psyche, being both a life-saving operation in some cases but also being seen as 'convenient' and 'easier' than a vaginal birth [22]. The pre-existing tensions between the medical and midwifery professions around the role of medical intervention in pregnancy and birth are arguably exacerbated in the case that a medical intervention is used but without a clear medical reason. Organisationally, these women trasverse organisational boundaries during their pregnancy, in particular, between the community health system and the hospital and changes to the pathway require the co-ordination and commitment of both systems.

A recent review, of how co-design had been used, found it had been used in at least 57 projects in many specialities within medicine and across multiple countries [18]. The review also demonstrated that the approach has been adapted by those to have used it, with this being done on the basis that the process, as outlined in the toolkit, takes too long. Most commonly, this resulted in not undertaking non participant observation and not holding the celebration event and, while over 80 % of projects reported undertaking interviews, many dispensed with the filmed component. While using film may be challenging to those planning any future project, recent evidence has suggested that use of national archive of patient experience, rather than developing local interviews was a rigorous and cost effective alternative [23]. The strength of the approach for our purposes was that it held the experience of women (and staff) at the centre of the project and required collaboration throughout. This was a powerful approach given the controversies about maternal request for Caesarean section and professional rivalries that were embedded in the context.

There were limitations to the project, which was carried out in a single hospital and with a group of women that were only partially illustrative of the diversity of women living locally and using the service (particularly in relation to socio-economic status and ethnicity). As a result, some of the emergent themes from the interviews may only be applicable to the hospital where the project was carried out. We were not able to use to most appropriate quotes to demonstrate the 'touch points' in the audio tape due to the requirement by the Ethics committee that we gain explicit written informed consent for the use of these. In addition, the learning about patient experience and interprofessional discussions that came from participating in the project could only be replicated by undertaking the whole process. For instance, some staff were surprised to find out that women could sense their disapproval of their choice to have a Caesarean section even when they had tried to 'hide' their feelings.

However, we would argue that the experience-based principles around, for instance, ensuring mode of birth is discussed early in the pregnancy were be transferable to other contexts. The new pathway and the leaflet on mode of birth could certainly be used or adapted for other maternity care contexts. We are not alone in not fulfilling all the objectives of the project or in not undertaking a formal or systematic evaluation [18]. While the research and co-design phases of the project were underway we were leading the project and so able to keep the momentum moving forward but once it passed back to the health care professionals, who have the pressure of clinical commitments as well as the researchers competing priorities, this lost its impetus. This was compounded by staff changes. Researchers considering using Experience-Based Co-Design should not underestimate the time it takes or the multi-level support required and should build in a formal evaluation, but they should be reassured of the value of this collaborative process in agreeing changes that are acceptable to all parties.

Abbreviations

BWNFT: Birmingham Women's NHS Foundation Trust; CLAHRC: Collaboration for Leadership in Applied Health Research and Care; NHS: National Health Service; NICE: National Institute of Health and Care Excellence; NRES: National Research Ethics Service

Acknowledgements

Thank you to all the women and health care professionals who were interviewed; to Pam Nayyar, Fiona Cross Sudworth and Sophie Dann who provided support to the project; and to members of the Advisory and Project Management Group Matthew Parsons, Paula Clarke, Ellen Knox, Jenny Henry (co-investigator) and Jo Naylor Smith (Midwifery Community Services Manager) and Claire Bellows (service user).

Funding

Sara Kenyon is supported by the National Institute for Health Research (NIHR) Collaboration for Leadership in Applied Health Research and Care West Midlands. This paper presents independent research and the views expressed are those of the author(s) and not necessarily those of the NHS, the NIHR or the Department of Health.

Authors' contributions

SK was the overall lead for the study, co-designed the study, contributed to data analysis, was involved in running the co-design workshops, and contributed to writing the first draft of the paper. NJ was the clinical lead for the study, contributed to data analysis, was involved in running the workshops. SD undertook the data collection and contributed to data analysis and was involved in running the co-design workshops. RH was a user representative on the study, contributed to study design and data analysis, and was involved in running the co-design workshops. NG was the methodological lead for the study, co-designed the study, was involved in running the workshops, led the data analysis and contributed to writing the first draft of the paper. All authors commented on the draft paper, contributed intellectually to its development and approved the final version.

Competing Interests

The authors declare that they have no competing interests.

Author details

[1]Institute of Applied Health Research, University of Birmingham, Edgbaston, Birmingham B15 2TT, UK. [2]Birmingham Women's NHS Foundation Trust, Mindelsohn Way, Birmingham, West Midlands B15 2TG, UK. [3]Research Fellow, Institute of Applied Health Research, University of Birmingham, 255 Walmley Road, Walmley, Sutton Coldfield, West Midlands B76 2PN, UK. [4]Health Services Management Centre, University of Birmingham, Park House, 40 Edgbaston Park Road, Edgbaston, Birmingham B15 2RT, UK.

References

1. Fenwick J, Staff L, Gamble J, Creedy DK, Bayes S. Why do women request cesarean section in a normal, healthy first pregnancy? Midwifery. 2010;26: 394–400.
2. McCourt C, Weaver J, Statham H, Beake S, Gamble J, Creedy D. Elective cesarean section and decision making: a critical review of the literature. Birth. 2007;34:65–79.
3. Kalish RB, McCullough LB, Chervenak FA. Decision-making about caesarean delivery. Lancet. 2006;367:883–5.
4. Wiklund I, Edman G, Ryding EL, Andolf E. Expectations and experiences of childbirth in primiparae with caesarean section. BJOG. 2007;115:324–31.
5. Wiklund I, Edman G, Andolf E. Cesarean section on maternal request: reasons for the request, self-estimated health, expectations, experience of birth and signs of depression among first-time mothers. Acta Obstet Gynecol Scand. 2007;86:451–6.
6. Minkoff H, Chervenak FA. Elective primary cesarean delivery. N Engl J Med. 2003;348:946–50.
7. Green JM, Baston HA. Feeling in control during labor: concepts, correlates, and consequences. Birth. 2003;30:235–47.
8. Melender HL. What constitutes a good childbirth? A qualitative study of pregnant Finnish women. J Midw Women's Health. 2006;51:331–9.
9. Karlström A, Nystedt A, Hildingsson I. A comparative study of the experience of childbirth between women who preferred and had a caesarean section and women who preferred and had a vaginal birth. Sex Reprod Healthc. 2011;2(3):93–9. Epub 2011 Apr 3.
10. Greenhalgh T, Humphrey C, Woodard F. (Eds.). (2010). *User involvement in health care.* John Wiley & Sons.

11 Greenhalgh T, Woodard F, Humphrey C. Where next for User Involvement? In: Greenhalgh T, Humphrey C, Woodard F, editors. User Involvement in Health Care. Oxford: Wiley-Blackwell; 2010. doi:10.1002/9781444325164.ch8.

12 Bate P, Robert G. Experience-based design: from redesigning the system around the patient to co-designing services with the patient. Qual Saf Health Care. 2006;15:307–10. doi:10.1136/qshc.2005.016527.

13 Piper D, Iedema R, Gray J, Verna R, Holmes L, Manning N. Utilizing Experience-based Co-design to improve the experience of patients accessing emergency departments in New South Wales public hospitals: an evaluation study. Health Serv Manage Res. 2012;25:162–72.

14 Tsianakas V, Robert G, Maben J, Richardson A, Dale C, Wiseman T. Implementing patient centred cancer care: using experience-based co-design to improve patient experience in breast and lung cancer services. J Support Care Cancer. 2012;20(11):2639–47.

15 Larkin M, Boden ZVR, Newton E. 'On the brink of genuinely collaborative care: experience-based codesign in mental health' Qualitative Health Research. 10.1177/1049732315576494

16 National Institute for Health and Clinical Excellence. Caesarean section. (Clinical guideline 13). 2004. http://guidance.nice.org.uk/CG13

17 National Institute for Health and Clinical Excellence. Caesarean section (update). (Clinical guideline 132). 2011. http://guidance.nice.org.uk/CG132

18 Donetto S, Tsianakas V, Robert G. Using Experience-based Co-design to improve the quality of healthcare: mapping where we are now and establishing future directions. London: King's College London; 2014.

19 Gale NK, Heath G, Cameron E, Rashid S, Redwood S. Using the framework method for the analysis of qualitative data in multi-disciplinary health research. BMC Med Res Methodol. 2013;13(1):117.

20 Cotzias C, Paterson-Brown S, Fisk N. Obstetricians say yes to maternal request for elective caesarean section: a survey of current opinion. Eur J Obstet Gynaecol. 2001;97:15–6.

21 Churchill H, Francome C. British midwives' views on rising caesarean section rates. Br J Midwifery. 2009;17(12):774–8.

22 Douché J, Carryer J. Caesarean section in the absence of need: a pathologising paradox for public health. Nurs Inq. 2009;18(2):143–53.

23 Locock L, Robert G, Boaz A, Vougioukalou S, Shuldham C, Fielden J, et al. Testing accelerated experience-based co-design: a qualitative study of using a national archive of patient experience narrative interviews to promote rapid patient-centred service improvement. Health Serv Deliv Res. 2014;2(4). http://dx.doi.org/10.3310/hsdr02040.

21

Why women bleed and how they are saved: a cross-sectional study of caesarean section near-miss morbidity

S. Maswime[1*] and E. J. Buchmann[2]

Abstract

Background: Maternal deaths from 'bleeding during and after caesarean section' (BDACS) have increased in South Africa, and have now become the largest sub-cause of deaths from obstetric haemorrhage. The aim of this study was to describe risk factors and causes of near-miss related to BDACS and interventions used to arrest haemorrhage and treat its effects.

Methods: Cross-sectional prospective study in 13 urban public hospitals in South Africa, from July to December 2014.

Results: There were 93 cases of near-miss related and 7 maternal deaths related to BDACS. The near-miss rate was 2.1/1000 live births, and the case fatality rate was 3.5/10 000 caesarean sections. Associated near-miss risk factors were previous caesarean section in 60% of multiparas, pre-operative anaemia (55%), abruptio placentae (20%) and placenta praevia and/or accreta (20%). Atonic uterus (43%) was the most frequent anatomical cause of bleeding for near-miss, followed by surgical trauma (29%). The median duration of the operations resulting in near-miss was 90 min, with 81% noted as difficult by the surgeon. Interventions in cases of near-miss included second-look laparotomy (46%), hysterectomy (41%), B-Lynch brace suture (9%), intensive care unit admission (32%) and red cell transfusion ≥3 units (21%).

Conclusion: Cases from maternal near-miss from BDACS were frequently associated with pre-operative risk factors. Extensive life-saving interventions were required during and after the operations. An important factor in initiating the sequence of interventions is the realisation by the surgeon that the caesarean section is difficult, so that the progression from uneventful operation to near-miss to death can be arrested.

Keywords: Near-miss, Caesarean section related haemorrhage, Bleeding during and after caesarean section

Background

The safety of caesarean sections has recently come into question in South Africa. Maternal death resulting from 'bleeding during and after caesarean section' (BDACS) is becoming increasingly frequent. The triennial reports of the government's confidential enquiries into maternal deaths recorded 78 such deaths in 2002–2004, 140 in 2005–2007, 180 in 2008–2010, and 221 in 2011–2013 [1–4]. Maternal death from BDACS is now the largest sub-cause of death from obstetric haemorrhage in South Africa [4]. The increase in maternal deaths has been attributed to a rising national caesarean section rate, but this increase exceeded the rise in caesarean section rate, which increased from 12.7% in 2001/02 to 20.8% in 2012/13 [5]. Other possible reasons, for which data are lacking, related to changes in health care quality, such as a lower standard of surgical skill with increased risk of bleeding [6], failure to detect antepartum risk factors, and possibly substandard labour management, anaesthesia and post-operative care.

Globally, there are insufficient data on maternal deaths related to BDACS, especially in terms of clinical and surgical detail. Even with the recent increase in deaths, these events are so rare that meaningful prospective studies are difficult to do. A helpful alternative is to study 'near-miss' related to BDACS. A maternal near-miss is a woman who survives severe complications

* Correspondence: Tumishang.Maswime@wits.ac.za
[1]Wits Obstetrics and Gynaecology Clinical Research Division, Johanesburg, South Africa
Full list of author information is available at the end of the article

during pregnancy, childbirth or postpartum. The study of near-miss is an increasingly useful tool in obstetric clinical audit, because of the larger number of cases available for study compared with maternal deaths, and because valuable information can be obtained on how clinical and surgical and clinical management obstacles are overcome after the onset of an acute complication [7].

To our knowledge, there has been no published scientific work focusing on maternal near-miss related to BDACS. Studies or audits on near-miss could improve understanding of the evolution of severe bleeding at caesarean section, and describe opportunities taken and missed to control the bleeding and treat its consequences. The information gained may inform quality improvement and interventions to reduce near-miss and death from BDACS.

The aim of this study was to determine the risk factors and causes of near-miss related to BDACS and to describe the clinical and surgical interventions undertaken.

Methods

This was a cross-sectional prospective study in 13 government hospitals in southern Gauteng province, South Africa, from July to December 2014. Ethical approval was obtained to conduct this study from the University of the Witwatersrand's Human Research Ethics Committee. Informed written consent was obtained from the participants.

The city of Johannesburg is the geographic and economic centre of southern Gauteng province. There are 18 government hospitals with maternity services in southern Gauteng, with about 100 000 births per annum. Three of these hospitals are university-attached tertiary referral hospitals. The 13 hospitals in the study included the three tertiary hospitals, as well as seven regional referral hospitals, and three district hospitals. The district hospitals are staffed by non-specialist doctors and have relatively small case loads. The regional hospitals all have at least one specialist, as well as medical officers who are responsible for most of the daily clinical activities. The tertiary hospitals are better resourced in terms of equipment and facilities, and include university faculty staff and residents training to become specialists.

The World Health Organization (WHO) Intervention criteria were used to identify cases of near-miss, and were modified to suit this population [7]. Only near-misses related to BDACS were included in this study. A near-miss related to BDACS was any woman with a gestational age ≥24 weeks, or who delivered a baby weighing ≥500 g, who had a caesarean section with a combined intraoperative and postoperative blood loss ≥1000 mL, and at least one of the following: red cell blood transfusion ≥3 units, emergency hysterectomy, repeat laparotomy, transfer to a higher level of care, started or restarted postoperative ventilation, use of inotropic drugs, acute dialysis, cardiopulmonary resuscitation and admission to an intensive care unit. Women with ruptured uterus, extra-uterine pregnancy, and where another cause of haemorrhage was the primary reason for bleeding, were excluded.

The researcher trained obstetric staff in each hospital on how to identify a near-miss from BDACS. Each time such a case was identified, a staff member notified the researcher telephonically. The researcher then travelled to the hospital and screened the file for study eligibility. Data were collected from maternal case records, and supplemented, where necessary, from patients themselves or from staff. Informed consent was obtained from the patients. Data collected from the clinical notes were antenatal history, details about the previous pregnancy and blood test results, reason for admission, clinical management, and events leading to the decision for caesarean section. Details about the caesarean section, the findings and the complications were recorded, as well as postnatal observations and interventions. The researcher made regular visits to all hospitals to ensure ongoing surveillance. Numbers of maternal deaths related to BDACS were also recorded.

A sample of 100 near-misses related to BDACS was envisaged to provide reasonable confidence intervals for observed percentage frequencies. With a sample of 100 subjects, an observed percentage has 95% confidence limits that are not more than 10% above and below it. Data analysis employed quantitative techniques, using Stata version 11 software (Statacorp, College Station, TX, USA). Descriptive data were analysed using medians, ranges and interquartile ranges for continuous variables, and proportions with percentages for categorical variables. Comparisons of categorical variable frequencies were made using Fisher's exact test. A p-value <0.05 was used to determine statistical significance.

Results

The hospitals reported 93 near-misses related to BDACS, as well as 7 maternal deaths. The total number of deliveries at all the hospitals was 46 775, of which 20527 were caesarean sections (43%). The near-miss related to BDACS rate was therefore 2.1 per 1000 (93/43474) live births, and the BDACS- related case fatality rate was 3.4 per 10 000 caesarean sections.

Obstetric data and risk factors for near-misses are shown in Table 1. Teen pregnancy ($n = 2$) and parity ≥4 ($n = 5$) were infrequent. Twenty women were nulliparous and 73 were multiparous. Forty-four (60.3%) of the multiparous women had previous caesarean sections. Anaemia prior to caesarean section (haemoglobin level <11.0 g/dL) was found in 49 of 89 women tested (55.1%). Thirty-six women (40.4%) were HIV

Table 1 Obstetric characteristics and risk factors for maternal near-miss from bleeding during or after caesarean section ($n = 93$, unless otherwise specified because of missing data)

	Number	Percent
Maternal age (years):		
< 20	2	2.2
20–34	69	74.2
≥ 35	22	23.7
Parity:		
0	20	21.5
1–3	68	73.1
4	5	5.4
Attended antenatal clinic	83	89.2
Previous caesarean section	44	47.3
Haemoglobin level prior to caesarean section (g/dL) ($n = 89$):		
< 8.0	11	12.4
8.0–10.9	38	42.7
≥ 11.0	40	43.0
HIV infection ($n = 89$)	36	40.4
Antenatal weight ≥90 kg ($n = 79$)	8	10.1
Caesarean section ($n = 91$):		
Elective (planned)	11	12.1
Emergency not in labour	28	30.8
Emergency in first stage	44	48.4
Emergency in second stage	8	8.8
Hypertensive disorder of pregnancy	26	28.0
Abruptio placentae	19	20.4
Placenta praevia/accreta:		
Placenta praevia	7	7.5
Placenta accreta	9	9.7
Placenta praevia and accreta	3	3.2
Birth weight (g) ($n = 85$):		
< 1000	6	7.1
1000–2499	33	38.8
≥ 2500	46	54.1

infected. Clinical risk factors included hypertensive disorders in pregnancy in 26 (28.0%), abruptio placentae in 19 (20.4%), and placenta praevia and/or accreta in 19 women (20.4%) Nine of the 19 women with abruptio placentae had a hypertensive disorder. The main primary indications for caesarean section were fetal distress ($n = 14$; 15.1%), abruptio placentae ($n = 13$; 14.0%) and placenta praevia ($n = 12$; 12.9%). Eleven women had caesarean section for prolonged labour, 7 in the first stage of labour (7.5%) and 4 in the second stage (4.3%). Twenty-four infants were stillborn, 17 of them in association with abruptio placentae. The surgeons who started the caesarean sections were non-specialists in 29 cases (31.2%), residents in 54 cases (58.1%) and specialists in 7 cases (7.5%). Seven caesarean sections (7.5%) were done in district hospitals, 22 (23.7%) in regional hospitals and 64 (68.9%) in tertiary hospitals.

The most frequent cause (anatomical site) of haemorrhage was atonic uterus ($n = 40$; 43.0%), followed by uterine incisional bleeding ($n = 27$; 29.0%), placental site bleeding ($n = 16$; 17.2%), bleeding at the bladder reflection ($n = 8$; 8.6%), pampiniform venous plexus bleeding ($n = 5$; 5.4%) and abdominal wall bleeding ($n = 4$; 4.3%). Two or more causes of bleeding occurred in some women. In 14 women (15.1%), the cause of haemorrhage was not specified. The causes of bleeding were compared between women with previous caesarean section, placenta praevia/accreta, abruptio placentae, and the remainder (considered as having no surgical risk). There were significant associations between placenta praevia/accreta and placental site bleeding ($p < 0.01$), and between abruptio placentae and atonic uterus ($p = 0.04$). There was a trend to more frequent pampiniform plexus and abdominal wall bleeding in women with previous caesarean section (Table 2).

The surgeons noted difficulty in 76 operations (81.7%). The duration of surgery was estimable in 80 cases, and was <60 min in 14 (17.5%), 60–119 min in 34 (42.5%) and ≥120 min in 32 (40.0%). The median duration was 90 min, with a range of 23–345 min. Forty-nine women (52.7%) received blood transfusions during their caesarean sections. Medications and procedures used to arrest bleeding (in addition to routine intravenous oxytocin) included ergometrine, misoprostol, prostaglandin F2-alpha, tranexamic acid, B-Lynch brace suture, systematic uterine vessel ligation (devascularisation), and intrauterine balloons (Table 3). The median blood loss at caesarean section (estimated by the surgeons in 69 cases) was 1000 mL, with a range of 250–3600 mL. Second-look emergency laparotomy was performed in 43 women, of whom 18 underwent hysterectomy (total hysterectomies: $n = 38$; 40.9%) and 8 had B-Lynch compression sutures (of which 4 failed, requiring hysterectomy). Fourteen women had only resuturing or uterine vessel ligation done, and 5 required no specific haemostatic procedure. Seventy-four women (79.6%) received three or more units of red cell transfusion during their hospital stay. The median lowest postoperative haemoglobin level was 6.05 g/dL ($n = 90$), with a range of 2.8–12.5 g/dL. Thirty-six of 78 women in whom the platelet count was measured had a postoperative thrombocytopenia <100 000/μL. Seven women had severe acute kidney injury (serum creatinine ≥250 μmol/L), and 6 required dialysis. Thirty women (32.3%) were admitted to intensive care units postoperatively. Eleven women (11.8%)

Table 2 Caesarean section near-miss haemorrhage anatomical sites, according to presence or absence of specific prior surgical risk factors

	Previous caesarean section only ($n = 23$)	Placenta praevia/accreta ($n = 19$) – includes 13 previous caesarean sections	Abruptio placentae ($n = 19$) – includes 8 previous caesarean sections	No surgical risks anticipated ($n = 32$)
Uterine incision	5	5	3	14
Atonic uterus	9	4	14*	13
Placental site	1	14*	0	1
Bladder reflection	1	3	2	2
Pampiniform plexus	3	0	1	1
Abdominal wall	3	1	0	0
Not specified	3	1	2	8

*Comparison for placental site bleeding, placenta praevia/accreta v. no surgical risks: $p < 0.01$
*Comparison for atonic uterus, abruptio placentae v. no surgical risks: $p = 0.04$

received inotropic drugs. Ten women (10.8%) were transferred by ambulance to higher levels of care.

The seven maternal deaths included a case of placenta accreta with previous caesarean section, who required a hysterectomy, and one woman with placental abruption who died four days postoperatively from multi-organ dysfunction. The remaining five women had no surgical risk factors, and all had intraoperative blood loss ≤700 mL.

Discussion

This study, from a middle-income urban setting, found that about one in 216 caesarean sections are complicated by severe morbidity from bleeding, and that about 1 in 14 women with severe morbidity progress to maternal death. The near-miss definition seemed appropriate as applied in this study, providing a sample of women severely affected by bleeding, evidenced by a very low median postoperative haemoglobin level of 6.05 g/dL.

Table 3 Intraoperative interventions during caesarean section in cases of near-miss haemorrhage ($n = 93$ unless otherwise specified because of missing data). Multiple interventions were used in some cases

	Number	Percent
Red cell blood transfusion ($n = 89$)		
None	40	44.9
1 unit	8	9.0
2 unit	22	24.7
≥ 3 units	19	21.3
Intramuscular or intravenous ergometrine	19	20.4
Oral or rectal misoprostol	8	8.6
Intramyometrial prostaglandin-F2-alpha	10	10.8
Intravenous tranexamic acid	6	6.5
Systematic uterine vessel ligation (devascularisation)	7	7.5
Intrauterine balloon[a]	4	4.3
B-Lynch compression suture[a]	15	16.1
Hysterectomy	20	21.5

[a]Three of the intrauterine balloons failed to stop the bleeding, and two of the B-Lynch compression sutures (in whom balloons were not used) failed. All five failures went on to hysterectomy

The most important common risk factors for near-miss related to BDACS were preoperative anaemia (over half had haemoglobin <11.0 g/dL), and previous caesarean section (in over half of multiparas). A rising caesarean section rate increases not only the number of caesarean sections currently, but adds women with previous caesarean section to those who will become pregnant in future. This is one of the reasons for calls to prevent the first caesarean section in women [8]. The HIV infection rate, while high, is not statistically significantly higher than the 28.7% prevalence in pregnant women in this part of South Africa ($p = 0.05$) [9]. Anaemia limits the body's response to blood loss, and makes any caesarean section potentially hazardous. Previous caesarean section is well known as a cause of overall surgical difficulty [10]. Accordingly, multiple causes of bleeding were found in women with previous caesarean sections, including extrauterine causes such as pampiniform plexus and abdominal wall injury. The other two important risk factor categories, abruptio placentae and placenta previa/accreta, are uncommon conditions, yet occurred in large numbers in this series. The published literature supports our finding of uterine atony being the most common cause of post-partum haemorrhage, and placental site bleeding associated with placenta praevia/accreta [11]. Previous caesarean section itself is also associated with placenta praevia/accreta [12]. A number of women had no specific surgical risk factors, and bled severely from a variety of sources. The absence of risk factors gives no guarantee of an uncomplicated caesarean section and postoperative course.

In 76% of near-misses related to BDACS, the caesarean sections were noted by the surgeons as difficult, and early interventions were made intra-operatively. A range of life-saving options was used, usually in combination, to manage the source and effects of bleeding. Medical management included utero-tonics, tranexamic acid, inotropic support and blood transfusion, with recourse to emergency transport if needed, and intensive care, suggesting the elements of a well-resourced functional health service. Surgical options included frequent use of uterine vessel ligation, B-Lynch compression sutures and hysterectomy, both at caesarean section and at second-look emergency laparotomy, suggesting the presence of skilled obstetric surgeons. The few attempts at intra-uterine balloon tamponade were mostly unsuccessful, but this may reflect the characteristics of this group of women. Balloon tamponade works best when placed early in severe postpartum haemorrhage after vaginal birth [13].

This study has certain strengths and limitations. Strengths were a robust near-miss definition and a sample size that allowed description of prevalence and relationships. Another strength is the clinical detail obtained from inspection of all women's clinical notes by a specialist obstetrician. The reliance on record review for clinical information is also a limitation, with some data missing. Limitations include the possibility that some near-miss cases were not included, because the researcher and the trained contacts at the hospitals could not be in attendance at all births. However, it is certain that all maternal deaths from BDACS were included, because these are subject to compulsory confidential enquiries.

Further research should focus on detail in risk factors, surgical findings and interventions. An ideal design would be a case-control study, in which near-miss cases are compared with non-near-miss caesarean sections for risk factors, surgical findings and interventions. A similar study should also be done in a resource-poor setting, where access to technological and specialist interventions is restricted, and where there are likely to be more maternal deaths.

Conclusion

Our findings show that maternal near-miss from BDACS is uncommon, but severe enough to necessitate extensive life-saving interventions. These require skilled or specialist health professionals, and a functional obstetric service with access to medication, blood transfusion, emergency transport and intensive care units. An important factor in initiating the sequence of interventions is the realisation by the surgeon that the caesarean section is difficult, so that the progression from uneventful operation to near-miss to death can be arrested.

Abbreviations

BDACS: Bleeding during and after caesarean section; g: Gram; g/dl: Gram/decilitre; HIV: Human immunodeficiency virus; mL: Millilitre; n: Number; p: Probability; v.: Versus; WHO: World Health Organization

Acknowledgements

Not applicable

Funding

- Carnegie Corporation of New York, Grant B8749.R01.
- Research submitted in this report was supported by the South African Medical Research Council under a Self-Initiated Research Grant.

The work as supported by the Carnegie Corporation of New York, and the, SA MRC, the views and opinions expressed, however, are not those of the Carnegie Corporation or the SA MRC, but of the authors.

Authors' contributions

SM: Made substantial contributions to conception and design, acquisition of data, and interpretation of data; Was involved in drafting the manuscript, revising it critically for important intellectually content; Acquired funding for the study. EB: Made substantial contributions to conception and design, and analysis and interpretation of data; Supervised the study. SM and EB: Gave final approval of the version to be published; Agreed to be accountable for all aspects of the work in ensuring that questions related to the accuracy or integrity of any part of the work are appropriately investigated and resolved.

Authors' information

Not applicable.

Competing interests

This study was done as part of a PhD with the University of the Witwatersrand. Funding to do a full-time PhD was received from the Carnegie Corporation of New York. Funding for the research was received from the Carnegie Corporation of New York and the South African Medical Research Council.

Author details

[1]Wits Obstetrics and Gynaecology Clinical Research Division, Johanesburg, South Africa. [2]Department of Obstetrics and Gynaecology, University of the Witwatersrand, Johannesburg, South Africa.

References

1. Department of health. Saving Mothers 2002–2004: Third report on the confidential enquiries into maternal deaths in South Africa. Pretoria: Department of Health; 2006.
2. Department of health Department of health. Saving Mothers 2005–2007: Fourth report on the confidential enquiries into maternal deaths in South Africa. Pretoria: Department of Health; 2009.
3. Department of health. Saving Mothers 2008–2010: Fifth report on the confidential enquiries into maternal deaths in South Africa. Pretoria: Department of Health; 2011.
4. Department of health. Saving Mothers 2011–2013: Sixth report on the confidential enquiries into maternal deaths in South Africa. Pretoria: Department of Health; 2015.
5. Massyn N, Day C, Dombo M, et al. District health Barometer 2012/13. Durban: Health Systems Trust; 2013.
6. Gebhart G, Fawcus S, Moodley X, et al. Maternal death and caesarean section in South Africa: Results from 2011 to 2013 Saving mothers report of the national committee for confidential enquiries into maternal deaths. S Afr Med J. 2015;105(4):287–91.
7. Say L, Souza J, Pattinson R. Maternal near miss – towards a standard tool for monitoring quality of maternal health care. Best Pract Res Clin Obstet Gynaecol. 2009;23:287–96.

8. Spong C, Berghella V, Wenstrom K, Mercer B, Saade G. Preventing the first cesarean delivery. Obstet Gynecol. 2012;120:1181–93.
9. Deirdre J, Lyell M. Adhesions and perioperative complications of repeat cesarean delivery. Am J Obstet Gynecol. 2011;205(6 Suppl):S12–7.
10. Avert. South Africa HIV and statistics. http://www.avert.org/south-africa-hiv-aids-statistics.htm. Accessed 7 Oct 2015.
11. Walfish M, Neuman A, Wlody D. Maternal haemorrhage. Br J Anaesth. 2009; 103(suppl 1):i47–56.
12. De Souza R. Caesarean section on maternal request for non-medical reasons: putting the UK national institute of health and clinical excellence guidelines in perspective. Best Prac Res Clin Obstet Gynaecol. 2013;27:165–77.
13. Bakri Y, Arulkumaran S. Intrauterine balloon tamponade for control of postpartum hemorrhage. UpToDate, Post TW (Ed), UpToDate, Waltham, MA; 2015. https://www.uptodate.com/contents/intrauterine-balloon-tamponade-for-control-of-postpartum-hemorrhage. Accessed 12 Dec 2016.

22

Rates and trends in cesarean sections between 2008 and 2012 in Iraq

Nazar P. Shabila

Abstract

Background: The prevalence of cesarean sections is increasing globally; however, it can lead to significant increases in maternal and infant morbidity and mortality. This study aimed to determine the rates and trends of cesarean sections in Iraq.

Methods: The cesarean section rates of all births and public and private hospital-based births were calculated from the data on births provided by the annual reports of the Iraqi Ministry of Health for the years 2008 and 2012. The comparable rates for the Center/South and Kurdistan Region and the individual governorates were determined. The cesarean section rates for all births in 2008 were computed and compared with the 2012 rates.

Results: The cesarean section rate for all births in Iraq was 24.4% in 2012, which was similar to the rates in the Iraqi Kurdistan Region (25.4%) and the Center/South of Iraq (24.3%). The cesarean section rates were specifically high in the governorates containing a larger number of private hospitals, and there was a significant positive relationship between the number of private hospitals and the cesarean section rate (beta = 0.671; $r = 0.671$; $P < 0.002$). The hospital-based cesarean section rate was 34.7%. The cesarean section rate in private hospitals (77.9%) was remarkably higher than the rate in public hospitals (29.3%). The overall rate of cesarean sections in Iraq increased from 18.0% in 2008 to 24.4% in 2012.

Conclusions: The cesarean section rate in Iraq is far above the recommended rate. Iraq witnessed a rapid upward trend in the cesarean section rate from 2008 to 2012, with most of this trend attributable to the Kurdistan Region. There is a potential relationship between the expansion of the private health sector and the increasing cesarean section rate, and further studies of this relationship are necessary. Future research should consider an audit of the indications for a cesarean section rather than measuring the cesarean section rate alone.

Background

Cesarean sections are a commonly performed operation for women. The procedure is associated with significant increases in maternal and infant morbidity and mortality, particularly in low-income countries. Increases in maternal morbidity are particularly prevalent after an emergency cesarean section or a cesarean section performed during the second stage of labor [1–3].

The prevalence of cesarean sections is increasing globally each year where the rates have increased beyond the recommended level of 10%. Cesarean section rates beyond this level do not further reduce maternal and perinatal mortality [4, 5]. There is considerable variation in the rates of cesarean sections, particularly between high- and low-income countries and between different institutions within these countries [1, 6]. Many factors have contributed to the increasing rates of cesarean sections including medical and non-medical factors. Examples of medical factors include increases in maternal age and body mass index and changes in obstetric practices and technologies. Examples of non-medical factors include cesarean sections requested by the mother, fear of litigation among caregivers, the inappropriate organization of maternity care and physician-induced demand for cesarean sections [7, 8].

There is significant variation in the cesarean section rate in terms of socioeconomic status. However, research has suggested that the increasing rate is attributed to structural factors related to service supply and compensation structure and not a woman's ability to pay [9]. A systematic review and meta-analysis of observational

Correspondence: nazarshabila@gmail.com
Department of Community Medicine, College of Medicine, Hawler Medical University, Erbil, Iraq

studies revealed that the preference for a cesarean section in women is greater than 15% [10]. The same review concluded that the actual contribution of women demanding the procedure to the rising cesarean section rates is not well studied. Recent evidence also shows that the demand for a cesarean section among young, educated women residing in urban areas has increased [11].

According to the limited available research, the cesarean section rate in Iraq is considerably higher than the recommended upper limit of 10% [12, 13]. Research concerning the factors contributing to the increased rate of cesarean sections in Iraq is very scarce. The private healthcare sector in Iraq has witnessed a rapid unguided expansion during the last decade [14]. The poor governmental oversight and regulation of this sector have raised concerns about a possible increase in the physician-induced demand for healthcare including cesarean sections [15–17]. The aim of this study was to determine the rates and trends of cesarean sections in Iraq. This study also sought to determine any differences in the cesarean section rates according to the governorates and regions as well as the size of the private healthcare sector.

Methods

This descriptive study is based on the data on births provided by the Iraqi Ministry of Health. The data on total births, public and private hospital-based births and births by cesarean section were extracted from the 2012 Annual Report of the Iraqi Ministry of Health, which is the latest published report. The report, which is publicly available on the ministry's website, is primarily a compilation of institutional and administrative records submitted by the directorates of health of the Iraqi governorates [18]. The annual report of the Ministry of Health contains summary tables that include the data on all births registered during the reporting year distributed by the place of occurrence such as homes, public hospitals or private hospitals. These data are also segregated at the governorate levels. The data from the annual report is considered adequately reliable because birth registration in Iraq was almost universal in 2006 and 2011. The Multiple Indicator Cluster Survey (MICS) 3 and 4 showed that the completeness of birth registration in Iraq was 95% in 2006 [19] and 99.2% in 2011 [20]. In 2012, there were no specific areas in Iraq outside of the control of the government that might have lacked proper registration of births. This study was approved by the Research Ethics Committee of Hawler Medical University, and authorization of the Ministry of Health was obtained to use the data from the annual reports.

The cesarean section rates for all births and hospital-based births were calculated for each governorate. The comparable rates for the Center/South of Iraq and Iraqi Kurdistan Region were determined. The segregated rates of public hospitals and private hospitals were also calculated for each governorate with the exception of the three governorates of the Iraqi Kurdistan Region because these segregated data were not provided in the report and could not be obtained from the respective directorates of health.

The data on all births and total births by cesarean section were also extracted from the 2008 Annual Report of the Iraqi Ministry of Health [21], which is the earliest published report providing detailed data. The cesarean section rates of all births in 2008 were calculated for each governorate and the rates were compared with the 2012 rates to determine the trend in the cesarean section rate from 2008 to 2012. The relative change between the two time periods was computed for each governorate ((cesarean section rate 2012 − cesarean section rate 2008)/cesarean section rate 2008). The effect of the number of private hospitals in the different governorates on the cesarean section rate was examined using a linear regression. The data were analyzed using SPSS statistical software (version 19). A P value of ≤ 0.05 was considered statistically significant.

Results

Of the 1,300,103 births recorded in Iraq in 2012, 29.6% were home births and 70.4% were hospital-based births, 61.8% of which were in public hospitals and 8.6% in private hospitals. The overall cesarean section rate for all births in Iraq in 2012 was 24.4%. The cesarean section rates did not differ much between the Iraqi Kurdistan Region and the Center/South of Iraq (25.4 and 24.3%, respectively). The rate was specifically high in the governorates of Baghdad (38.9%), Al-Diwaniya (35.1%), Erbil (31.4%) and Al-Najaf (30.1%). The overall hospital-based cesarean section rate was (34.7%). The rate was slightly higher in the Center/South of Iraq compared to the Iraqi Kurdistan Region (34.9 and 33.8%, respectively). The cesarean section rate in public hospitals in the Center/South of Iraq ranged between 17.4 and 38.8%. This rate was the highest in Baghdad (38.8%), followed by Al-Diwaniya (35.7%) and Al-Anbar (33.8%). The cesarean section rate in private hospitals ranged between 35% and 100%. The segregated data for the hospital-based cesarean section rate in the Iraqi Kurdistan Region was not available. The details of the distribution of all births and hospital-based cesarean section rates in the different governorates of Iraq are shown in Table 1. The cesarean section rates were significantly higher in the governorates that had a larger number of private hospitals compared to those with a smaller number or no private hospitals (beta = 0.671; $r = 0.671$; $P < 0.002$).

The overall rate of cesarean section increased remarkably from 18.0% in 2008 to 24.4% in 2012. The increase

Table 1 Distribution of all births and hospital-based cesarean section rates according to the governorates for the year 2012

Governorates	All births		Public hospitals		Private hospitals		No. of private hospitals
	No. of births	CS rate %	No. of births (%)	CS rate %[a]	No. of births (%)	CS rate %[a]	
Baghdad	254,862	38.9	136,531 (53.6)	38.8	60,679 (23.8)	76.2	36
Basrah	102,386	22.9	83,011 (81.1)	26.2	4798 (4.7)	35.0	4
Nineveh	147,917	15.2	97,951 (66.2)	22.3	680 (0.5)	100.0	3
Maysan	42,566	9.5	23,238 (54.6)	17.4	0 (0.0)	-	0
Al-Diwaniya	41,761	35.1	26,955 (64.5)	35.7	5100 (12.2)	98.6	3
Diyala	61,400	20.1	33,087 (53.9)	32.1	1725 (2.8)	100.0	3
Al-Anbar	58,096	24.0	34,908 (60.1)	33.8	3710 (6.4)	57.5	2
Babylon	64,563	21.0	44,249 (68.5)	26.9	1696 (2.6)	100.0	4
Kerbala	44,693	26.7	30,770 (68.8)	24.4	4925 (11.0)	89.4	2
Kirkuk	55,078	19.0	32,940 (59.8)	28.0	1262 (2.3)	98.4	2
Wasit	58,527	18.5	31,461 (53.8)	34.4	0 (0.0)	-	0
Thi-Qar	66,034	16.6	38,898 (58.9)	23.3	1905 (2.9)	99.8	2
Al-Muthanna	35,461	17.1	25,960 (73.2)	23.4	0 (0.0)	-	0
Salah Al-Deen	55,202	14.0	21,767 (39.4)	26.1	2274 (4.1)	88.9	2
Al-Najaf	50,762	30.1	40,029 (78.9)	31.1	3114 (6.1)	91.2	3
Centre/South	1,139,308	24.3	701,755 (61.6)	29.3	91,868 (8.1)	77.9	66
Erbil	55,864	31.4	37,666 (67.4)	NA	9012 (16.1)	NA	13
Dohouk	52,569	15.9	27,909 (53.1)	NA	5117 (9.7)	NA	3
Al-Sulaimaniya	52,362	27.5	35,626 (68.0)	NA	6118 (11.7)	NA	14
Kurdistan	160,795	25.4	101,201 (62.9)	-	20,247 (12.6)	-	30
Total Iraq	1,300,103	24.4	802,956 (61.8)	-	112,115 (8.6)	-	96

CS cesarean section, *NA* data not available
[a]The distribution for the Iraqi Kurdistan Region is not included because the segregated data for the public/private hospitals was unavailable. The cesarean section rates for all hospital births were Erbil: 37.6%, Dohouk: 26.6%, Al-Sulaimaniya: 34.5%, Kurdistan: 33.8%, Centre/South: 34.9%, and total Iraq: 34.7%

was higher in the Iraqi Kurdistan Region compared to the rest of Iraq (from 14.6 to 25.4% versus from 18.4 to 24.3%). The rate increased in all of the governorates during this period except Maysan. The increase was highest for Erbil, Basrah, Al-Sulaimaniya and Kirkuk with a relative change of 116.6, 90.8, 58.0 and 52.0%, respectively (Table 2).

Discussion

The overall cesarean section rate in Iraq in 2012, as revealed by this study (24.4%), is far higher than the recommended level of 10% [5]. The Iraq MICS 2011 showed a slightly lower cesarean section rate (22.2%) than that revealed by the present study [20]. The cesarean section rate in Iraq is greater than the rate in some neighboring countries such as Jordan (18.5%) [22], but it is considerably lower than the rate in Iran (40%) [23]. In general, Western Asia, including Iraq, is one of the regions of the world with high cesarean section rates, which are on an average of 26.8%. However, this rate varies widely among the countries of the region ranging from 4.8% in Yemen to 47.5% in Turkey [24].

The rates of cesarean section in the different governorates of Iraq are in line with the findings of the Iraq MICS 2011, which revealed variations in the rates ranging from 16 to 38% with the governorates of Al-Sulaimaniya, Al-Diwaniya, Erbil, Kerbala, Najaf and Baghdad showing the highest rates [20].

The overall hospital-based cesarean section rate in Iraq was considerably high and exceeded the rates of many other Arab countries. A review of the hospital-based cesarean section rates in 18 Arab countries, not including Iraq, reported lower rates ranging from 5.3% in Mauritania (2003) to 26.2% in Egypt (2000) [25]. The high hospital-based cesarean section rate might be indirectly attributed to having many low-risk pregnancies delivered at home, whereas the high-risk pregnancies and the elective or planned cesarean sections are referred to hospitals. Thus, the rate of cesarean sections in hospitals increases proportionally.

The private hospital-based cesarean section rates in most of the governorates in the Center/South of Iraq were very high. It is expected that these rates would be higher in the Iraqi Kurdistan Region; however, these segregated data are unfortunately not available. The very

Table 2 Change in the cesarean section rates in the different governorates from 2008 to 2012

Governorates	2008		2012		Relative change in %[a]
	No. of births	CS rate %	No. of births	CS rate %	
Baghdad	216,883	28.5	254,862	38.9	36.5%
Basrah	96,137	12.0	102,386	22.9	90.8%
Nineveh	117,967	12.6	147,917	15.2	20.6%
Maysan	39,092	9.5	42,566	9.5	0.0%
Al-Diwaniya	39,022	28.7	41,761	35.1	22.3%
Diyala	42,676	17.0	61,400	20.1	18.2%
Al-Anbar	38,693	17.0	58,096	24.0	41.2%
Babylon	70,488	20.7	64,563	21.0	1.4%
Kerbala	39,331	19.8	44,693	26.7	34.8%
Kirkuk	45,887	12.5	55,078	19.0	52.0%
Wasit	47,513	16.0	58,527	18.5	15.6%
Thi-Qar	66,971	11.3	66,034	16.6	46.9%
Al-Muthanna	31,498	14.7	35,461	17.1	16.3%
Salah Al-Deen	45,093	11.0	55,202	14.0	27.3%
Al-Najaf	46,999	24.2	50,762	30.1	24.4%
Centre/South	984,250	18.4	1,139,308	24.3	32.1%
Erbil	40,667	14.5	55,864	31.4	116.6%
Dohouk	41,364	11.7	52,569	15.9	35.9%
Al-Sulaimaniya	41,935	17.4	52,362	27.5	58.0%
Kurdistan	123,966	14.6	160,795	25.4	74.0%
Total Iraq	1,108,216	18.0	1,300,103	24.4	35.6%

CS cesarean section
[a](Cesarean section rate last time period – cesarean section rate first time period)/cesarean section rate first time period

high cesarean section rate in private hospitals is the main contributor to the high hospital-based cesarean section rate in Iraq. Private hospitals in Iraq are primarily surgical hospitals that provide cesarean section services, and many of these facilities do not provide normal vaginal delivery services. This could be the reason why some of the governorates showed private hospital-based cesarean section rates of up to 100%.

The trend of an increasing cesarean section rate is not limited to Iraq because most countries follow a similar or a more rapidly rising trend. The global average cesarean section rate increased from 6.7% in 1990 to 19.1% in 2014 with an average annual rate of increase of 4.4%. The increasing trend was remarkable in Western Asia where the cesarean section rate increased from 6.3 to 28.1% with an average annual rate of increase of 6.4% [24].

The recent global increase in the cesarean section rate can be largely attributed to different factors including advances in technologies to detect fetal distress and the attitudes of clinicians and women toward cesarean sections such as the avoidance of labor pain [26]. In Iraq, there is a lack of clear evidence of the main factors attributing to the reported high cesarean section rate. However, a previous study showed that 11% of cesarean sections in a public hospital in Baghdad were conducted for non-medical reasons such as the fear of vaginal delivery (45.7%), choosing the right timing for security reasons (31.4%), avoiding delivery pain (14.3%) and performing a tubal ligation (8.6%) [12].

Another important potential factor for the high cesarean section rate is provider-induced demand because there is clear evidence of an association between private care and an increased rate of cesarean sections [26]. This factor could be relevant to the Iraqi context since governorates with a larger number of private hospitals had increased rates of cesarean sections. This factor could also explain the larger increase in the cesarean section rate in the Kurdistan Region because this region has recently witnessed a rapid expansion of a poorly regulated private healthcare sector [14]. Iraq may potentially be prone to the problem of provider-induced demand due to a lack of consumer organizations and patients' rights groups to protect patients' interests and the absence of health insurance agencies to scrutinize providers and prevent the easy abuse of these services.

In addition, Iraq relies on the fee-for-service or out-of-pocket payment for private healthcare services, which increases the risk of provider-induced demand [8, 15].

The present study only assessed the cesarean section rate, which, alone, is not a proper indicator to monitor the quality of emergency obstetric care. Heemelaar et al. [27] conducted a criteria-based audit of cesarean sections by measuring the prevalence of substandard quality of care that led to unnecessary cesarean sections and a delay in performing interventions to prevent cesarean sections. They identified high rates of unnecessary and potentially preventable cesarean sections. Another study also showed that a clinical audit is an effective strategy for reducing the cesarean section rate and recommended strict monitoring of the indications for cesarean sections to reduce the cesarean section rate [28]. Therefore, future research needs to consider conducting an audit of the indications for cesarean sections rather than measuring the cesarean section rate alone.

This study is limited by being a descriptive study based on already available data. This study provides information about the rates and trends of cesarean sections in Iraq, but does not look at the actual reasons for the increasing trend. It does not show whether this trend is related to medical reasons or non-medical reasons such as the women's preferences or provider-induced demand. This study is based on data extracted from the annual reports of the Ministry of Health. These reports are primarily dependent on the completeness of birth registration and the accurate reporting of births by the civil registration offices and the directorates of health at the governorate level. According to UNICEF, birth registration is nearly universal in Iraq [19, 20]. However, the issue of accuracy of reporting birth records remains a concern, which adds another limitation to this study.

Conclusions

The overall cesarean section rate in Iraq of 24.4% is far above the recommended rate of 10%. Iraq has witnessed a rapid upward trend in the cesarean section rate from 2008 to 2012, with much of this trend being attributed to the Kurdistan Region. The hospital-based rate of cesarean sections, particularly in private hospitals, is extremely high. There is a potential relationship between the expansion of the private health sector and the increasing rate of cesarean sections, particularly in the Kurdistan Region. Further research is needed to monitor the indications for cesarean sections and explore the determinants of this rapid upward trend of cesarean sections in Iraq.

Abbreviations

CS: Cesarean section; MICS: Multiple Indicator Cluster Survey

Acknowledgments

The author would like to thank Valeria Cetorelli and Tariq Al-Hadithi for their help in reviewing the manuscript.

Funding

This study was not supported by any funding source to be declared.

Author's contributions

NPS conceptualized and designed the study, carried out the data analyses and interpretation and prepared the manuscript.

Author's information

NPS has a MSc degree in Public Health in Developing Countries from the London School of Hygiene and Tropical Medicine and a Ph.D. in Community Medicine from Hawler Medical University. He is an assistant professor of public health at Hawler Medical University, Erbil, Iraq. His current research interest is primarily related to health services research, women's health and violence against women in the Iraqi Kurdistan Region.

Competing interests

The author declares that he has no competing interests.

References

1. Althabe F, Sosa C, Belizán J, Gibbons L, Jacquerioz F, Bergel E. Caesarean section rates and maternal and neonatal mortality in low-, medium- and high-income countries: an ecological study. Birth. 2006;33(4):270–7.
2. Oladapo O, Lamina M, Sule-Odu A. Maternal morbidity and mortality associated with elective caesarean delivery at a university hospital in Nigeria. Aust N Z J Obstet Gynaecol. 2007;47(2):110–4.
3. MacDorman M, Declercq E, Menacker F, Malloy M. Infant and neonatal mortality for primary caesarean and vaginal births to women with "no indicated risk," United States, 1998–2001 birth cohorts. Birth. 2006;33(3):175–82.
4. Stanton C, Holtz S. Levels and trends in caesarean birth in the developing world. Stud Fam Plann. 2006;37(1):41–8.
5. Ye J, Zhang J, Mikolajczyk R, Torloni MR, Gülmezoglu AM, Betran AP. Association between rates of caesarean section and maternal and neonatal mortality in the 21st century: a worldwide population-based ecological study with longitudinal data. BJOG. 2016;123(5):745–53.
6. Villar J, Valladares E, Wojdyla D, Zavaleta N, Carroli G, Velazco A, et al. Caesarean delivery rates and pregnancy outcomes: the 2005 WHO global survey on maternal and perinatal health in Latin America. Lancet. 2006; 367(9525):1819–29.
7. Tollånes MC. Increased rate of caesarean sections - causes and consequences. Tidsskr Nor Laegeforen. 2009;129(13):1329–31.
8. Mossialos E, Allin S, Karras K, Davaki K. An investigation of caesarean sections in three Greek hospitals: the impact of financial incentives and convenience. Eur J Public Health. 2005;15(3):288–95.
9. Feng XL, Xu L, Guo Y, Ronsmans C. Factors influencing rising caesarean section rates in China between 1988 and 2008. Bull World Health Organ. 2012;90(1):30–9A.
10. Mazzoni A, Althabe F, Liu NH, Bonotti AM, Gibbons L, Sánchez AJ, et al. Women's preference for caesarean section: a systematic review and meta-analysis of observational studies. BJOG. 2011;118(4):391–9.
11. Lei H, Wen SW, Walker M. Determinants of caesarean delivery among women hospitalized for childbirth in a remote population in China. J Obstet Gynaecol Can. 2003;25(11):937–43.
12. Habib HA, Abdulla MM, Yacoub SE. Knowledge and preference of mothers delivering at ALKadhumyia Teaching Hospital regarding caesarean section and normal vaginal delivery. Iraqi Postgrad Med J. 2011;10(4):512–8.
13. Jarjees YT. Cesarean section rates at Al-Batool Maternity Teaching Hospital. Al-Kindy Col Med J. 2011;7(1):1–4.
14. Anthony CR, Moore M, Hilborne LH, Mulcahy AW. Health sector reform in

the Kurdistan Region-Iraq: financing reform, primary care, and patient safety. Santa Monica: RAND Corporation; 2014.

15. Shabila NP. Provider-induced demand in healthcare market: the case of Iraqi Kurdistan region. Zanco J Med Sci. 2013;17(3):482–3.
16. Maternal Health Task Force. Maternal health and c-sections in Iraq. Massachusetts: Harvard School of Public Health; 2011.
17. Rise in Iraqi c-sections worries doctors. NY: Fox News Network; 2011. http://www.foxnews.com/world/2011/08/16/rise-in-iraqi-c-sections-worries-doctors. Accessed 14 Apr 2014.
18. Iraq's Ministry of Health. Annual report for 2012. Baghdad: Ministry of Health; 2013.
19. Central Organization for Statistics, Kurdistan Regional Statistics Office, UNICEF. Iraq Multiple Indicator Cluster Survey 2006. Geneva: UNICEF; 2007.
20. Central Organization for Statistics, Kurdistan Regional Statistics Office, UNICEF. Iraq Multiple Indicator Cluster Survey 2011. Geneva: UNICEF; 2012.
21. Iraq's Ministry of Health. Annual report for 2008. Baghdad: Ministry of Health; 2009.
22. Gibbons L, Belizán JM, Lauer JA, Betrán AP, Merialdi M, Althabe F. The global numbers and costs of additionally needed and unnecessary caesarean sections performed per year: overuse as a barrier to universal coverage. Geneva: World Health Organization; 2010.
23. Yazdizadeh B, Nedjat S, Mohammad K, Rashidian A, Changizi N, Majdzadeh R. Cesarean section rate in Iran, multidimensional approaches for behavioral change of providers: a qualitative study. BMC Health Serv Res. 2011;11:159.
24. Betrán AP, Ye J, Moller AB, Zhang J, Gülmezoglu AM, Torloni MR. The increasing trend in caesarean section rates: Global, regional and national estimates: 1990–2014. PLoS One. 2016;11(2):e0148343.
25. Khawaja M, Choueiry N, Jurdi. Hospital-based caesarean section in the Arab region: an overview. East Mediterr Health J. 2009;15(2):458–69.
26. Roberts CL, Algert C, Ford JB, Todd AL, Morris JM. Pathways to a rising caesarean section rate: a population-based cohort study. BMJ Open. 2012; 2(5):e001725.
27. Heemelaar S, Nelissen E, Mdoe P, Kidanto H, van Roosmalen J, Stekelenburg J. Criteria-based audit of caesarean section in a referral hospital in rural Tanzania. Trop Med Int Health. 2016;21(4):525–34.
28. Peng FS, Lin HM, Lin HH, Tu FC, Hsiao CF, Hsiao SM. Impact of clinical audits on cesarean section rate. Taiwan J Obstet Gynecol. 2016;55(4):530–3.

23

Trial of labour after caesarean section and the risk of neonatal and infant death

Sinéad M. O'Neill[1,2*], Esben Agerbo[3], Ali S. Khashan[1,4], Patricia M. Kearney[4], Tine Brink Henriksen[5], Richard A. Greene[2] and Louise C. Kenny[1]

Abstract

Background: Caesarean section (CS) rates are increasing worldwide and as a result repeat CS is common. The optimal mode of delivery in women with one previous CS is widely debated and the risks to the infant are understudied. The aim of the current study was to evaluate if women with a trial of labour after caesarean (TOLAC) had an increased odds of neonatal and infant death compared to women with an elective repeat CS (ERCS).

Methods: A population register-based cohort study was conducted in Denmark between 1982 and 2010. All women with two deliveries [in which the first was a CS, and the second was an uncomplicated, term delivery ($n = 61{,}626$)] were included in the study. Logistic regression models were used to report adjusted odds ratios (AOR) and 95% confidence intervals (CI) of the odds of death according to mode of delivery. The main outcome measures were neonatal death (early and late) and infant death.

Results: Women with a TOLAC had an increased odds of neonatal death (AOR 1·87, 95% CI 1·12 to 3·12) due to an increased risk of early neonatal death (AOR 2·06, 95% CI 1·19 to 3·56) and no effect on late neonatal death (AOR 0·97, 95% CI 0·22 to 4·32), or infant death (AOR 1·12, 95% CI 0·79 to 1·59) when compared to the reference group of women with an ERCS. There was evidence of a cohort effect as the increased odds of neonatal death (AOR 3·89, 95% CI 1·33 to 11·39) was most significant in the earlier years (1982–1991) and gradually disappeared (AOR 1·01, 95% CI 0·44 to 2·31) in the later years (2002–2010).

Conclusions: Although an increased risk of neonatal death was found in women with a TOLAC, there was evidence of a cohort effect, which showed this increased odds disappearing over time. Advances in modern healthcare including improved monitoring and earlier detection of underlying pregnancy complications may explain the findings.

Keywords: Trial of labour, Neonatal death, Repeat Caesarean section

Background

Caesarean section (CS) rates are increasing worldwide, and currently CS is the most commonly performed surgical procedure in women of childbearing age in the United States (US) [1]. Proposed driving forces include increasing maternal age at first pregnancy [2], increasing body mass index (BMI) [3], elective CS for breech presentation and more recently maternal request for a CS [4, 5], as well elective repeat CS (in women with a first CS) [ERCS] [6]. Trial of labour after Caesarean section (TOLAC) rates have decreased significantly in some countries [7], largely due a reported increased risk of uterine rupture and perinatal asphyxia in women undergoing a TOLAC compared to a planned ERCS [8–11], whilst remaining unchanged in others [12, 13]. Rising CS rates have generated much debate on the benefits and risks to the mother and her offspring attributable to mode of delivery, particularly whether or not to attempt a TOLAC in the subsequent

* Correspondence: sinead.oneill@ucc.ie
[1]The Irish Centre for Fetal and Neonatal Translational Research (INFANT), Cork University Maternity Hospital, University College Cork, Wilton, Cork, Ireland
[2]National Perinatal Epidemiology Centre (NPEC), Department of Obstetrics and Gynaecology, Cork University Maternity Hospital, 5th Floor Wilton, Cork, Ireland
Full list of author information is available at the end of the article

delivery [14]. Numerous studies have focused on maternal outcomes reporting an increased risk of uterine rupture, placenta accreta and placenta previa [15–17]. Evidence remains to be explored regarding infant outcomes in the subsequent pregnancy following first CS delivery particularly early and late neonatal death [18, 19]. Controversy remains on whether a TOLAC or an ERCS is preferable for women with one prior CS. In the absence of clinical trials on the topic which are difficult to conduct, population register-based research incorporating detailed obstetric information remains the optimum study design to address this important question.

The objective of the current study was to examine the odds of neonatal death, early and late neonatal death and infant mortality in a cohort of women with an uncomplicated term delivery who had a TOLAC or ERCS following a first CS.

Methods

Study design, data source and population studied

A cohort study design using the Danish Civil Registration System (CRS) data was used to identify all women with their first two deliveries in Denmark between January 1st 1982 and December 31st 2010 (of which the first was a CS, and the second an ERCS or TOLAC). In order to be eligible for inclusion in this study the second delivery had to be an uncomplicated, term delivery (i.e. a singleton, cephalic delivery between 37 and 42 weeks' gestation). After removal of ineligible women and deaths due to congenital anomalies, there were 61,626 women eligible for inclusion in the analyses (Fig. 1).

The Danish CRS was established in 1968 originally for administrative purposes but has since become an invaluable source of population-based data for use in epidemiological research [20, 21]. The CRS uses a unique identifier known as the civil person register (CPR) which enables researchers to link data from different registers as well as the continuous follow-up of individuals living in Denmark. For the current study data from the CRS were linked to the Danish Medical Birth Registry (MBR) [22, 23], the National Hospital Register (NHR) [24], the Danish Causes of Death Register [25] and socioeconomic data were obtained from *Statistics Denmark* [26] using the unique CPR number.

Exposure

Mode of delivery was categorised as follows: 1) first CS and subsequent ERCS [reference group] ($n = 20{,}941$), 2) first CS and subsequent TOLAC ($n = 40{,}685$). For the purposes of this study the TOLAC group included any patient with a previous CS who did not have an ERCS. It therefore includes patients who have a vaginal birth after Caesarean (VBAC, i.e. a successful TOLAC) or an emergency CS (which may have arisen from a failed TOLAC or may have been done for women with a planned CS who attends in labour, with ruptured membranes not in labour, etc. and had an 'emergency/semi-emergency' CS). The groups represent what happens in a real life situation, i.e. ERCS (planned) versus all other modes of delivery.

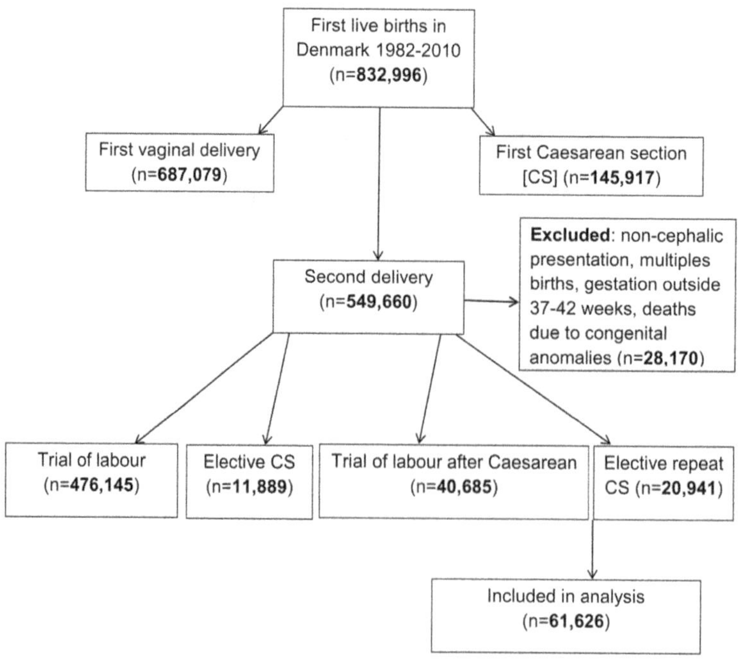

Fig. 1 Flowchart of the study population

Mode of delivery recorded in the Danish registers is the 'actual' mode of delivery (which may differ from the woman's intended mode of delivery). For example, a woman may attempt a TOLAC and fail, ending up with an emergency CS delivery. In the Danish registries, an elective CS is defined as a pre-planned (before initiation of labour) procedure whilst an emergency CS is unplanned. In this study, we only have information on the final 'actual' mode of delivery recorded in the registry using the appropriate codes (elective CS *DO820*; emergency CS *DO821*).

Main outcome measures

The primary outcome was neonatal death: death of a live new born within ≤28 days. Secondary outcomes included: 1) Early neonatal death: death of a live new born within ≤7 days; 2) Late neonatal death: death of a live new born > 7 days ≤ 28 days and 3) Infant death: the death of a child within ≤365 days.

Statistical analyses

Crude and adjusted logistic regression models were computed to estimate the odds of each outcome in women with a TOLAC compared to women with an ERCS using crude odds ratios (ORs) or adjusted ORs (AORs) and 95% confidence intervals (CIs). Adjusted models were *a priori* defined as follows:

Model 1: key potential confounders available for the entire study period from the second live birth including maternal age, country of origin, educational attainment, mother and father's gross income, marital status, infant birthplace, infant birth weight, birth year and history of pregnancy loss (1982–2010, cohort n = 61,626).

Testing for a cohort effect

In order to test for the cohort effect and temporal changes over time, the cohort was split into three different time periods (1982–1991, 1992–2001, 2002–2010) and the analyses repeated.

Subgroup and sensitivity analyses

A subgroup analysis restricted to women delivering between 38 and 40 weeks' gestation was conducted to investigate the effect of gestational age on the outcomes of interest in overdue or induced pregnancies with a TOLAC. In addition, data for smoking, co-morbidities and BMI were only available for specific time periods. Sensitivity analyses were conducted restricting the cohort to the specific time periods for which data were available on smoking, co-morbidities and BMI (with and without adjusting for these covariates).

Model 1: adjusted for key potential confounders available for the entire study period including maternal age, country of origin, educational attainment, mother and father's gross income, marital status, infant birthplace, infant birth weight, birth year and history of pregnancy loss plus smoking status (1991–2010, cohort n = 50,880).
Model 2: adjusted for Model 1 plus comorbidities in the second live birth including hypertension, eclampsia, preeclampsia, fetal distress and gestational diabetes (1994–2010, cohort n = 45,979).
Model 3: adjusted for Model 2 plus BMI (2004–2010, cohort n = 22,672).

Where a variable had missing data, the variable was re-coded to include missing data as a separate category (for example, for maternal smoking, 1 = smoker, 2 = non-smoker, 3 = missing) and included in the various analyses. As outlined by Vach and Blettner, adding missing data as a separate category where the proportion of missing data is small (as in this study) should not impact greatly on the effect estimates [27]. All analyses were conducted using SAS© version 9.4 software (SAS Institute, Inc., Cary, NC, USA) and the PROC LOGISTIC [28] command. Approval to use the data was obtained from the Danish National Board of Health and *Statistics Denmark* for the current study.

Results

Characteristics of the study population

The study included 61,626 women with at least two live births. These women were subdivided into 40,685 women with a TOLAC (66%), and 20,941 (34%) women with an ERCS, (Fig. 1). Maternal characteristics of the study group are outlined in [Table 1] and infant characteristics are outlined in [Table 2].

The rate of successful TOLAC (VBAC) did not vary significantly over the entire study period ranging from 5 to 8% (see Additional file 1).

Neonatal death, early neonatal death, late neonatal death and infant death

Neonatal death (≤28 days): An increased odds of neonatal death was found in women with a TOLAC (AOR 1 · 87, 95% CI 1 · 12, 3.12) compared to the reference group of women with an ERCS. Early neonatal death (≤7 days after birth): Compared to the reference group of women with an ERCS, women with a TOLAC had more than twice the odds of early neonatal death (AOR 2 · 06, 95% CI 1 · 19, 3 · 56), (see Table 3).

Late neonatal death (>7 days, ≤ 28 days after birth): Compared to the reference group, women with a TOLAC had no increased odds of late neonatal death (AOR 0 · 97, 95% CI 0 · 22, 4 · 32). Infant death (≤365 days after birth): There was no association (AOR 1.12, 95%

Table 1 Maternal characteristics in the second live birth in Denmark, 1982–2010

	First CS		
	Elective repeat CS	Trial of labour after CS	Total
Maternal characteristics of the second delivery			
Age in years, <20	24 (0%)	133 (0%)	157 (0%)
20–25	1,920 (9%)	5,655 (14%)	7,575 (12%)
26–30	6,997 (33%)	16,582 (41%)	23,579 (38%)
31–35	8,096 (39%)	14,349 (35%)	22,445 (36%)
36–40	3,423 (16%)	3,660 (9%)	7,083 (11%)
41+	481 (2%)	306 (1%)	787 (1%)
Origin, Denmark	18,685 (89%)	36,757 (90%)	55,442 (90%)
Other	2,183 (10%)	3,834 (9%)	6,017 (10%)
Unknown	73 (0%)	94 (0%)	167 (0%)
Marital status, Married	7,514 (36%)	13,567 (33%)	21,081 (34%)
Divorced/separated/widowed	573 (3%)	748 (2%)	1,321 (2%)
Co-habiting	12,633 (60%)	25,917 (64%)	38,550 (63%)
Unknown	221 (1%)	453 (1%)	674 (1%)
Educational attainment, Primary	4,496 (21%)	9,817 (24%)	14,313 (23%)
High school	10,193 (49%)	20,057 (49%)	30,250 (49%)
Third level degree	4,183 (20%)	7,432 (18%)	11,615 (19%)
Masters/PhD	1,447 (7%)	2,183 (5%)	3,630 (6%)
Unknown	622 (3%)	1,196 (3%)	1,818 (3%)
Mother's gross income (quartiles), 25	2,997 (14%)	5,766 (14%)	8,763 (14%)
50	3,954 (19%)	7,789 (19%)	11,743 (19%)
75	9,513 (45%)	19,299 (47%)	28,812 (47%)
100	4,339 (21%)	7,514 (18%)	11,853 (19%)
Unknown	138 (1%)	317 (1%)	455 (1%)
[a]Smoker, No	14,387 (82%)	25,814 (78%)	40,201 (79%)
Yes	2,665 (15%)	6,733 (20%)	9,398 (18%)
Unknown	566 (3%)	715 (2%)	1,281 (3%)
Characteristic of the second delivery			
Father's gross income (quartiles), 25	1,497 (7%)	3,156 (8%)	4,653 (8%)
50	2,264 (11%)	4,765 (12%)	7,029 (11%)
75	6,266 (30%)	12,702 (31%)	18,968 (31%)
100	10,582 (51%)	19,412 (48%)	29,994 (49%)
Unknown	332 (2%)	650 (2%)	982 (2%)
[b]BMI (kg/m^2) <18.5	523 (5%)	638 (5%)	1,161 (5%)
18.5–25	5,849 (55%)	7,412 (62%)	13,261 (58%)
26–30	2,198 (21%)	2,092 (18%)	4,290 (19%)
31–35	1,064 (10%)	753 (6%)	1,817 (8%)
36+	643 (6%)	347 (3%)	990 (4%)
Unknown	439 (4%)	714 (6%)	1,153 (5%)
[c]Preeclampsia, eclampsia	342 (2%)	613 (2%)	955 (2%)
[d]Fetal distress	98 (1%)	6,358 (22%)	6,456 (14%)
[e]Gestational diabetes	645 (4%)	504 (2%)	1,149 (3%)
[f]Hypertension	203 (1%)	337 (1%)	540 (1%)

Table 1 Maternal characteristics in the second live birth in Denmark, 1982–2010 *(Continued)*

Previous stillbirth	494 (2%)	371 (1%)	865 (1%)
Previous miscarriage	3,288 (16%)	6,675 (16%)	9,963 (16%)
Previous ectopic pregnancy	863 (4%)	1,681 (4%)	2,544 (4%)

Data are n (%).[a]Smoking data available from 1991 to 2010 (cohort $n = 50{,}880$). [b]BMI: Body mass index, data available from 2004 to 2010 only (cohort $n = 22{,}672$). [c, d, e, f] Preeclampsia, eclampsia; fetal distress; gestational diabetes, hypertension: data available from 1994 to 2010 (cohort $n = 45{,}979$). *CS* Caesarean section

CI 0.79, 1.59) between women with a TOLAC and infant death compared to women with an ERCS (see Table 3).

Testing for a cohort effect

To test for the cohort effect, the cohort was split into three time periods. The increased odds of neonatal death among women with a TOLAC was greatest in the earliest years (1982–1991) with an AOR of 3 · 89 (95% CI 1 · 33, 11 · 39) compared to women with an ERCS (see Table 4).

This decreased over time to an AOR of 2 · 87 (95% CI 0 · 85, 9 · 70) between 1992 and 2001, and disappeared in the most recent years of 2002–2010 (AOR 1 · 01, 95% CI 0 · 44, 2 · 31). This decreasing trend is displayed graphically (see Fig. 2).

Subgroup and sensitivity analyses

A subgroup analysis restricted to include women delivering between 38 and 40 weeks was conducted to assess the effect of gestational age on overdue or induced women with a TOLAC compared to the reference group of women with an ERCS (see Additional file 2). Women with a TOLAC had an increased odds of neonatal death (AOR 1 · 78, 95% CI 1 · 03, 3 · 08) and early neonatal death (AOR 1 · 99, 95% CI 1 · 11, 3 · 58). No association was found for late neonatal death (AOR 0 · 71, 95% CI 0 · 13, 3 · 76) or infant death (AOR 1 · 11, 95% CI 0 · 76, 1 · 63) in women with a TOLAC compared to women with an ERCS (see Additional file 2). Further sensitivity analyses were conducted restricting the cohort to the specific time period for which certain covariates were available (smoking, co-morbidities, BMI) but without adjusting for them specifically. For example, smoking data were available from 1991 to 2010 and the cohort was restricted to this time period without adjustment for the effects of smoking. The increased risk of neonatal death overall disappeared in these additional analyses, but did not explain the overall findings (see Additional files 3 and 4).

Table 2 Infant characteristics in the second live birth in Denmark, 1982–2010

Infant characteristics of the second delivery	First CS	
	Elective repeat CS	Trial of labour after CS
Infant sex, male	10,845 (52%)	20,472 (50%)
Female	10,096 (48%)	20,213 (50%)
Birthplace, Capital (Copenhagen)	3,809 (18%)	6,352 (16%)
Capital suburbs	2,224 (11%)	5,409 (13%)
Provincial city	2,641 (13%)	4,852 (12%)
Provincial town	5,846 (28%)	11,184 (27%)
Rural area	6,369 (30%)	12,807 (31%)
Unknown	52 (0%)	81 (0%)
Apgar score <7 at 5 min	190 (1%)	1,016 (3%)
Birth weight (g), <2,500	1,440 (7%)	6,165 (15%)
2500–3500	8,179 (39%)	18,805 (46%)
3500–4500	9,556 (46%)	14,358 (35%)
4500+	1,569 (7%)	1,129 (3%)
Unknown	197 (1%)	228 (1%)
Gestational age, weeks, mean ± standard deviation	39.06 (1.2)	40.28 (1.3)
Admission to NICU[a]	645 (5%)	414 (3%)

Data are n (%) or mean ± standard deviation unless otherwise stated. *CS* Caesarean section, *NICU* Neonatal intensive care unit. [a]Admission to NICU: data available from 2002 to 2010 ($n = 27{,}868$)

Discussion

Main findings

In the present study the odds of delivery-related neonatal and infant death were assessed in a large cohort of more than 61,000 women. We found evidence of a cohort effect over time, where in the earliest years the increased odds of neonatal death were greatest (over three times higher than that of the women with an ERCS), gradually disappearing over time. Post-hoc analyses summarising the case-mix of TOLAC women according to cohort time were conducted (see Additional file 5). Overall, there was no change in the percentage of women having a TOLAC across the study period as well as in the characteristics of these women including age, educational attainment, gross income and origin. Advances in obstetrics and changes in practice, as well as perhaps changes in the women having a TOLAC are some of the driving forces behind this finding, meaning that the neonatal death rate is now not significantly different with TOLAC, making it a reasonable choice for pregnant women. We found no increased odds of late neonatal death or infant death. It must be acknowledged however that there were only six late neonatal deaths in women with a TOLAC. The association disappeared in additional adjusted analyses accounting for smoking, co-

Table 3 Neonatal death and infant death according to mode of delivery in a Danish cohort, 1982–2010

Mode of delivery 1st and 2nd birth (Number of events)	Neonatal death (≤28 days) $n = 95$	
	OR (95% CI)	[a]Model 1 AOR (95% CI)
CS – ERCS ($n = 21$)	Ref	Ref
CS – TOLAC ($n = 74$)	1.82 (1.12, 2.95)	1.87 (1.12, 3.12)
Mode of delivery 1st and 2nd birth (Number of events)	Early neonatal death (≤7 days) $n = 86$	
	OR (95% CI)	[a]Model 1 AOR (95% CI)
CS – ERCS ($n = 18$)	Ref	Ref
CS – TOLAC ($n = 68$)	1.95 (1.16, 3.27)	2.06 (1.19, 3.56)
Mode of delivery 1st and 2nd birth (Number of events)	Late neonatal death (>7 days, ≤28 days) $n = 9$	
	OR (95% CI)	[a]Model 1 AOR (95% CI)
CS – ERCS ($n = 3$)	Ref	Ref
CS – TOLAC ($n = 6$)	1.03 (0.26, 4.12)	0.97 (0.22, 4.32)
Mode of delivery 1st and 2nd birth (Number of events)	Infant death (≤365 days) $n = 171$	
	OR (95% CI)	[a]Model 1 AOR (95% CI)
CS – ERCS ($n = 49$)	Ref	Ref
CS – TOLAC ($n = 122$)	1.28 (0.92, 1.79)	1.12 (0.79, 1.59)

Data are crude and adjusted odds ratios with 95% confidence intervals. *OR* odds ratio, *AOR* adjusted odds ratio, *CI* confidence interval, *ERCS* Elective repeat caesarean section, *TOLAC* Trial of labour after caesarean section

[a]Model 1: adjusted for key covariates in the second birth including maternal age, maternal country of origin, educational attainment, mother and father's gross income, marital status, infant birthplace and infant birth weight, history of pregnancy loss and birth year (cohort $n = 61{,}626$)

morbidities and BMI, suggesting that generally safety is improving and that better case selection is vital and could make TOLAC even safer. When the cohort was restricted to include women with term deliveries (38–40 weeks gestation), the findings remained the same.

The improved safety in terms of outcomes following TOLAC could be for a multitude of reasons including improvements in CS as an abdominal surgery (for example changes in uterine incision which came into effect in Denmark) and advances in the diagnosis and management of pregnancy and pregnancy-related co-morbidities. Confounding by indication for underlying medical conditions may also explain the increased odds of early neonatal death found in women with a TOLAC due to acute events during delivery for example.

Strengths and limitations

Our study used population-based registry data which are regularly updated and validated for epidemiological research. The unique CPR identifier enables accurate linkage between the various registers and as a result detailed obstetric data were available for the current study allowing us to adjust for a large number of clinical

Table 4 Neonatal death and infant death according to mode of delivery by time period (cohort effect)

Mode of delivery 1st and 2nd births	Neonatal death (≤28 days) $n = 95$ in entire cohort 1982–2010		
	[a]Model 1 AOR (95% CI) (35 deaths)	[b]Model 2 AOR (95% CI) (34 deaths)	[c]Model 3 AOR (95% CI) (26 deaths)
CS – ERCS	Ref	Ref	Ref
CS – TOLAC	3.89 (1.33, 11.39)	2.87 (0.85, 9.70)	1.01 (0.44, 2.31)
Mode of delivery 1st and 2nd birth	Infant death (≤365 days) $n = 171$ in entire cohort 1982–2010		
	[a]Model 1 AOR (95% CI) (69 deaths)	[b]Model 2 AOR (95% CI) (64 deaths)	[c]Model 3 AOR (95% CI) (38 deaths)
CS – ERCS	Ref	Ref	Ref
CS – TOLAC	1.24 (0.70, 2.21)	1.37 (0.70, 2.69)	0.81 (0.42, 1.59)

Data are adjusted odds ratios with 95% confidence intervals. *AOR* adjusted odds ratio, *CI* confidence interval, *ERCS* Elective repeat caesarean section, *TOLAC* Trial of labour after caesarean

[a]Model 1: Cohort restricted to first time period (1982–1991, cohort $n = 11{,}698$) and adjusted for key covariates in the second birth including maternal age, maternal country of origin, educational attainment, mother and father's gross income, marital status, infant birthplace and infant birth weight, history of pregnancy loss and birth year

[b]Model 2: Cohort restricted to second time period (1992–2001, cohort $n = 22{,}060$) and adjusted for key covariates as in Model 1

[c]Model 3: Cohort restricted to last time period (2002–2010, cohort $n = 27{,}868$) and adjusted for key covariates as in Model 1

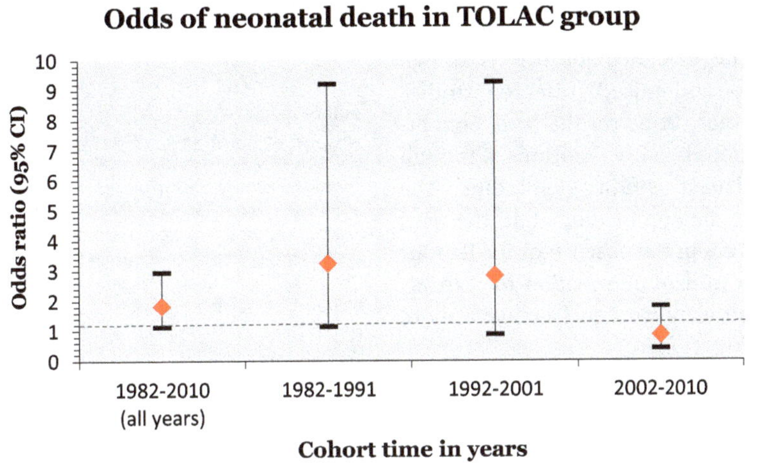

Fig. 2 Odds ratio of neonatal death in the trial of labour after caesarean section (TOLAC) group

and demographic potential confounders. The cohort included more than 61,000 women and spanned almost three decades. Therefore, we were also able to test for evidence of a cohort effect over time. We focused on infant mortality as most of the research to date has prioritised outcomes for mothers.

Limitations to this study and the majority of studies conducted prior to this include that we only have data on the actual mode of delivery recorded rather than the 'planned' mode of delivery. Although 'maternal request for a CS' has been recorded in the Danish registry data since 2002, the number of neonatal deaths was too few in this subgroup to assess whether any association exists in the data. Clinical trials will likely not be forthcoming as women will decline to be randomised according to mode of delivery. Therefore, large-scale observational studies like the current study detailed here remain the best way to study the effects of mode of delivery on subsequent pregnancy outcomes. In addition, we did not have access to data on type of stillbirth (antepartum or intrapartum). This calls for more delicate registrations of events and series of events, indications and procedures, etc. related to reproduction, pregnancy and delivery to enable more detailed analyses of potential associations between e.g. procedures such as CS and adverse events. The study was also carried out using registry data that contain no specific information on the clinical indication for CS. We tried to reduce this problem by adjusting for a number of medical conditions but this could not cover all possible indications. In addition to this, data were only available for certain covariates for specific time periods as outlined earlier. Unmeasured confounders are also a limitation of this study and all observational studies.

Interpretation

Our findings are in contrast to a previous study conducted in Scotland [29] which found that women with a first CS undergoing a TOLAC had 11 times the odds of delivery-related perinatal death (AOR 11·7, 95% CI 1·4–101·6) compared to women with an ERCS. The confidence intervals reported in the Scottish study are very broad and must be interpreted with caution. Furthermore, the Scottish study included intrapartum stillbirths and did not adjust for medical conditions in addition to BMI as was the case in the current study. The first and only nested randomised control trial (RCT) to date which divided women according to patient preference ($n = 2{,}323$) or randomisation ($n = 22$) to planned TOLAC or planned ERCS found that among women with one prior CS, planned ERCS compared with planned TOL was associated with a lower risk of fetal death and infant death or serious infant outcome (relative risk [RR] 0·39, 95% CI 0·19–0·80) [30]. Although strengthened by the process of randomisation, very few women actually consented to randomisation.

Ideally further research into the effect of mode of delivery on subsequent pregnancy outcome should incorporate a woman's 'intended' mode of delivery. This is the best way to assess any risks as one would know whether or not a woman was truly eligible to attempt a TOLAC. RCTs would be the optimal method of answering this question however they are difficult to conduct as it is hard to randomise a woman according to mode of delivery and unfeasible for rare outcomes such as perinatal death. Currently however, large population-based data such as the Danish registry data used in this study are the best methods for assessing the effects of mode of delivery and there is a continuous call for improvements in the quality and amount of data collected.

Conclusions

There are benefits and harms associated with each mode of delivery and the evidence for this is drawn from observational (non-randomised) research studies that may be prone to bias. Any results and conclusions must be interpreted with caution although large-scale population-based studies including the present one offer the best method of estimating the risks in women with one prior CS in the absence of RCTs. Our data provide essential, up to date information for expectant parents as well as healthcare workers to make a more informed decision regarding TOLAC.

Additional files

Additional file 1: Trial of Labour after Caesarean Section (TOLAC) Rates in Denmark: 1983–2010.

Additional file 2: Neonatal and infant death according to mode of delivery – subgroup analysis restricted to women delivering between 38 and 40 weeks gestation.

Additional file 3: Neonatal and infant death according to mode of delivery – sensitivity analyses with adjustment for smoking, co-morbidities and body mass index.

Additional file 4: Neonatal and infant death according to mode of delivery – sensitivity analyses without adjustment for smoking, co-morbidities and body mass index.

Additional file 5: Post-hoc analyses investigating characteristics of women with a TOLAC in Denmark according to cohort time

Abbreviations

AOR: Adjusted Odds Ratio; BMI: Body Mass Index; CI: Confidence Interval; CPR: Central Person Number; CRS: Civil Registration System; CS: Caesarean Section; ERCS: Elective Repeat Caesarean Section; MBR: Medical Birth Register; NHR: National Hospital Register; NICU: Neonatal Intensive Care Unit; OR: Odds Ratio; RCT: Randomised Control Trial; TOL: Trial Of Labour; TOLAC: Trial Of Labour After Caesarean; US: United States

Acknowledgements

Malene Thygesen and Michael Pedersen for preparing the data and Professor Preben Bo Mortensen for his advice on this study (NCRR, Aarhus, Denmark).

Funding

The National Perinatal Epidemiology Centre, Cork, Ireland provided funding to SON as part of the Health Research Board, Ireland PhD Scholars programme in Health Services Research (Grant No. PHD/2007/16). LCK is a Science Foundation Ireland Principal Investigator (08/IN.1/B2083) and the Director of the SFI funded Centre, INFANT (12/RC/2272).

Authors' contributions

All authors (SON, EA, AK, PK, TH, RG and LK) were involved in the conception and design of the study. EA acquired data approval. SON analysed the data and drafted the manuscript. All authors (SON, EA, AK, PK, TH, RG and LK) commented on the manuscript and approved the final version for submission to the journal.

Competing interests

The authors declare that they have no competing interests.

Author details

[1]The Irish Centre for Fetal and Neonatal Translational Research (INFANT), Cork University Maternity Hospital, University College Cork, Wilton, Cork, Ireland. [2]National Perinatal Epidemiology Centre (NPEC), Department of Obstetrics and Gynaecology, Cork University Maternity Hospital, 5th Floor Wilton, Cork, Ireland. [3]Centre for Integrated Register-based Research (CIRRAU), National Centre for Register-based Research (NCRR), Aarhus University, Aarhus, Denmark. [4]Department of Epidemiology and Public Health, University College Cork, Western Gateway Building, Cork, Ireland. [5]Perinatal Epidemiology Research Unit, Department of Paediatrics, Aarhus University Hospital, Skejby, Aarhus N DK-8200, Denmark.

References

1. Kozhimannil KB, Law MR, Virnig BA. Cesarean delivery rates vary tenfold among US hospitals; reducing variation May address quality and cost issues. Health Aff. 2013;32(3):527–35.
2. Kenny LC, Lavender T, McNamee R, O'Neill SM, Mills T, Khashan AS. Advanced maternal Age and adverse pregnancy outcome: evidence from a large contemporary cohort. PLoS One. 2013;8(2):e56583.
3. Crane JM, Murphy P, Burrage L, Hutchens D. Maternal and perinatal outcomes of extreme obesity in pregnancy. J Obstet Gynaecol Can. 2013; 35(7):606–11.
4. Biswas A, Su LL, Mattar C. Caesarean section for preterm birth, and breech presentation and twin pregnancies. Best Pract Res Clin Obstet Gynaecol. 2013;27(2):209–19.
5. Fabri R, Murta E. Socioeconomic factors and cesarean section rates. Int J Gynaecol Obstet. 2013;76:87–8.
6. Glavind J, Kindberg SF, Uldbjerg N, Khalil M, Moller AM, Mortensen BB, Rasmussen OB, Christensen JT, Jorgensen JS, Henriksen TB. Elective caesarean section at 38 weeks versus 39 weeks: neonatal and maternal outcomes in a randomised controlled trial. BJOG. 2013;120(9):1123–32.
7. Fong A, King E, Duffy J, Wu E, Pan D, Ogunyemi D. Declining VBAC rates despite improved delivery outcomes compared to repeat Cesarean delivery [20Q]. Obstet Gynecol. 2016;127:144S.
8. Uddin SF, Simon AE. Rates and success rates of trial of labor after cesarean delivery in the United States, 1990–2009. Matern Child Health J. 2013;17(7): 1309–14.
9. Rosenstein MG, Kuppermann M, Gregorich SE, Cottrell EK, Caughey AB, Cheng YW. Association between vaginal birth after cesarean delivery and primary cesarean delivery rates. Obstet Gynecol. 2013;122(5):1010–7.
10. Simon AE, Uddin SG. National trends in primary cesarean delivery, labor attempts, and labor success, 1990–2010. Am J Obstet Gynecol. 2013;209(6): 554 e551–558.
11. Fitzpatrick KE, Kurinczuk JJ, Alfirevic Z, Spark P, Brocklehurst P, Knight M. Uterine Rupture by Intended Mode of Delivery in the UK: A National Case-control Study. PLoS Med. 2012;9(3):e1001184. doi:10.1371/journal.pmed. 1001184.
12. Lundgren I, Evelien vL, Vehvilainen-Julkunen K, Nicoletti J, Lalor J, Matterne A, Begley C, Nilsson C: Clinicians views of factors of importance for improving the rate of vaginal births after caesarean section (VBAC)-A study from countries with high and low VBAC-rates. Optimising Childbirth Across Europe, 9–10 April 2014 Brussels, Belgium 2014.
13. Lundgren I, van Limbeek E, Vehvilainen-Julkunen K, Nilsson C. Clinicians' views of factors of importance for improving the rate of VBAC (vaginal birth after caesarean section): a qualitative study from countries with high VBAC rates. BMC Pregnancy Childbirth. 2015;15(1):196.
14. Spong CY. To vbac or not to vbac. PLoS Med. 2012;9(3):e1001191. doi:10. 1371/journal.pmed.1001191.
15. Barger MK, Nannini A, Weiss J, Declercq ER, Stubblefield P, Werler M, Ringer S. Severe maternal and perinatal outcomes from uterine rupture among women at term with a trial of labor. J Perinatol. 2012;32(11):837–43.
16. Gurol-Urganci I, Cromwell DA, Edozien LC, Smith GC, Onwere C, Mahmood TA, Templeton A, van der Meulen JH. Risk of placenta previa in second birth

after first birth cesarean section: a population-based study and meta-analysis. BMC Pregnancy Childbirth. 2011;11(1):95.
17. Sumigama S, Sugiyama C, Kotani T, Hayakawa H, Inoue A, Mano Y, Tsuda H, Furuhashi M, Yamamuro O, Kinoshita Y. Uterine sutures at prior caesarean section and placenta accreta in subsequent pregnancy: a case–control study. BJOG. 2014;121(7):866–75.
18. Guise J, Denman M, Emeis C, Marshall N, Walker M, Fu R, Janik R, Nygren P, Eden K, McDonagh M. Vaginal birth after Cesarean: New insights on maternal and neonatal outcomes. Obstetric Anesthesia Digest. 2011;31(3): 159–60.
19. Signore C. VBAC: what does the evidence show? Clin Obstet Gynecol. 2012; 55(4):961–8.
20. Pedersen CB. The Danish civil registration system. Scand J Public Health. 2011;39(7):22–5.
21. Erlangsen A, Fedyszyn I. Danish nationwide registers for public health and health-related research. Scand J Public Health. 2015;43(4):333–9.
22. Kristensen J, Langhoff-Roos J, Skovgaard LT, Kristensen FB. Validation of the Danish Birth Registration. J Clin Epidemiol. 1996;49(8):893–7.
23. Knudsen LB, Olsen J. The Danish Medical Birth Registry. Dan Med Bull. 1999; 45(3):320–3.
24. Lynge E, Sandegaard JL, Rebolj M. The Danish National Patient Register. Scand J Public Health. 2011;39(7):30–3.
25. Helweg-Larsen K. The Danish Register of Causes of Death. Scand J Public Health. 2011;39(7):26–9.
26. Petersson F, Baadsgaard M, Thygesen LC. Danish registers on personal labour market affiliation. Scand J Public Health. 2011;39(7 suppl):95–8.
27. Vach W, Blettner M. Biased estimation of the odds ratio in case-control studies due to the use of ad hoc methods of correcting for missing values for confounding variables. Am J Epidemiol. 1991;134(8):895–907.
28. Peng C-YJ, Lee KL, Ingersoll GM. An introduction to logistic regression analysis and reporting. J Educ Res. 2002;96(1):3–14.
29. Smith G, Pell JP, Cameron AD, Dobbie R. Risk of perinatal death associated with labor after previous cesarean delivery in uncomplicated term pregnancies. JAMA. 2002;287(20):2684.
30. Crowther CA, Dodd JM, Hiller JE, Haslam RR, Robinson JS. Planned vaginal birth or elective repeat caesarean: Patient preference restricted cohort with nested randomised trial. PLoS Med. 2012;9(3):e1001192. doi:10.1371/journal.pmed.1001192.

24

Caesarean section following induction of labour in uncomplicated first births - a population-based cross-sectional analysis of 42,950 births

Mary-Ann Davey[1,3*] and James King[2]

Abstract

Background: The impact of elective induction of labour at term on the increasing caesarean section (CS) rate is unclear. A Cochrane Systematic Review that concluded that elective induction was associated with a reduction in CS was based on trials that mostly reflect outdated obstetric care, or were flawed.
The findings of other studies vary widely in the magnitude and direction of the relationship between elective induction and CS. This inconsistency may be due to the heterogeneity in the methods used to induce or augment labour, such that the relationship with CS is not constant across methods.

Methods: Using validated, routinely-collected data on all births in Victoria in 2000–2005, all singleton, cephalic, first births following uncomplicated pregnancies at 37–40 completed weeks' gestation ('standard primiparae') were identified ($n = 42{,}950$). As well as comparing induced with non-induced labour, method of birth was compared between those women experiencing spontaneous labour without augmentation, and women undergoing each method of augmentation or induction using adjusted multinomial logistic regression. Proportions, chi-square tests, adjusted Relative Risk Ratios (aRRR) and 95 % confidence intervals are presented.

Results: Ten percent of "standard primiparae" had labour induced for no apparent medical indication. Women whose labour was induced were significantly more likely than those who laboured spontaneously to have a CS (26.5 and 12.5 % respectively (OR 2.54, 95 % CI 2.4, 2.7, $p < 0.001$). After adjustment for maternal age, epidural analgesia, birthweight, gestation, and public/private admission status, each method of induction or augmentation remained associated with a significant increase in the risk of CS (adjusted ORs range 1.48 to 4.13, p-values all <0.0001). Perinatal death did not differ by onset of labour.

Conclusion: Induction of labour in medically uncomplicated nulliparous women at term carries a more than doubling of risk of emergency CS, compared with spontaneous labour, with no impact on perinatal mortality. All methods of induction and augmentation of labour were associated with an increase in the rate of CS. Women included in this study had no apparent medical indication for induction of labour or any complication of pregnancy, so the increase in CS was not due to identifiable underlying risk factors. These results suggest that, in the absence of direction from well-designed, contemporary RCTs, minimising unindicated inductions before 41 weeks' gestation has the potential to reduce the rate of CS.

Keywords: Caesarean, Induction, Elective, Primipara, Augmentation, Low risk

* Correspondence: mary-ann.davey@monash.edu
[1]Department of Obstetrics and Gynaecology, Monash University, 246 Clayton Rd, Clayton 3186, Australia
[3]Judith Lumley Centre, La Trobe University, 215 Franklin St, Melbourne 3000, Australia
Full list of author information is available at the end of the article

Background

The high caesarean section (CS) rate in developed countries is causing widespread concern. In 2011, 32.3 % of women giving birth in Australia did so by CS (33.2 % of first births) [1]. The CS rate in the state of Victoria doubled from 15.3 % in 1985 to 30.6 % in 2006 [1], and was 32.0 % in 2011 [2]. Although CS can be life-saving for the mother and/or baby when used judiciously, it also carries risks for: higher rates of maternal morbidity, mortality and delayed recovery from the birth [3, 4]; difficulty establishing breastfeeding [5]; neonatal morbidity and admission to nursery care [4]; serious placental complications in subsequent pregnancies [6, 7]; and increased costs for the health system [8].

Coinciding with the increase in CS was an increase in the proportion of labours that were induced, from 20 % in Victoria in 1992 to 28 % in 2002 [9] and it has since stabilised at around 25 % [2]. Other countries share this trend. Zhang found a doubling of the induction rate in the United States between 1990 and 1998 [10] though this also appears to have plateaued [11].

Concerned clinicians and policy-makers are keen to identify evidence-based, appropriate strategies to safely reduce the CS rate. Vaginal birth after CS is relatively uncommon with 84.1 % of women in Australia who had a prior CS doing so again in the next birth in 2011 [12] along with 86.5 % of women giving birth in Victorian public hospitals in 2011 whose only prior birth was a CS [13], so strategies that would safely prevent a first CS show great promise for reducing the overall CS rate in the longer term.

The literature on the association between induction of labour and CS is divided. Some observational studies found no increase in the rate of CS following induction of labour [14, 15] while others have found an increase [16–21].

The Cochrane systematic review on this topic [22] was updated in 2012 with a total of 22 randomised controlled trials (RCTs), most of which were conducted in an era before RCT methods were developed to current standards and so have fundamental flaws. The authors reported a reduction in perinatal death with a policy of induction of labour and a lower rate of CS (RR 0.89) and no difference in the rate of admission to SCN/NICU. Other systematic reviews of studies that included indicated and non-indicated inductions of labour found a similar reduction in CS overall in those randomised to induction [23–25]. However the trials in the Mishanina review that looked separately at first births and subsequent births found no difference in CS between those randomised to induction or expectant management [23]. Saccone conducted a review of RCTs of induction or expectant management in uncomplicated multiparous and primiparous women and found no difference in the rate of CS [24].

During the period of this study, three techniques were commonly used individually or in combination to induce labour in Victoria: application of prostaglandins to the cervix if unfavourable, artificial rupture of the fetal membranes (amniotomy), and continuous intravenous infusion of synthetic oxytocin [1]. As well as being used to induce labour, oxytocin infusion and amniotomy were also used to augment labour that had begun spontaneously. Even though some of the same agents are used to induce or augment labour, it is plausible that their effect might differ when used at these different times depending on whether known and unknown pre-labour changes have occurred in the woman's body.

The overall aim in this study is to describe and analyse the events that follow induction of labour in uncomplicated nulliparous pregnancies. This information would be expected to improve the knowledge of identified risks and benefits, so that pregnant women expecting their first baby at term and their caregivers will be better informed as they consider whether to induce or await spontaneous labour. This paper examines the risk of CS in this low risk group following the induction of labour overall, and following the various individual methods of induction or augmentation of labour in uncomplicated pregnancies at term.

Methods

Maternal and perinatal data were collected by the midwife attending every birth in the state of Victoria, Australia, of at least 20 weeks' gestation, or, if gestation was unknown, of at least 400 g birth weight. These were reported using a standard perinatal statistics form to the Victorian Perinatal Data Collection (VPDC), which collects this information on behalf of the Consultative Council on Obstetric and Paediatric Mortality and Morbidity (CCOPMM).

The perinatal form contained information on maternal age, parity, gestation, presentation, plurality, birthweight, sex of the baby, pre-existing maternal medical conditions, complications of pregnancy, onset of labour, indication for induction, agents or techniques used to induce or augment labour, analgesia used, method of birth, public or private admission status, as well as many other variables not used in this analysis.

The accuracy of the VPDC items used in these analyses was previously validated on a random sample of cases in the 2003 data set [26].

Use of the data for the calendar years 2000–2005 inclusive for this project was approved by the Consultative Council on Obstetric and Paediatric Mortality and Morbidity, and the project was approved by the Faculty of Health Sciences, Ethics in Human Research Committee, La Trobe University (approval number FHEC03/146).

In order to compare women with similar levels of risk and no medical indication for induction, according to whether they had labour induced or augmented or a spontaneous onset of labour, cases that did not meet the definition of the "standard primipara" were excluded. For the purpose of this study, a "standard primipara" was defined as being between 20 and 44 years of age, having no complications of pregnancy and no pre-existing diabetes, hypertension, heart disease or mental illness, giving birth for the first time, to a singleton, cephalic-presenting infant with a birthweight between the 10th and 90th centile for sex and gestation, at 37–40 weeks' gestation. The standard local definition of standard primipara excludes women aged 35 years or older, but given the increasing maternal age at first birth, we extended the definition to include women aged 35–44 years who otherwise met the criteria for the standard primipara. The upper gestational limit was set at 286 days (40 weeks and 6 days) because induction for post-dates at 41 weeks is standard practice in many settings. In order to clarify that we have made these modifications to the local standard primipara definition, we have enclosed the words "standard primipara" in quotes. All births to "standard primiparae" in Victoria from January 2000-December 2005 were included in the study.

Age, parity, plurality, presentation, birthweight and gestation were reported on the perinatal form and entered verbatim into the dataset. The specified maternal medical conditions, as well as pre-eclampsia, gestational diabetes mellitus, pre-labour rupture of the membranes, placental abruption and 'other APH' (antepartum haemorrhage) were reported by midwives by ticking a box on the form. The ICD10 code for each of these conditions appeared on the form and was entered into the dataset. Other complications of pregnancy, and indication for induction of labour, were reported as free text in response to the fields 'other obstetric complications' and 'specify indication for induction' on the form. This text was coded by a health information manager according to ICD10, and the code entered. Up to ten complications of pregnancy could be included. One indication for induction was specified. Forms submitted with missing data, including those with no specified indication for an induced labour, were queried with the hospital, and the data obtained and entered. Women with an entry in any of the ten 'obstetric complications' fields were excluded from the "standard primipara" set. Women were also excluded if the indication for induction was an obstetric complication or one of the specified maternal medical conditions.

When labour was induced (e.g. with amniotomy), then an oxytocin infusion commenced some time later, this labour was defined as induced, with the later oxytocin considered to be part of the induction process. When labour began spontaneously, and an oxytocin infusion or amniotomy (or both) were performed some time later, this was considered an augmentation of labour. If the membranes ruptured spontaneously and labour did not follow, an oxytocin infusion administered to stimulate labour was considered by VPDC to be an induction of labour, because there had been no spontaneous onset of labour.

Planned caesarean sections were those that had been arranged before the onset of labour (even if they needed to be moved forward when labour began unexpectedly). Unplanned caesareans were those that took place in response to an emergent problem, whether before labour (e.g. cord prolapse) or during labour.

The small number of women with failed induction of labour were classified as unplanned CS before the onset of labour.

Perinatal mortality included babies who were stillborn and those who died within 28 days of birth. Babies with congenital anomalies are not excluded unless the anomaly was reported as a complication of pregnancy, or as the indication for induction of labour.

In order to explore the effect of each method of induction or augmentation separately in multivariate analysis, a new variable was created with mutually exclusive and exhaustive categories for each combination of onset of labour and method of induction or augmentation. These categories were:

- spontaneous onset, no augmentation;
- spontaneous onset, augmented with amniotomy;
- spontaneous onset, augmented with oxytocin infusion;
- spontaneous onset, augmented with amniotomy and oxytocin infusion;
- labour induced with prostaglandin gel only;
- labour induced with amniotomy only;
- labour induced with oxytocin infusion only;
- labour induced with prostaglandin and amniotomy;
- labour induced with prostaglandin and oxytocin infusion;
- labour induced with amniotomy and oxytocin infusion;
- labour induced with prostaglandin, amniotomy and oxytocin infusion.

Those who had a CS without labour were excluded from multivariate analysis. Descriptive statistics were used to describe the characteristics of the women included in the study. Proportions were compared using Pearson Chi-square and Fisher's exact tests.

The association between each of these induction/augmentation methods or combination of methods and method of birth was analysed via multinomial logistic regression, adjusting for potential confounders selected a priori. Adjusted relative risk ratios and their 95 % confidence intervals are reported. Maternal age and birthweight were linearly and positively related to CS, so they were included in the model as continuous variables. Gestation, public/private admission status and use of epidural analgesia were included as categorical variables. The very small number of cases with missing data were excluded from multivariate analysis.

Multinomial logistic regression was used because there are three possible outcomes for method of birth – unassisted vaginal birth, operative vaginal birth or CS. This paper presents the results for caesarean compared with unassisted vaginal birth. The Relative Risk Ratio is the output of multinomial logistic regression but is mathematically equivalent to an Odds Ratio.

Results

There were a total of 381,751 births to 375,077 women in Victoria in 2000–2005 of whom 158,402 were first births, and 42,950 met all "standard primipara" inclusion criteria (Figure 1). Fewer than half had a spontaneous labour without augmentation and one in ten had labour induced (Table 1).

Increasing maternal age and admission as a private patient were associated with induction of labour and pre-labour CS (Table 2).

Overall, 18.2 % of all "standard primiparae" gave birth by CS ($n = 7834$); and 13.9 % of "standard primiparae" who experienced labour gave birth by CS ($n = 5675$).

Women whose labour was induced were significantly more likely to have a CS than those whose labour was entirely spontaneous (26.5 and 12.5 % respectively) (unadjusted Odds Ratio 2.54, 95 % CI 2.4, 2.7, $p < 0.0001$) (Table 3). Those with a spontaneous onset of labour that was later augmented were significantly more likely to have a CS than those who did not have labour augmented (18.5 and 7.5 % respectively) (Table 4).

At a bivariate level each individual method of induction or augmentation of labour was associated with an increased odds of CS compared with spontaneous labour (Table 4). The greatest increase was seen in labours that were induced with both prostaglandin and oxytocin, with or without amniotomy.

CS was also positively associated with a number of other factors: higher maternal age, admission as a private patient, higher birthweight, use of epidural analgesia for pain relief in labour, and use of oxytocin infusions to induce or augment labour (Table 4). The relationship between gestation and CS differed in that babies born at 38 weeks (266 to 272 days) were more likely than any other gestation to be born by CS. The majority of CS performed at 38 weeks were planned procedures (14.3 % of all births in this group at 38 weeks, compared with 9.3 % unplanned). These variables are likely to influence each other in complex ways. For example, women who had labour induced or augmented were three times as likely to use epidural analgesia as those in spontaneous labour (52.2 and 52.4 % for those with induced and augmented labour respectively compared with 18.0 % of those whose labour was neither induced nor augmented –data not shown).

Adjusting for all of the other variables in the model reduced the magnitude of the risk but each method of induction and augmentation of labour remained

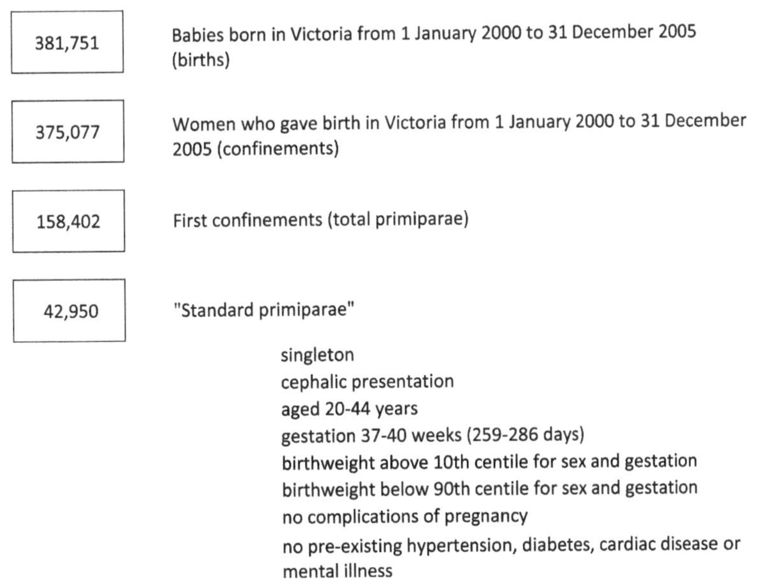

Fig. 1 Flow chart in selection of "Standard primiparae"

Table 1 Maternal characteristics and birth details of participants

	n	%
Total	42,950	
Maternal age		
20–24 years	7781	18.1
25–29 years	15,290	35.6
30–34 years	14,637	34.1
35–39 years	4534	10.6
40–44 years	708	1.6
Gestation (completed weeks)		
37	1941	4.5
38	6085	14.2
39	12,186	28.4
40	22,738	52.9
Admission status		
Public	24,110	56.1
Private	18,840	43.9
Type of labour		
Spontaneous with no augmentation	20,117	46.8
Spontaneous and augmented	16,492	38.4
Induced	4182	9.7
No labour	2159	5.0
Type of birth		
Unassisted vaginal	23,407	54.5
Vacuum	5727	13.3
Forceps	5981	13.9
Planned no-labour caesarean	1984	4.6
Planned in-labour caesarean	93	0.2
Unplanned no-labour caesarean	275	0.6
Unplanned in-labour caesarean	5482	12.8
Unknown	1	0
Epidural analgesia in labour (of those who experienced labour, $n = 40{,}791$)		
No	26,752	65.6
Yes	14,039	34.4

significantly associated with CS. Women who had labour induced using prostaglandin or oxytocin, alone or in combination with each other without amniotomy, or with a combination of prostaglandin gel, oxytocin infusion and amniotomy, had a more than three-fold increase in the adjusted Relative Risk Ratio of a CS compared with those in spontaneous labour. Augmentation with oxytocin was associated with a more than doubling of the risk of CS, while a 'simple' amniotomy augmentation was accompanied by a 48 % increase in risk, though this was probably not a causal relationship (Table 4).

After adjustment there remained strong evidence that use of epidural analgesia in labour was associated with a large increase in CS, and that higher birthweight, older maternal age and admission as a private patient were also associated with an increased risk of caesarean.

Giving birth at 38 and 39 weeks (266 to 279 days) gestation was associated with a significant but slight reduction in the risk of CS, while birth at 37 weeks (259 to 265 days) did not differ from 40 weeks (280 to 286 days) in terms of the risk of CS.

The relationship between onset of labour and CS was graphed separately for those who used, and did not use, epidural analgesia, for public and private patients, and for each week of gestation (not shown). Inspection revealed no interactions.

Infant outcomes will be reported separately, but for "standard primiparae", perinatal mortality for labour that was induced did not differ from that for spontaneous or augmented labour or pre-labour CS (0.24 per thousand, 0.80 per thousand, 0.97 per thousand and 0.46 per thousand respectively, Fisher's exact test $p = 0.537$) though the study was not powered to detect a difference in this outcome.

Discussion

This paper examines the association between the various methods of induction and augmentation of labour and CS in nulliparous women free of existing medical complications ("standard primiparae") in Victoria, Australia, between January 2000 and December 2005. These women had no apparent medical reason for induction, so could reasonably have had induction withheld or delayed. This analysis provides strong evidence for an increase in CS associated with all methods of elective induction or augmentation of labour. The increase persisted after adjustment for maternal age, use of epidural analgesia in labour, birthweight, gestation and admission as a public or private patient. This information may assist decision-making for women considering induction of labour in the absence of medical indications, as it balances the perceived benefits of induction against the increased risk of CS.

Importantly, perinatal mortality was very rare in this low-risk group and there were no differences between spontaneous, augmented, induced onset of labour or pre-labour CS. Given that we excluded women with identifiable risk factors for stillbirth (those with any complication of pregnancy, those with fetal growth restriction and those who had reached 41 weeks' gestation), we think it unlikely that the primary aim of these inductions of labour would have been prevention of perinatal mortality. The sample size required to demonstrate a difference in perinatal mortality would have been very large, and it was not the primary aim of the

Table 2 Onset of labour by maternal characteristics

	Spontaneous and not augmented		Spontaneous and augmented		Induced		No labour		Total	
	n	%	n	%	n	%	n	%		*p*-value
Maternal age										<0.001
20–24 years	4129	*53.1*	2912	*37.4*	580	*7.5*	160	*2.1*	7781	
25–29 years	7521	*49.2*	5864	*38.4*	1402	*9.2*	503	*3.3*	15,290	
30–34 years	6482	*44.3*	5778	*39.5*	1564	*10.7*	813	*5.6*	14,637	
35–39 years	1751	*38.6*	1756	*38.7*	534	*11.8*	493	*10.9*	4534	
40–44 years	234	*33.1*	182	*25.7*	102	*14.4*	190	*26.8*	708	
Gestation (completed weeks)										<0.001
37	1213	*62.5*	520	*26.8*	68	*3.5*	140	*7.2*	1941	
38	2986	*49.1*	1893	*31.1*	299	*4.9*	907	*14.9*	6085	
39	6171	*50.6*	4703	*38.6*	613	*5.0*	699	*5.7*	12,186	
40	9747	*42.9*	9376	*41.2*	3202	*14.1*	413	*1.8*	22,738	
Admission status										<0.001
Public	12,975	*53.8*	9054	*37.6*	1484	*6.2*	597	*2.5*	24,110	
Private	7142	*37.9*	7438	*39.5*	2698	*14.3*	1562	*8.3*	18,840	

analysis. In light of the small number of deaths in this low risk cohort, it would not be justified to draw conclusions about apparent differences between groups.

The findings are generalisable in contemporary practice with similar approaches to induction and CS. Importantly, the rate of induction of labour has not increased in Australia since these data were collected, and the CS rate has changed little, indicating that the threshold for deciding on CS has not altered appreciably. The results are not generalisable to women who have a medical indication for induction of labour as they were excluded from this analysis.

These findings are at odds with a number of systematic reviews of RCTs of induction of labour and CS [22–25, 27] and consistent with a review of observational studies [27]. Reviews of RCTs are all dominated by the very large trial in Canada [28]. The protocol for this trial specified that women randomised to induction could have prostaglandin gel to ripen the cervix if needed, but women randomised to expectant management who developed an indication for induction could not. This means that women in the expectant arm with an indication for induction and an unfavourable cervix needed CS for delivery. Around one third of women randomised to induction entered labour spontaneously, and one third of those randomised to expectant management needed to be induced. The finding of a reduction in CS with a policy of induction at 41 weeks is therefore not surprising.

Table 3 Caesarean section in "standard primiparae" by type of labour

	Caesarean section			Odds ratio	95 % CI	
	n	%	Total			p
Overall	7834	18.2	42,950			
Women who experienced labour	5675	13.9	40,791			
Type of labour						<0.001
Spontaneous (all)	4565	*12.5*	36,609	1.00	ref	
(not augmented)	*(1507)*	*(7.5)*	*(20,117)*			
(augmented)	*(3058)*	*(18.5)*	*(16,492)*			
Induced	1110	*26.5*	4182	2.54	(2.4, 2.7)	

Though not as persuasive as well-conducted randomised controlled trials (which are lacking), large population-based datasets provide an opportunity to investigate questions in maternity care with some confidence because their completeness ensures representativeness and minimises bias, unlike voluntary surveys where non-response is seldom random.

A strength of this study is the high level of accuracy of the variables used in the analysis as assessed in a validation study of a random sample of births in 2003. Indication for induction was reported accurately in 95 % of cases and other variables used here were reported accurately in 95–99 % of cases [26].

Analyses of routinely-collected data are limited by the variables available in the dataset. This analysis benefits from the inclusion of the indication for induction of labour in the VPDC. This data set also has the advantage of allowing separate identification of those whose labour was induced and those whose labour was augmented. Although some of the same techniques are used in both cases (amniotomy and oxytocin infusion) the effect when used for induction could differ from augmentation because in the case of induction, the body has not undergone

Table 4 Relative risk ratios for caesarean section in "standard primiparae" who experienced labour

	RRR	95 % CI	aRRR[b]	95 % CI	*p*-value
Type of labour					
Spontaneous	1	ref gp[a]	1	ref gp[a]	
Aug amniotomy	1.76	(1.6, 1.9)	1.48	(1.3, 1.6)	<0.0001
Aug oxytocin	6.17	(5.7, 6.7)	2.89	(2.6, 3.2)	<0.0001
Aug amniotomy & oxytocin	6.51	(5.9, 7.2)	2.55	(2.3, 2.8)	<0.0001
IOL PG	5.84	(5.0, 6.9)	3.86	(3.2, 4.6)	<0.0001
IOL amniotomy	3.08	(1.8, 5.2)	2.73	(1.6, 4.7)	<0.0001
IOL oxytocin	7.37	(4.4, 12.2)	4.13	(2.4, 7.0)	<0.0001
IOL PG & amniotomy	5.05	(3.9, 6.5)	2.78	(2.1, 3.6)	<0.0001
IOL PG & oxytocin	11.83	(8.4, 16.6)	4.06	(2.8, 5.8)	<0.0001
IOL amniotomy & oxytocin	3.86	(3.3, 4.6)	1.82	(1.5, 2.2)	<0.0001
IOL PG&amniotomy&oxytocin	10.19	(8.8, 11.9)	3.79	(3.2, 4.5)	<0.0001
Mother's age in years					
per year older	1.132	(1.12, 1.14)	1.088	(1.08, 1.10)	<0.0001
Epidural analgesia in labour					
No	1	ref gp[a]	1	ref gp[a]	
Yes	4.47	(4.2, 4.7)	5.68	(5.3, 6.1)	<0.0001
Birthweight					
per 100 g increase	1.086	(1.08, 1.1)	1.101	(1.09, 1.11)	<0.0001
Gestation (completed weeks)					
37	0.72	(0.6, 0.8)	0.94	(0.8, 1.1)	0.523
38	1.31	(1.2, 1.4)	0.85	(0.8, 0.95)	0.005
39	0.87	(0.8, 0.9)	0.83	(0.8, 0.9)	<0.0001
40	1	ref gp[a]	1	ref gp[a]	
Admission status of mother					
Public	1	ref gp[a]	1	ref gp[a]	
Private	2.47	(2.3, 2.6)	1.11	(1.03, 1.2)	0.003

Aug augmented, *IOL* induction of labour, *PG* prostaglandins
[a] ref gp = reference group
[b] Relative Risk Ratios after adjustment for all other variables in the table

any known or unknown changes that occur physiologically in preparation for labour. The multivariate analysis demonstrated that there were considerably different risks of CS associated with the same techniques according to whether they were used to augment or induce labour.

There are a number of factors that might have been influential but were not available in the VPDC for this analysis including method of fetal monitoring in labour, maternal body mass index, length of labour, preferences of the mother and maternity care providers, time of day and day of the week and model of maternity care.

Some of these items have been added to the perinatal data collection in Victoria at the beginning of 2009, which will enhance future similar analyses.

Induction of labour without medical indication was able to be accurately identified from this detailed and validated dataset, but one limitation of this analysis is that the indication for augmentation of labour was not collected. As a result, we were not able to distinguish a labour that was inco-ordinate, prolonged, or otherwise in undisputed need of augmentation from one that had no such indication for augmentation. For this reason, the results related to induction are more persuasive than those for augmentation.

This analysis compares outcomes for "standard primiparae" who had labour induced with those who did *not* have labour induced (adjusting for important confounders including gestation). This provides evidence of the outcomes of the induction techniques, which is useful information akin to a *per protocol* analysis. Another analysis method could provide a comparison between induction at a particular point in time compared with not inducing at that time (which could result in spontaneous labour on that or a later date, or in induction on a later date). Since gestation was reported only in completed weeks in this dataset, it was not possible to accurately conduct this analysis. Such analysis is planned now that gestation is reported in days.

Like all observational studies, there may well be other unmeasured factors affecting the association between these variables.

The possible mechanism/s for the relationship between induction of labour and CS are beyond the scope of this descriptive paper.

Conclusion

Using a population dataset with demonstrated accuracy, we found strong evidence of association between elective induction of labour by any of the commonly used methods and birth by CS, which remained significant after adjustment for important confounders. Augmentation of labour that began spontaneously was also associated with an increased risk of CS. Women in this study had no apparent indication for induction of labour, so the increase in CS is not due to underlying risk factors identifiable in the Victorian perinatal data collection. These results suggest that, in the absence of well-designed, contemporary RCTs, minimising unindicated inductions of labour before 41 weeks' gestation has the potential to reduce the rate of CS without increasing adverse perinatal outcomes.

Competing interests

In addition to her university appointment, Dr Davey also has a part-time appointment at the Department of Health, Victoria, working with the Victorian Perinatal Data Collection.
Associate Professor King is a past Chairman of the Consultative Council on Obstetric and Paediatric Mortality and Morbidity (CCOPMM).
Neither the Health Department nor the CCOPMM had input into the manuscript.

Authors' contributions

M-AD conceived and designed the study, analysed the data, wrote the first draft of the manuscript; JFK participated in the design of the study, provided advice on analysis and interpretation and critically revised the manuscript. Both authors read and approved the final manuscript.

Acknowledgements

The authors are grateful to the Consultative Council on Obstetric and Paediatric Mortality and Morbidity for authorising access to the data for this research, and for the assistance of staff who compiled the Victorian Perinatal Data Collection. The care with which midwives in Victoria provided these data to the VPDC is greatly appreciated.
Dr Davey was supported by an Australian Postgraduate Award.
The support and counsel of Emerita Professor Judith Lumley in the early design of this project is greatly appreciated.

Author details

[1]Department of Obstetrics and Gynaecology, Monash University, 246 Clayton Rd, Clayton 3186, Australia. [2]Department of Obstetrics and Gynaecology, University of Melbourne, Parkville 3052, Australia. [3]Judith Lumley Centre, La Trobe University, 215 Franklin St, Melbourne 3000, Australia.

References

1. Davey M-A, Taylor O, Oats J, Riley M. Births in Victoria, 2005 and 2006. Melbourne: Consultative Council on Obstetric and Paediatric Mortality and Morbidity, Victorian Department of Human Services; 2008.
2. Consultative Council on Obstetric and Paediatric Mortality and Morbidity. 2010 and 2011,Victoria's Mothers and Babies; Victoria's Maternal, Perinatal, Child and Adolescent Mortality. Melbourne: State Government of Victoria; 2014.
3. Deneux-Tharaux C, Carmona E, Bouvier-Colle M-H, Breart G. Postpartum maternal mortality and cesarean delivery. Obstet Gynecol. 2006;108(3 Pt 1):541–8.
4. Villar J, Carroli G, Zavaleta N, Donner A, Wojdyla D, Faundes A, Velazco A, Bataglia V, Langer A, Narvaez A, et al. Maternal and neonatal individual risks and benefits associated with caesarean delivery: multicentre prospective study. BMJ. 2007;335(7628):1025.
5. Davey M, Gibson K. PD.02 Intervention in labour and early breastfeeding outcomes. Arch Dis Child Fetal Neonatal Ed. 2014;99 Suppl 1:A81.
6. Hemminki E, Merilainen J. Long-term effects of cesarean sections: ectopic pregnancies and placental problems. Am J Obstet Gynecol. 1996;174(5):1569–74.
7. Yang Q, Wen SW, Oppenheimer L, Chen XK, Black D, Gao J, Walker MC. Association of caesarean delivery for first birth with placenta praevia and placental abruption in second pregnancy. BJOG. 2007;114(5):609–13.
8. Allen VM, O'Connell CM, Farrell SA, Baskett TF. Economic implications of method of delivery. Am J Obstet Gynecol. 2005;193(1):192–7.
9. Riley M, King J. Births in Victoria 2001–2002. Melbourne: Victorian Perinatal Data Collection Unit, Victorian Government Department of Human Services; 2003.
10. Zhang J, Yancey MK, Henderson CE. U.S. national trends in labor induction, 1989–1998. J Reprod Med. 2002;47(2):120–4.
11. Osterman MJ, Martin JA. Recent declines in induction of labor by gestational age. NCHS Data Brief. 2014;155:1–8.
12. Li Z, Zeki R, Hilder L. Australia's mothers and babies 2011. In: Perinatal statistics series. Canberra: AIHW; 2013.
13. Victorian Government Department of Health. Victorian Maternity Services Performance Indicators: Complete set for 2010–2011, and 2011–2012. Melbourne: Victorian Government Department of Health; 2014.
14. Roberts CL, Algert CS, Douglas I, Tracy SK, Peat B. Trends in labour and birth interventions among low-risk women in New South Wales. Aust N Z J Obstet Gynaecol. 2002;42(2):176–81.
15. Stock SJ, Ferguson E, Duffy A, Ford I, Chalmers J, Norman JE. Outcomes of elective induction of labour compared with expectant management: population based study. BMJ. 2012;344:e2838.
16. Dublin S, Lydon-Rochelle M, Kaplan RC, Watts DH, Critchlow CW. Maternal and neonatal outcomes after induction of labor without an identified indication. Am J Obstet Gynecol. 2000;183(4):986–94.
17. Grivell RM, Reilly AJ, Oakey H, Chan A, Dodd JM. Maternal and neonatal outcomes following induction of labor: a cohort study. Acta Obstet Gynecol Scand. 2012;91(2):198–203.
18. Heimstad R, Romundstad PR, Eik-Nes SH, Salvesen KA. Outcomes of pregnancy beyond 37 weeks of gestation. Obstet Gynecol. 2006;108(3 Pt 1):500–8.
19. Seyb ST, Berka RJ, Socol ML, Dooley SL. Risk of cesarean delivery with elective induction of labor at term in nulliparous women. Obstet Gynecol. 1999;94(4):600–7.
20. Tracy SK, Sullivan E, Wang YA, Black D, Tracy M. Birth outcomes associated with interventions in labour amongst low risk women: A population-based study. Women Birth. 2007;20(2):41–8.
21. Roberts CL, Algert CS, Carnegie M, Peat B. Operative delivery during labour: trends and predictive factors. Paediatr Perinat Epidemiol. 2002;16(2):115–23.
22. Gülmezoglu AM, Crowther CA, Middleton P, Heatley E. Induction of labour for improving birth outcomes for women at or beyond term. Cochrane Database Syst Rev. 2012;6:CD004945.
23. Mishanina E, Rogozinska E, Thatthi T, Uddin-Khan R, Khan KS, Meads C. Use of labour induction and risk of cesarean delivery: a systematic review and meta-analysis. CMAJ. 2014;186(9):665–73.
24. Saccone G, Berghella V. Induction of labor at full term in uncomplicated singleton gestations: a systematic review and metaanalysis of randomized controlled trials. Am J Obstet Gynecol. 2015;213(5):629–36.
25. Wood S, Cooper S, Ross S. Does induction of labour increase the risk of caesarean section? A systematic review and meta-analysis of trials in women with intact membranes. BJOG. 2014;121(6):674–85. discussion 685.

26. Davey MA, Sloan ML, Palma S, Riley M, King J. Methodological processes in validating and analysing the quality of population-based data: a case study using the Victorian Perinatal Data Collection. HIM J. 2013;42(3):12–9.
27. Caughey AB, Sundaram V, Kaimal AJ, Gienger A, Cheng YW, McDonald KM, Shaffer BL, Owens DK, Bravata DM. Systematic review: elective induction of labor versus expectant management of pregnancy. Ann Intern Med. 2009; 151(4):252–63. W253-263.
28. Hannah ME, Hannah WJ, Hellmann J, Hewson S, Milner R, Willan A. Induction of labor as compared with serial antenatal monitoring in post-term pregnancy. A randomized controlled trial. The Canadian Multicenter Post-term Pregnancy Trial Group. N Engl J Med. 1992;326(24):1587–92.

Permissions

All chapters in this book were first published in P&C, by BioMed Central; hereby published with permission under the Creative Commons Attribution License or equivalent. Every chapter published in this book has been scrutinized by our experts. Their significance has been extensively debated. The topics covered herein carry significant findings which will fuel the growth of the discipline. They may even be implemented as practical applications or may be referred to as a beginning point for another development.

The contributors of this book come from diverse backgrounds, making this book a truly international effort. This book will bring forth new frontiers with its revolutionizing research information and detailed analysis of the nascent developments around the world.

We would like to thank all the contributing authors for lending their expertise to make the book truly unique. They have played a crucial role in the development of this book. Without their invaluable contributions this book wouldn't have been possible. They have made vital efforts to compile up to date information on the varied aspects of this subject to make this book a valuable addition to the collection of many professionals and students.

This book was conceptualized with the vision of imparting up-to-date information and advanced data in this field. To ensure the same, a matchless editorial board was set up. Every individual on the board went through rigorous rounds of assessment to prove their worth. After which they invested a large part of their time researching and compiling the most relevant data for our readers.

The editorial board has been involved in producing this book since its inception. They have spent rigorous hours researching and exploring the diverse topics which have resulted in the successful publishing of this book. They have passed on their knowledge of decades through this book. To expedite this challenging task, the publisher supported the team at every step. A small team of assistant editors was also appointed to further simplify the editing procedure and attain best results for the readers.

Apart from the editorial board, the designing team has also invested a significant amount of their time in understanding the subject and creating the most relevant covers. They scrutinized every image to scout for the most suitable representation of the subject and create an appropriate cover for the book.

The publishing team has been an ardent support to the editorial, designing and production team. Their endless efforts to recruit the best for this project, has resulted in the accomplishment of this book. They are a veteran in the field of academics and their pool of knowledge is as vast as their experience in printing. Their expertise and guidance has proved useful at every step. Their uncompromising quality standards have made this book an exceptional effort. Their encouragement from time to time has been an inspiration for everyone.

The publisher and the editorial board hope that this book will prove to be a valuable piece of knowledge for researchers, students, practitioners and scholars across the globe.

List of Contributors

Kyoko Yoshioka-Maeda and Mariko Kuroda
Department of Community Health Nursing, School of Nursing, Faculty of Medicine, Tokyo Medical University, Tokyo, Japan

Erika Ota and Rintaro Mori
Department of Health Policy, National Center for Child Health and Development, Tokyo, Japan

Togoobaatar Ganchimeg
Department of Health Policy, National Center for Child Health and Development, Tokyo, Japan
Faculty of Medicine, University of Tsukuba, Ibaraki, Japan

Fatimat M. Akinlusi, Kabiru A. Rabiu, Idayat A. Durojaiye, Adeniyi A. Adewunmi, Tawaqualit A. Ottun and Yusuf A. Oshodi
Department of Obstetrics and Gynaecology, Lagos State University College of Medicine/Lagos State University Teaching Hospital, Ikeja, Lagos, Nigeria

Shuang Liu, Liang Zhang and Xiang Zhang
Department of Health Management, School of Medicine and Health Management, Tongji Medical College, Huazhong University of Science and Technology, Wuhan, Hubei 430030, China

Jing Wang
Department of Health Management, School of Medicine and Health Management, Tongji Medical College, Huazhong University of Science and Technology, Wuhan, Hubei 430030, China
The Key Research Institute of Humanities and Social Science of Hubei Province, Huazhong University of Science and Technology, Wuhan, Hubei 430030, China

Theresa Morris
Department of Sociology, Texas A&M University, MS4351, College Station, TX 77843, USA

Amanda Gomez
Independent Scholar, Bryan, TX, USA

Miriam Naiman-Sessions
Independent Scholar, Helena, MT, USA

Christine H. Morton
Independent Scholar, Redwood City, CA, USA

Maaike Fobelets and Koen Putman
I-CHER (Interuniversity Centre for Health Economics Research), Faculty of Medicine and Pharmacy, Vrije Universiteit Brussels, Laarbeeklaan 103, 1090 Brussels, Belgium
Department of Public Health, Faculty of Medicine and Pharmacy, Vrije Universiteit Brussel, Laarbeeklaan 103, 1090 Brussels, Belgium

Katrien Beeckman
Department of Public Health, Faculty of Medicine and Pharmacy, Vrije Universiteit Brussel, Laarbeeklaan 103, 1090 Brussels, Belgium
Department of Nursing and Midwifery, Nursing and Midwifery research group, Universitair Ziekenhuis Brussel, Laarbeeklaan 103, 1090 Brussels, Belgium

Gilles Faron
Department of Obstetrics, Universitair Ziekenhuis Brussel, Vrije Universiteit Brussel, Laarbeeklaan 101, 1090 Brussels, Belgium

Déirdre Daly
School of Nursing and Midwifery, Trinity College Dublin, 24 D'Olier Street, Dublin D02 T283, Ireland

Cecily Begley
School of Nursing and Midwifery, Trinity College Dublin, 24 D'Olier Street, Dublin D02 T283, Ireland
Institute of Health and Care Sciences, Sahlgrenska Academy, University of Gothenburg, Gothenburg, Sweden

Reihaneh Pirjani
Obstetrics and Gynecology Department, Arash Women's Hospital, Tehran University of Medical Sciences, Tehran, Iran
Research development center, Arash Women's Hospital, Tehran University of Medical Sciences, Tehran, Iran

Motahareh Afrakhteh
School of medicine, Tehran University of Medical Sciences, Tehran, Iran

Mahdi Sepidarkish
Department of Epidemiology and Reproductive Health, Reproductive Epidemiology Research Center, Royan Institute for Reproductive Biomedicine, ACECR, Tehran, Iran

Shahin Nariman
Department of Pediatrics, Arash women's Hospital, Tehran University of Medical Sciences, Tehran, Iran

Mahboobeh Shirazi
Maternal, Fetal and Neonatal Research Center, Tehran University of Medical Sciences, Tehran, Iran

Ashraf Moini
Obstetrics and Gynecology Department, Arash Women's Hospital, Tehran University of Medical Sciences, Tehran, Iran
Department of Endocrinology and Female Infertility, Reproductive Biomedicine Research Center, Royan Institute for Reproductive Biomedicine, ACECR., Tehran, Iran

Ladan Hosseini
Research development center, Arash Women's Hospital, Tehran University of Medical Sciences, Tehran, Iran

IY Park and MR Kim
Department of Obstetrics and Gynecology, College of Medicine, Seoul St. Mary's Hospital, The Catholic University of Korea, Seoul, Republic of Korea

HN Lee, Y Gen and MJ Kim
Department of Obstetrics and Gynecology, College of Medicine, Bucheon St. Mary's Hospital, The Catholic University of Korea, 327 Sosa-ro, Bucheon, Gyeonggi-do 14647, Republic of Korea

Hong-Tao Hu, Jing-Jing Xu, Jing Lin and Cheng Li
Department of Obstetrics and Gynecology, International Peace Maternity and Child Health Hospital, School of Medicine, Shanghai Jiao Tong University, Shanghai, China

Yan-Ting Wu
Department of Reproductive Medicine, International Peace Maternity and Child Health Hospital, School of Medicine, Shanghai Jiao Tong University, Shanghai, China

Jian-Zhong Sheng
Department of Pathology and Pathophysiology, School of Medicine, Zhejiang University, Zhejiang, China

Xin-Mei Liu
Institute of Embryo-Fetal Original Adult Disease, Shanghai Key Laboratory for Reproductive Medicine, School of Medicine, Shanghai Jiao Tong University, Shanghai, China
International Peace Maternity and Child Health Hospital, School of Medicine, Shanghai Jiao Tong University, 910 Hengshan Road, Shanghai 200030, China

He-Feng Huang
Department of Reproductive Medicine, International Peace Maternity and Child Health Hospital, School of Medicine, Shanghai Jiao Tong University, Shanghai, China
Institute of Embryo-Fetal Original Adult Disease, Shanghai Key Laboratory for Reproductive Medicine, School of Medicine, Shanghai Jiao Tong University, Shanghai, China
International Peace Maternity and Child Health Hospital, School of Medicine, Shanghai Jiao Tong University, 910 Hengshan Road, Shanghai 200030, China

Ahmad Sameer Sanad, Ahmad E. Mahran, Mahmoud Elmorsi Aboulfotouh, Hany Hassan Kamel, Hashem Fares Mohammed, Haitham A. Bahaa, Reham R. Elkateeb, Alaa Gamal Abdelazim, Mohamed Ahmed Zeen El-Din and Hossam El-Din Shawki
Obstetrics and Gynecology, Faculty of Medicine, Minia Maternity University Hospital, Minia University, Minia, Egypt

Tahmina Begum, Aminur Rahman and Iqbal Anwar
Health Systems and Population Studies Division, International Centre for Diarrhoeal Disease Research Bangladesh (icddr,b), Dhaka, Bangladesh

Cathryn Ellis and Jean-Francois Rostoker
Department of Family Practice, University of British Columbia, Vancouver, BC, Canada

Malabika Sarker
James P Grant School of Public Health, BRAC University, Dhaka, Bangladesh
Institute of Public Health University, Heidelberg, Germany

Laura Reichenbach
Population Council, Washington, DC, USA

Sunita Panda
School of Nursing and Midwifery, Trinity College Dublin, 2 Clare Street, D02 CK80 Dublin, Ireland

Deirdre Daly
School of Nursing and Midwifery, Trinity College Dublin, 24 D'Olier Street, Dublin D02 T283, Ireland

Cecily Begley
School of Nursing and Midwifery, Trinity College Dublin, 24 D'Olier Street, Dublin D02 T283, Ireland
Sahlgrenska Academy, University of Gothenburg, Gothenburg, Sweden

Annika Karlström, Birgitta Larsson and Lena Bäck
Department of Nursing, Mid Sweden University, 86170 Sundsvall, Sweden

Ingegerd Hildingsson
Department of Nursing, Mid Sweden University, 86170 Sundsvall, Sweden
Department of Women's and Children's health, Uppsala University, Uppsala, Sweden

Aireen Wingert and Cydney Johnson
Alberta Research Centre for Health Evidence, Department of Pediatrics, University of Alberta, Edmonton, AB, Canada

Robin Featherstone and Lisa Hartling
Alberta Research Centre for Health Evidence, Department of Pediatrics, University of Alberta, Edmonton, AB, Canada
Alberta Strategy for Patient-Oriented Research (SPOR) SUPPORT Unit Knowledge Translation Platform, University of Alberta, Edmonton, AB, Canada

Meghan Sebastianski
Alberta Strategy for Patient-Oriented Research (SPOR) SUPPORT Unit Knowledge Translation Platform, University of Alberta, Edmonton, AB, Canada

R. Douglas Wilson
Department of Obstetrics and Gynecology, Cumming School of Medicine, University of Calgary, 1403 - 29 Street NW, Calgary, AB T2N 2T9, Canada

Emily White VanGompel
Department of Family Medicine, The University of Chicago, Pritzker School of Medicine, NorthShore University HealthSystem Research Institute, 1001 University Place, Evanston, IL 60201, USA
Department of Obstetrics and Gynecology, The University of Chicago, Pritzker School of Medicine, NorthShore University HealthSystem Research Institute, 1001 University Place, Evanston, IL 60201, USA

Elliott K. Main
California Maternal Quality Care Collaborative, Stanford University, Stanford Medical School Office Building, 1265 Welch Road, MS 5415, Stanford, CA 94305, USA

Daniel Tancredi
Center for Healthcare Policy and Research and Department of Pediatrics, University of California Davis School of Medicine, 2103 Stockton Blvd, Sacramento, CA 95817, USA

Joy Melnikow
Center for Healthcare Policy and Research and Department of Family and Community Medicine, University of Clifornia Davis School of Medicine, 2103 Stockton Blvd, Sacramento, CA 95817, USA

Eileen A. Curran and Louise C. Kenny
Department of Obstetrics and Gynaecology, The Irish Centre for Fetal and Neonatal Translational Research (INFANT), University College Cork, Cork, Ireland

Christina Dalman
Department of Public Health Sciences, Division of Public Health Epidemiology, Karolinska Institutet, Stockholm, Sweden

Ali S Khashan
Department of Obstetrics and Gynaecology, The Irish Centre for Fetal and Neonatal Translational Research (INFANT), University College Cork, Cork, Ireland
Department of Epidemiology and Public Health, University College Cork, Cork, Ireland

Patricia M. Kearney
Department of Epidemiology and Public Health, University College Cork, Cork, Ireland

John F. Cryan
Department of Anatomy and Neuroscience, APC Microbiome Institute, University College Cork, Cork, Ireland

Timothy G. Dinan
Department of Psychiatry, APC Microbiome Institute, University College Cork, Cork, Ireland

Zhi-Da Qian, Yue Weng, Yong-Jiang Du and Li-Li Huang
Women's Hospital, School of Medicine, Zhejiang University, 1 Xueshi Road, Hangzhou, Zhejiang Province 310006, People's Republic of China

Chun-Fen Wang
Maternal and Child Health Institute of Lin'an City, 25 Jiangnan Road, Lin'an, Zhejiang Province 311300, People's Republic of China

Phocas Biraboneye S
Department of Obstetrics and Gynaecology, Jeanne de Navarre Hospital Center, Château-Thierry, France

Omondi Ogutu
Department of Obstetrics and Gynaecology, University of Nairobi, Nairobi, Kenya

Jos van Roosmalen
Athena Institute, VU University Amsterdam, Amsterdam, The Netherlands

Samson Wanjala
Department of Obstetrics and Gynaecology, University of Nairobi, Nairobi, Kenya

Kizito Lubano
Kenya Medical Research Institute, Nairobi, Kenya

John Kinuthia
Department of research and programs, Kenyatta National Hospital, Nairobi, Kenya

Mei Yang, Qiong Fang and Lixin Jiang
Futian District Center for Disease Control and Prevention of Shenzhen China, Futian District, Shenzhen 518000, China

Qin Qin
Department of Health Prevention and Care, Zhongshan Hospital, Xiamen University, Xiamen 361004, China
Department of Epidemiology and Biostatistics, School of Public Health, Tongji Medical College, Huazhong University of Science and Technology, 13 Hangkong Road, Wuhan 430030, China

Shaofa Nie
Department of Epidemiology and Biostatistics, School of Public Health, Tongji Medical College, Huazhong University of Science and Technology, 13 Hangkong Road, Wuhan 430030, China

Chinta Annie Jyothirmayi and Anil Kuruvilla
Department of Neonatology, Christian Medical College, Vellore, India

Ajay Halder and Ruby Jose
Department of Obstetrics and Gynecology Unit IV, Christian Medical College, Vellore, India

Bijesh Yadav
Department of Biostatistics, Christian Medical College,Vellore, India

Santosh Thomas Samuel
MLL Hospital, Madanapalle, Chittoor, Andhrapradesh, India

Rami H. Al Rifai
Institute of Public Health, College of Medicine and Health Sciences, United Arab Emirates University, Al-Ain, United Arab Emirates

Sara L. Kenyon and Sandhya Duggal
Institute of Applied Health Research, University of Birmingham, Edgbaston, Birmingham B15 2TT, UK

Nina Johns
Birmingham Women's NHS Foundation Trust, Mindelsohn Way, Birmingham, West Midlands B15 2TG, UK

Ruth Hewston
Research Fellow, Institute of Applied Health Research, University of Birmingham, 255 Walmley Road, Walmley, Sutton Coldfield, West Midlands B76 2PN, UK

Nicola Gale
Health Services Management Centre, University of Birmingham, Park House, 40 Edgbaston Park Road, Edgbaston, Birmingham B15 2RT, UK

S. Maswime
Wits Obstetrics and Gynaecology Clinical Research Division, Johanesburg, South Africa

E. J. Buchmann
Department of Obstetrics and Gynaecology, University of the Witwatersrand, Johannesburg, South Africa

Nazar P. Shabila
Department of Community Medicine, College of Medicine, Hawler Medical University, Erbil, Iraq

Louise C. Kenny
The Irish Centre for Fetal and Neonatal Translational Research (INFANT), Cork University Maternity Hospital, University College Cork, Wilton, Cork, Ireland

Richard A. Greene
National Perinatal Epidemiology Centre (NPEC), Department of Obstetrics and Gynaecology, Cork University Maternity Hospital, 5th Floor Wilton, Cork, Ireland

Sinéad M. O'Neill
The Irish Centre for Fetal and Neonatal Translational Research (INFANT), Cork University Maternity Hospital, University College Cork, Wilton, Cork, Ireland
National Perinatal Epidemiology Centre (NPEC), Department of Obstetrics and Gynaecology, Cork University Maternity Hospital, 5th Floor Wilton, Cork, Ireland

Esben Agerbo
Centre for Integrated Register-based Research (CIRRAU), National Centre for Register-based Research (NCRR), Aarhus University, Aarhus, Denmark

Ali S. Khashan
The Irish Centre for Fetal and Neonatal Translational Research (INFANT), Cork University Maternity Hospital, University College Cork, Wilton, Cork, Ireland

Patricia M. Kearney
Department of Epidemiology and Public Health, University College Cork, Western Gateway Building, Cork, Ireland

Tine Brink Henriksen
Perinatal Epidemiology Research Unit, Department of Paediatrics, Aarhus University Hospital, Skejby, Aarhus N DK-8200, Denmark

Mary-Ann Davey
Department of Obstetrics and Gynaecology, Monash University, 246 Clayton Rd, Clayton 3186, Australia
Judith Lumley Centre, La Trobe University, 215 Franklin St, Melbourne 3000, Australia

James King
Department of Obstetrics and Gynaecology, University of Melbourne, Parkville 3052, Australia

Index

O

P

R

S

T

U

V

www.ingramcontent.com/pod-product-compliance
Lightning Source LLC
LaVergne TN
LVHW080704210926
848485LV00003B/419